The International Behavioural and

COMMUNITY AS DOCTOR

TAVISTOCK

MIND & MEDICINE
In 6 Volumes

COMMUNITY AS DOCTOR

New Perspectives on a
Therapeutic Community

ROBERT N RAPOPORT
WITH THE COLLABORATION OF
RHONA RAPOPORT AND
IRVING ROSOW

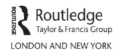

LONDON AND NEW YORK

First published in 1960 by
Tavistock Publications Limited

Published in 2001 by
Routledge
2 Park Square, Milton Park, Abingdon, Oxfordshire OX14 4RN
711 Third Avenue, New York, NY 10017

First issued in paperback 2014

Routledge is an imprint of the Taylor and Francis Group, an informa business

The publishers have made every effort to contact authors/copyright holders
of the works reprinted in the *International Behavioural and Social Sciences
Library*. This has not been possible in every case, however, and we would
welcome correspondence from those individuals/companies we have been
unable to trace.

These reprints are taken from original copies of each book. In many cases
the condition of these originals is not perfect. The publisher has gone to
great lengths to ensure the quality of these reprints, but wishes to point
out that certain characteristics of the original copies will, of necessity, be
apparent in reprints thereof.

British Library Cataloguing in Publication Data
A CIP catalogue record for this book
is available from the British Library

Community as Doctor
ISBN 0-415-26461-8
Mind & Medicine: 6 Volumes
ISBN 0-415-26512-6
The International Behavioural and Social Sciences Library
112 Volumes
ISBN 0-415-25670-4

ISBN 13: 978-1-138-88140-2 (pbk)
ISBN 13: 978-0-415-26461-7 (hbk)

Community as Doctor

NEW PERSPECTIVES ON A THERAPEUTIC COMMUNITY

ROBERT N. RAPOPORT

with the collaboration of

RHONA RAPOPORT AND IRVING ROSOW

INTRODUCTION BY MAXWELL JONES

SOCIAL SCIENCE PAPERBACKS
in association with
TAVISTOCK PUBLICATIONS

First published in 1960
by Tavistock Publications Limited
2 Park Square, Milton Park,
Abingdon, Oxon, OX14 4RN
First published in this series 1967
in 12 pt Bembo

SOCIAL SCIENCE PAPERBACKS
are published by members of
Associated Book Publishers Limited

A WORLD MENTAL HEALTH YEAR PUBLICATION

This book is dedicated to
World Mental Health Year
in recognition of the purposes for which
this world-wide effort was launched and
to which it is hoped that this book will
make some small contribution.

CONTENTS

ACKNOWLEDGEMENTS

This book is based on research sponsored by Dr Maxwell Jones conducted with the participation of the research and clinical staffs of the Belmont Hospital Social Rehabilitation Unit in 1953–7. We are grateful to all of them for their participation and help in the research. Footnotes in the text indicate where individual contributions are used in this book.

Research Staff

G. ELLES	psychiatric nurse, psychoanalyst
P. MORRIS	psychiatric social worker
T. MORRIS	sociologist
P. NOKES	anthropologist
S. PARKER	anthropologist
R. RAPOPORT	anthropologist
RHONA RAPOPORT	sociologist, psychoanalyst
G. ROPER	psychologist
I. ROSOW	sociologist
J. DE SMITH	statistician

Clinical Staff

C. BROOKS	instructor
G. BROWN	staff nurse
E. CANN	disablement resettlement officer
M. JONES	psychiatrist**
N. JETMALANI	psychiatrist
F. JACQUIST	instructor
N. McCULLOCH	psychiatrist
F. MATEER	nurse
B. POMRYN	psychiatrist
W. SHAW	disablement resettlement officer
E. SKELLERN	charge nurse**

H. SMITH staff nurse**
F. STRAUSS psychologist
F. STALLARD psychiatrist
J. STREET instructor
E. TAYLOR instructor
J. TUXFORD psychiatric social worker**
social therapists*

The research was made possible financially through the assistance of the Medical Research Council for initial exploratory work and of the Nuffield Foundation for the employment of a larger staff of investigators. During the period of final writing in the United States, the author was assisted by funds from the National Institute of Health and from Harvard University's Laboratory of Social Relations.

At Belmont (now Henderson) Hospital, the physician superintendent, Dr L. Minski, the nursing matron, Miss P. Arnold, and the executive secretary, Mr L. Walter, were all very helpful. Dr M. Desai of the Belmont Hospital psychology department also afforded valuable help. Mrs Marcella Davis, a visiting Fulbright scholar, collaborated in studies of the role of social therapist. The project benefited from the advice of Professors (Sir) Aubrey Lewis, G. Morris Carstairs, Richard Titmuss, and Adam Curle. Professor Raymond Firth, though not officially connected with the project, was most sympathetic and helpful. Representatives of the Royal Anthropological Institute and of the Tavistock Institute extended numerous courtesies to members of our group, and we thank them for their kindness. In the United States, we found discussions with Professor Morris Schwartz and Mrs Charlotte Schwartz most stimulating.

Secretarial assistance at various points was provided by Mrs Carolyn Accola, Mrs Maureen Davidson, Mrs Patricia Foley, Miss Cyrille Gell, Mrs Peggy McCarthy, Mrs Audrey Roper, Mrs Dorinthe Sacks, and Mrs Marie Scannell.

Thanks are due to the Editors of *Human Relations*, the *Lancet*, and *Psychiatry* for permission to reproduce material that first appeared in these journals.

* A large number of social therapists were of assistance in conducting the research, and only a few who were particularly helpful can be named here. Outstanding among these were Trudy Goebertus, Birte Hejnfeld, Ingrid Jonsson, Elsie Nokes, Sally Wong, and Frieda Wouterse.
** While all the members of the clinical staff were very helpful to the research, these individuals were particularly active, having participated in research and written reports, that are drawn on in the text of this volume.

INTRODUCTION

The concept of a therapeutic community has tended to be used in so many ways that its meaning has become vague and confused. Nevertheless it is becoming increasingly clear that the social environment of psychiatric patients whether in hospital or in the outside community can have a profound effect on their readjustment and eventual recovery. To study these social forces and apply them in therapeutically desirable ways calls for the closest collaboration between the psychiatric team and their social-science colleagues. It was in this context that we sought the help that was so generously afforded us by the Nuffield Foundation and the Medical Research Council.

Dr Rapoport spent four years in all (1953 to 1957) working with the staff of the Social Rehabilitation Unit at Belmont (now Henderson) Hospital. During the first year of his stay Dr Rapoport was on his own without other research assistance. He spent this year in familiarizing himself with the whole structure and functioning of the Social Rehabilitation Unit. In particular he made close contact with hospital patients, getting to know them more informally than most staff members are able to do. He also sought to view the staff as objectively as possible. It was during this time that Stanton and Schwartz's[1] book appeared, which emphasized the importance of staff interrelationships as affecting the treatment of patients. As the work developed, it was decided to add additional research staff to enlarge the Unit's understanding of its action experiment with treating personality disorders in a therapeutic community. Dr Rapoport worked in collaboration with his research colleagues for the two years that followed. This book draws on the findings of individuals in this group, though much of their work is published separately or is being developed in subsequent research in other organizations to which they have gone.

In order to place this research in perspective, a brief historical sketch of the Unit may be useful. The staff at the Social Rehabilitation Unit had long been interested in the problems of social psychiatry; the historical background to this has been given in our earlier book.[2] Our interest in the concept of the therapeutic community really started in 1940 at the beginning of the Second World War, when the problems of the treatment of cases of war neurosis with relatively similar clinical conditions and a small staff brought about an early awareness of the possibilities of community treatment. We soon came to realize that the development of community methods of treatment went beyond the skills at our disposal. Group treatment stemmed largely from psycho-analytic concepts, and was, we felt, within our range of competence to develop. Community treatment, however, made us aware of new problems that we felt incompetent to deal with unaided. We had the feeling that the social structure of a hospital could with advantage be changed, but to assess the effects of such changes on the patient population and on the culture of the whole community of staff and patients needed new skills.

The Social Rehabilitation Unit started in April 1947 with a population of patients who were primarily seen in terms of their poor employment records. They represented the hard core of the chronic unemployed, and were referred to us from medical sources and from the Ministry of Labour. The Unit was at that time called the Industrial Neurosis Unit. As time went on, more and more patients were referred to us from the courts, and our problems became much greater when we were faced by the problem of treating serious character disorders. We changed to the title Social Rehabilitation Unit in 1954. The type of patient observed by Dr Rapoport's group is now giving way in large degree to even more socially troublesome types. In the 1956 sample 10 per cent of the intake were referred by the courts. In the three following years the figure steadily increased to the point where in some months the courts send 30 per cent of all our referrals. In addition the whole scene in Britain has changed in a very remarkable way. The Royal Commission on the Law relating to Mental Illness and Mental Deficiency[3] made very important recommendations regarding the treatment of patients with character disorders, or psychopaths as they chose to call them. These recommendations were in favour of an active attempt to treat such patients, and, where practicable, to refer them to medical rather than penal institutions. The Royal Commission report was followed by the Mental Health Act[4] which became law in July 1959 and is undoubtedly a most revolutionary piece of legislation, enacting most of the recommendations of the Royal Commission's report.

Dr Rapoport's book was written at a time when the very existence of the Social Rehabilitation Unit was occasionally in jeopardy because there was a great deal of social disapproval regarding the permissive treatment of patients of this kind in an open hospital. The change for the better in the social climate since that time is presumably due in part to the effect of the Royal Commission report on public opinion. This change has of course affected the attitude of the staff and possibly to some extent of the patients in the Unit. There is much less fear regarding threats to survival of the Unit; indeed, the Act provides for the creation of more special units for the treatment of psychopaths. In addition it anticipates considerable development by local authorities in the provision of facilities for after-care and hostel accommodation for such patients.

Our own development is progressing on these lines, and to some extent parallels many of the points made in Dr Rapoport's book. Clearly we were very much influenced by the findings of the research team while they were with us, and we owe a great debt of gratitude to them for demonstrating to us many of the flaws in our treatment ideology and practice. We have come to realize that the great weakness in our treatment programme is the lack of sufficient attention to selective after-care. The provision for the past ten years of an out-patient club with sessions once a week is inadequate for the after-care needs of this type of patient. We have now approached the Ministry of Health with a view to having an after-care centre in London where intensive work could be done with selected cases. In addition we have worked towards developing a clearer concept of the type of patient who is amenable to treatment of the kind we can offer. We anticipate that improved screening of potential patients and the decision as to whether they should be admitted to a therapeutic community such as we provide or be treated on an out-patient basis, possibly in family groups or within the family structure itself, will greatly enhance the value of our work. To make such a service effective, the active collaboration of the local Medical Officer of Health and of the various medical and social service agencies within a circumscribed area would of course be needed. The mere bringing together of personnel in the social-work field, including general practitioners, who are in contact with patients and their families should do much to create a better understanding of the roles and role relationships of each of the trained personnel. The sharing of problems and their discussion is in itself an educational process, and it is in this setting that the psychiatrist interested in group work and in social dimensions of treatment may well play a valuable part in postgraduate education as well as in improving the rational basis for referral practice. A trend of this kind is already apparent in such training facilities as those offered by the Tavistock Clinic in London for general practitioners[5] and social workers.[6]

Everything that Dr Rapoport has said in his book would seem to fall into line with the development which has been taking place in Britain since the time when he and his team were working in this country. The changes brought about by the Royal Commission and the passing of the new Mental Health Act, while not directly influenced by the work of social scientists, have possibly been indirectly affected by this general type of approach, which has given so much to psychiatry by helping us to become more aware of the social dimensions in treatment.

Dr Rapoport has begun to study the concept of a therapeutic community by breaking it down into certain basic concepts. The gaps in our knowledge, of which we were dimly aware but which we tended to keep peripheral in our consciousness, are brought into sharp focus. The tendency amongst psychiatrists to cover confused thinking by words whose meaning is kept rather vague and general is commented on in various ways. Moreover, the fact that different treatment methods can be carried out with fervent enthusiasm on patients with similar diagnosis clearly illustrates the tentativeness with which even the most convinced (and convincing) viewpoints of present-day psychiatrists must be regarded. Like our colleagues we have been subject to such bias regarding our own particular line of thought. It has been suggested in the text of this book that the treatment method that we have developed over the past twenty years may have some anti-therapeutic aspects. The treatment milieu is seen to some extent as an atypical environment despite our efforts to make it more like conditions in the outside world than is usual in psychiatric hospitals. The norms of our therapeutic community are in many instances different from those found in the outside world, but we believe that they aid therapy, and we have come to use the term therapeutic culture. Though this may be a valuable learning process, Dr Rapoport argues that the incorporation of such ideas and values may be therapeutic in the sense of bringing about better social relationships and better understanding of the meaning of behaviour while in the hospital community, but that the same values and attitudes applied to the outside world may produce serious conflicts on return to the wider community. In fact, his analysis of the follow-up data indicated that those patients who tended to change their values in the direction of the values of the Unit community showed less satisfactory adjustment outside than those who did not. He suggests, on the basis of this finding, that we distinguish conceptually between our treatment goals and our rehabilitation goals— which may in some circumstances work at cross purposes.

Data such as these must cause one to reconsider the culture that the hospital community has developed in terms of the different ends it may serve. The data force one to a realization that while we have made strides towards understanding what socio-environmental elements of hospital culture tend to be therapeutic for character disorders, we know far too little as yet about how to apply these group and community methods most efficiently to problems of rehabilitation in the outside world. Presumably the same argument applies to any type of psychiatric patient exposed to hospital treatment. Perhaps the most thought-provoking finding of all is that in those patients who had improved on discharge—and this means the majority of patients treated—the relapse rate during the first few months after discharge was high. During the period of six to twelve months after discharge, however, there was partial recovery. Dr Rapoport quite understandably argues that this would be evidence in favour of a better after-care service; the critical period of adjustment being the first few months after discharge.

At the same time Dr Rapoport is very ready to admit the limitations of the study undertaken by himself and his colleagues. For example, the questionnaires on which the report on the values of patients and staff are based are clearly open to serious criticism. When asked about their attitude to various aspects of the Unit and its values, many patients might tend to display a kind of pseudo-identification with the Unit and say things that were meant to create a good impression. There are obvious difficulties too in studying staff attitudes; for example, I was frequently conscious when answering the questions of an acute desire to qualify or elaborate the sense in which I felt I could make one or another choice of response to the questionnaire used. Others, substantially in agreement with my values, might have chosen another response because of their implicit qualifications, whereas still other staff members might have chosen the same response, but for different reasons. Though it would be virtually impossible to incorporate all the qualifications required by scientific accuracy, one cannot help but wish that more could have been worked into the quantitative analysis.

This book raises and examines many of the problems associated with the concept of a therapeutic community. In this sense it does much to clarify what is meant by the term. However it does much more than this; by studying the individual in the social setting of both hospital and home it forces us to reconsider what are the relevant social forces that affect the course of patients' lives and how they can be used in a therapeutic way. Thus the concept of a therapeutic community as a somewhat artificial hospital social milieu gives way to the wider concept of socio-cultural therapy in all the relevant environments in which a patient must function as a social being.

MAXWELL JONES

NOTES AND REFERENCES

1. Stanton, Alfred H., and Schwartz, Morris S.; *The Mental Hospital*. New York, Basic Books, 1954.
2. Jones, Maxwell, *et al.: Social Psychiatry*. London, Tavistock Publications, 1952 (also published as *The Therapeutic Community*, New York, Basic Books, 1953).
3. Report of the Royal Commission on the Law Relating to Mental Illness and Mental Deficiency. London, H.M.S.O., 1957.
4. Mental Health Act, 1959.
5. Balint, Michael: *The Doctor, His Patient, and the Illness*. London, Pitman, 1956.
6. Family Discussion Bureau: *Social Casework in Marital Problems*. London, Tavistock Publications, 1955.

ABBREVIATIONS OF TITLES OF PERIODICALS
referred to in Notes and References

Admin. Sci. Quart.	*Administrative Science Quarterly*, Ithaca, N.Y.
Amer. J. Insan.	*American Journal of Insanity*, Utica, N.Y.
Amer. J. Psychiat.	*American Journal of Psychiatry*, Baltimore.
Amer. J. Psychother.	*American Journal of Psychotherapy*, Lancaster, Pa.
Amer. J. Sociol.	*American Journal of Sociology*, Chicago.
Behavioral Science	*Behavioral Science*, Ann Arbor, Mich.
Brit. J. Delinq.	*British Journal of Delinquency*, London.
Brit. J. med. Psychol.	*British Journal of Medical Psychology*, Cambridge.
Brit. J. Philos. Sci.	*British Journal for the Philosophy of Science*, London.
Brit. J. Sociol.	*British Journal of Sociology*, London.
Brit. med. J.	*British Medical Journal*, London.
Bull. Menninger Clin.	*Bulletin of the Menninger Clinic*, Topeka, Kansas.
Hum. Organiz.	*Human Organization*, New York.
Hum. Relations	*Human Relations*, London.
Int. J. Psycho-Anal.	*International Journal of Psycho-Analysis*, London.
Int. J. soc. Psychiat.	*International Journal of Social Psychiatry*, London.
J. abnorm. soc. Psychol.	*Journal of Abnormal and Social Psychology*, Boston.
J. Neurol. Psychiat.	*Journal of Neurology, Neurosurgery and Psychiatry*, London.
J. R. sanit. Inst.	*Journal of the Royal Sanitary Institute*, London.
J. soc. Issues.	*Journal of Social Issues*, New York.
Lancet	*The Lancet*, London.
Neuropsychiat.	*Neuropsychiatry*, Charlottesville, Va.
Nurs. Times	*Nursing Times*, London.
Occup. Ther.	*Occupational Therapy and Rehabilitation*, Baltimore.
Proc. R. Soc. Med.	*Proceedings of the Royal Society of Medicine*, London.
Psychiat. Quart.	*Psychiatric Quarterly*, Albany, N.Y.
Psychiatry	*Psychiatry*, Baltimore.
Publ. Hlth. Rep., Wash.	*Public Health Reports*, Washington.
Soc. Forces	*Journal of Social Forces*.
Soc. Problems	*Social Problems*, Washington.
World Mental Health.	*Bulletin of the World Federation for Mental Health*, London.

CHAPTER 1

Treatment and Rehabilitation

We are concerned with the problem of how best to help psychiatric patients. Individuals that we would now call the psychiatrically ill have been dealt with over the years in a great variety of ways. Before they were brought under the aegis of medicine, they tended to be treated as possessed by supernatural spirits, for better or worse, and handled accordingly. The transformation that occurred as medical care was substituted for other ways of handling the mentally ill was so great as to have been termed the first great 'revolution'[1] in the development of psychiatry. The second 'revolution' is marked by the development of the psychodynamic approach, in which therapy for the patient was based on a developmental and functional theory of personality. This change, marked by the work of Freud, brought into psychiatry a therapeutic method that was more than simply naturalistic classification and allowed more than simply sporadic, unexplained empirical success. Psychoanalysis introduced a system of thinking that conceived of psychiatric illness as an anomaly in personality development. It also developed a method for influencing or revising personality structure. This method, however, has remained expensive, time-consuming, practicable only by a few specialists whose training is so arduous as to preclude their widespread availability. Thus it has influenced psychiatry more through the ideas it has generated than through the actual numbers of patients it has dealt with.

At the present we are in the throes, many observers maintain, of a third 'revolution' in psychiatry,[2] one that is signalized by the use of group methods, milieu therapy, and administrative psychiatry. In general, *social* psychiatric approaches in therapy stress multi-person involvement in contrast to approaches aimed at affecting only one individual through the efforts of one other individual.[3]

9

One of the brightest stars in the social psychiatric firmament is the 'therapeutic community' idea. According to this approach, the hospital is seen not as a place where patients are classified and stored, nor a place where one group of individuals (the medical staff) gives treatment to another group of individuals (the patients) according to the model of general medical hospitals; but as a place which is organized as a community in which everyone is expected to make some contribution towards the shared goals of creating a social organization that will have healing properties. 'The therapeutic community views treatment as located not in the application by specialists of certain shocks, drugs, or interpretations, but in the normal interactions of healthy community life.'[4]

The present book is an attempt to describe and analyse some of the characteristics of one of the earliest and most vigorous pioneering attempts at the construction of a therapeutic community—the Social Rehabilitation Unit of Belmont Hospital in England—from a social science viewpoint. This is a 100-bed Unit within a neurosis centre that serves the United Kingdom under the National Health Service, and gears its programme to the treatment of patients with long-standing personality disorders. Dr Maxwell Jones, the Unit's director, and other members of the staff have presented numerous descriptions of their work as it has progressed,[5] and the present volume, which is based on work sponsored by them, must be seen as another attempt to illuminate the processes, pitfalls, and advantages of their approach.

The general movement of social psychiatry is best understood as a sub-movement within the awakening interest of medicine generally in the social dimensions of their problems.[6] Social scientists were used as collaborators early on in the practice of public health and in cross-cultural medical enterprises.[7] More recently they have been used in the investigation of hospitals—seen from various vantage points as a type of institution, a place where professional persons conduct much of their practice, a kind of 'small society', 'community', or 'social system'.[8] Today, there is an efflorescence of social science studies in medicine, encompassing almost every element in the medical situation that is recognized within social science as a field of investigation for which general social scientific experience has relevance. There have been studies of patients' families,[9] patterns of communications between patients and physicians,[10] ecological studies,[11] studies of ideology,[12] social status,[13] continuities and discontinuities in adult socialization experience,[14] structures of authority within the hospital seen as a kind of bureaucratic system,[15] studies of informal groupings within the hospital and their effect on the overall functioning,[16] ideal types of ward structures,[17] and studies of the studies.[18]

When these studies have been gathered together into book form they have either tended to cover a large range of illustrative materials excerpted from here and there to demonstrate the scope of the field,[19] or focused on a single institution to cover a range of topics illustrating the kinds of insights that the social science approach can facilitate.[20] We learn in either case that communication channels and processes have a relevance for patient care; that the structure of authority relations is relevant; that social processes occur that are unknown to the staff or undesired by them, but which cannot be overlooked if the *real* rather than the *ideal* social situation is to be coped with; and that any patient is involved in a network of relationships each of which has some influence on his emotional life and behaviour. In this context the patient's relationship with the psychiatric staff must be seen as only one in a field of forces, in which others may also be actively enlisted or otherwise advantageously dealt with in the therapeutic situation. While all these things have been long known, in a way, to perceptive practitioners, the systematization of ways of taking them into account is new.

Much ground has been cleared by these earlier studies so that it is no longer necessary to reiterate the fundamental new insights. The clinicians, administrators, and their cohorts are already aware of the therapeutic importance of communications channelling, authority, social class norms, and other aspects of institutional social structure as operative elements in their therapeutic situations. The new frontiers would seem to involve advancing in two somewhat different directions. The first of these is, in our view, the refinement and testing of hypotheses that come from the early insights through the use of structured research designs and the use of controlled experimentation. This kind of enterprise might be illustrated by considering how one would further develop the hypothesis associated with the 'Stanton-Schwartz effect'—viz., that covert disagreements between authority figures result in pathological excitement in patients within the joint jurisdiction of the figures in question. Would the same kind of pathological disturbance hold if the figures who disagreed were aware of their differences of opinion, but confirmed in them nevertheless? Are some kinds of patients more affected by this than others? Are other kinds of authority figures besides doctors (e.g., nurses, attendants) equally effective in provoking pathological excitement when they disagree about patients in their joint jurisdiction? To what extent and in what sense is the converse true—i.e., that harmony precludes pathological disturbance?

The second kind of need, we feel, is for more careful consideration of problems associated with implementing new ideas—whether they derive from the new insights brought through the application of social science concepts, from psychiatric thought itself, or from the inter-disciplinary stimulation. The task of working out ways of translating theoretical insights into practical programmes is still a vast one, and becomes in some ways more complex as ideas are generated in advance of their testing out in experience. The mind races ahead of the human organism (or organization) in its attempt to implement, test, and revise the idea. We are in a period of proliferation of ideas, and it would seem true to say that ideas as such are the proverbial 'penny a dozen'. One major task is the clarification, thinking through of implications, observing limitations and qualifications associated with particular ideas seriously put forth as valuable in psychiatric care.

The present book contains some elements in common with the earlier studies in that social science concepts are applied within this psychiatric setting in order to give the familiar phenomena a new perspective. It also has elements of *post hoc* experimentation in that a series of patients' careers is studied in a more rigorous framework than is usually possible in clinical reports. However, it is addressed primarily to the problems of clarification of certain *ideas*. The ideas are those of a particular variant of the 'therapeutic community', but more especially the ideas held about the relationship between 'treatment' and 'rehabilitation'.

The term rehabilitation was originally applied in psychiatry after the medical model. When patients had 'residual disabilities' (e.g., an amputee), or their hospitalization had led to new incapacitation (e.g., disuse atrophy in limb muscles), help was needed after the specific medical treatment had brought the patient to the best possible physical state with reference to the initial disease. 'Treatment' was designed to arrest, cure, or mitigate the disease, and 'rehabilitation' was an adjunctive measure to restore the patient to an extra-hospital social context given his bio-physiological condition at the end of treatment.

Richard Williams notes that one way that the term rehabilitation has been applied to psychiatry is as follows:[21]

'Rehabilitation is that form of therapy which is primarily concerned with assisting the patient to achieve an optimal social role (in the family, in a job, in the community generally) within his capacities and potentialities. Psychiatric rehabilitation is the application of rehabilitative therapy, thus defined, to mental and emotional disabilities.'

In psychiatry, however, the distinction in activity and division of labour could be kept clear only as long as the 'physical treatments' based on the medical model were the exclusive or primary forms of therapy. But as 'rehabilitation therapies' became incorporated into the patient's care from the beginning of treatment, and as treatment itself became psychotherapy, milieu therapy, or administrative therapy, the distinctiveness between 'treatment' and 'rehabilitation' began to break down, at least on the level of activity forms and division of labour. The comment of Burlingame summarized the situation.[22]

'Rehabilitation is an elastic term. Depending on its context it has come to mean everything from restoring to former capacity or condition, to making over in an improved form. Particularly in psychiatry, its connotation can be extremely broad, embracing all procedures that overcome the morbid patterns of mental illness, and restore the patient to effective personal and social functioning.'

A further step in this process of merging and overlap of the two terms has been the tendency to merge them *conceptually*. In some cases the terms were explicitly and self-consciously used as synonymous. Some advocates of the therapeutic community approach maintain this position—viz., that 'all treatment is (or should be) rehabilitation'.

The question of the relationship between treatment and rehabilitation is not confined to therapeutic communities, though they tend to exemplify one position taken in regard to it. With the growth of modern methods of psychiatric treatment, especially in chemical therapies, there is a decrease in the overall length of stay of patients in psychiatric hospitals. The staff, correspondingly, emphasize getting patients out. This occasions a reorientation in patterns of care and the concept of 'cure'. With the increased emphasis on cutting down on custodialism in mental hospitals, the tendency is to try to make it possible for the patient to live in an ordinary social environment, using the hospital only for those parts of his treatment that are not feasible in the outside context. Since many individuals who might have been hospitalized in earlier times are now encouraged to live outside, it is not surprising that the tendency is towards developing help measures of a different kind from the 'specific' psychiatric treatments characteristic of the hospital or consulting room settings. Some of the people who are leaving hospitals have been so 'institutionalized' that they have lost the facilities for participating in life according to outside norms, and in many cases social change has been so marked since the time of their entry to the hospital that whole new segments of the culture must be learned for the first time. In many cases the nature of the patients' persisting incapacities makes it necessary that they learn entirely new ways of fitting themselves into an ordinary social existence. The efforts to deal with these problems as distinct from the purely medical treatments administered by doctors in the hospital are sometimes called 'rehabilitation'.

In studying the social organization of the Belmont Social Rehabilitation Unit (which considers itself to be giving *treatment* to patients which is simultaneously rehabilitation) we felt that though the Unit staff did not include this among their problems, the lack of conceptual distinction between the two terms led to recurrent problematic situations. We feel, on the basis of this observation, that certain advantages accrue to the treatment-rehabilitation enterprise if the *conceptual* distinction is retained between all measures aimed at changing the patient's psycho-biological state (treatment) and all measures aimed at changing his performance in social roles (rehabilitation). The same kinds of activities may serve both purposes, individuals in the same social roles may be engaged in both kinds of enterprise, and the same kinds of processes may occur within the individual and within the social structure to bring about treatment goals or rehabilitation goals. We would suggest, however, that keeping rather than eliminating the conceptual distinction increases rationality in the selection and application of techniques that will be most effective in each individual case.

Since this is a problem for the field at large, with the Belmont Unit exemplifying one attempt at solution, we felt that our efforts could be placed in the most broadly applicable framework by addressing ourselves to this problem.

The implications of our present position can perhaps best be understood if we consider, in the rest of this chapter, the usages to which these two terms have been put in psychiatry. We can then state our own position with reference to them in greater detail.

THE HISTORY OF PSYCHIATRY: WITH SPECIAL REFERENCE TO USAGES OF THE TERMS 'TREATMENT' AND 'REHABILITATION'

For convenience, we can use the stages marked out by Zilboorg as broad phases in psychiatric history within which to trace the vicissitudes of the terms treatment and rehabilitation. Zilboorg[23] considered the first revolution in modern psychiatry to have occurred in the sixteenth century, as signified by the work of Agrippa and Weyer. Their efforts to reinstate a more humanistic attitude toward the insane made effective inroads into medieval superstition and brutality. The two centuries of the Renaissance and Reformation, through the time of Pinel's reforms in France, Tuke's in England, and Dorothea Dix's in the United States, he sees as essentially an unfolding and culmination of this same revolutionary upheaval. Dreikurs prefers to localize the series of massive revolutions in modern times (as against other effective reformist eras as with the Greeks) in the period beginning with the reformers of the eighteenth century.[24]

Medical treatments since the eighteenth century have been very varied. Blood-letting, cathartics, and emetics were very widespread in psychiatry as in general medicine. Benjamin Rush,[25] for example, based his endorsement of such practices on contemporary views that the disorders of the mind were due to diseases of the blood-vessels of the brain, indicating the need for reduction of blood congestion. Hydrotherapy, drugs of various kinds, surgery, the use of homeopathic and allopathic substances, endocrine extracts, and so on, were all tried during this period—each with partial and irregular success.

Moral treatment, which emphasized the adoption of kindly attitudes towards patients and involving them in constructive work—in a way superficially like the contemporary milieu therapy trend—was another line of development. Benjamin Rush used it as a kind of background for other treatments which he considered to be the essence of therapy, while the European reformers, notably Pinel and Tuke, used it more focally. In the United States, by the mid nineteenth century, moral treatment had become a well-defined method, though never a dominant one among hospital psychiatrists. Brigham defined moral treatment as 'the removal of the insane from home and former associations, with respectful and kind treatment under all circumstances, and in most cases manual labor, attendance on religious worship on Sunday, the establishment of regular habits and of self-control, diversion of the mind from morbid trains of thought. . . .'[26]

An enormous number of treatments were tried during this period, with what appears to the modern mind to be a remarkable proliferation of peculiar rationales. However, perhaps the greatest contribution was in the purely descriptive knowledge that was accumulated about the types of syndromes seen in the psychically ill. Whatever the therapeutic merits of the various measures in vogue, the energetic attendance on the psychically ill by men of biological training led to a naturalistic classification of the disorders, culminating in the work of Kraepelin. Chronic cases were thus separated from acute cases with greater accuracy. However, the classification of patients as 'chronic' types, along with the organic bias in psychiatry and negative public attitudes toward the insane, contributed to the development of the custodial mental hospital system. Here, with meagre staffing and pessimistic orientation, the most ill were kept in accumulating numbers to await their death or some unlikely apocalypse. Rehabilitation, as a concept or separate set of practices, had no place, since the 'acutes' were treated or spontaneously recovered, and the 'chronics' were simply stored away.

The apocalypse did not come from within the mental hospital system. Though Freud was stimulated by Charcot, the alpha and omega of his theories, which formed the foundation stone of the second revolution in psychiatry, were spelled out in the private treatment of neurotics. Freud did not see the psychically disordered individual simply as a carrier of diseased organs, pathogenic substances, or defective genes, but rather as a whole personality which had been malformed partly as a product of early emotional development within the family. Entrenched blockages to the expression of instinctual drives, infantile misconceptions about the attitudes and motivation of others, and other such personality malformations, were manifested in the variety of symptomatic patterns according to the age of trauma and other factors associated with the child's development. Therapy consisted partly in attempting to elucidate the covert and unrecognized layers of experience which underlay and determined contemporary behaviour, and in allowing the discharge of stored-up energies associated with the recollection of their original contexts.

At first, the Freudian movement, with all its derivatives which elaborated and developed one or another aspect of the original theory, had little to do with rehabilitation, though it was an active treatment method par excellence. In its classical form, psychoanalysis today represents the treatment method that is most focally concerned with the integration of the individual personality, to the exclusion of rehabilitation except insofar as the latter is considered to follow as a natural consequence of good treatment. The classical texts and reference books of psychoanalysis, of Freud,[27] Fenichel,[28] and Glover,[29] provide no reference to the concept of rehabilitation in their indexes.

During the period of the 'second revolution' in psychiatry, however, particularly towards its end in the mid twentieth century, the concept of rehabilitation began to be prominent.

In the dictionary sense, the term rehabilitation means to reinvest with some set of rights or privileges, to restore or re-establish a person, and in psychiatry its great period of development has come with the new interest in restoring hospitalized mental patients to 'normal' status in ordinary life. As Charlotte Schwartz has ably pointed out,[30] however, the term has come to have an enormous variety of meanings in different psychiatric contexts. In her own coverage of the meanings assigned to the term in the psychiatric and allied professions, she includes all measures that work toward the goal of restoring mental hospital patients to life outside the hospital. It has been used to indicate *what is done* to the patient, the *processes* that stem from this, the *goals* of the activity, or the measures taken at a particular *phase* in the patient's career.

To the extent that the active treatments aimed at restoring the mental patient to the community were clearly medical in form—e.g., the administration of insulin—the rehabilitative activities could be separated from the medical activities, phased to follow them and delivered into the responsibility of para-medical personnel. Rehabilitation was something that came into play after the medical measures that were possible had done as much as they were capable of by way of restoring the patient to contact with reality, stabilizing his emotional equilibrium, and so on. The growth of effective pharmacological measures served to keep the line clear between treatments and rehabilitation. Rehabilitation included all the other measures necessary to help the long-chronic patient 'bridge the gap' between hospital and community. The usual kind of thing that was necessary included education in such essential cultural elements as how to use modern public transport; how to shop in a supermarket; how to manage modern operations in a trade or domestic situation. The chronic patients who were involved in many of the rehabilitation programmes were veritable latter-day Rip van Winkels. Their own changed capacities—due to ageing, changes in family and other social network features—had to be taken into account, and social workers dealt with such problems. Aside from whatever treatment or care these patients were given, they were seen as needing 'rehabilitation' to help them adjust to the end-product of their hospital experience, whether it was something better, worse, different, or the same as that with which they came into the hospital.

In this context, rehabilitation in psychiatry was similar to rehabilitation in general medicine. It worked with 'residual' capacities after medical measures had brought the patient to the best possible biological state. In surgery, for example, a patient who had his leg amputated would receive rehabilitation therapies involving the retraining of muscles and psychological expectations in adaptation to an artificial leg. The rehabilitation measures were intermediate between the technical medical measures and the private matter of making a life outside the hospital. In these situations, 'treatment' is distinguished substantively and temporally as well as conceptually from 'rehabilitation'. It was in this sense that Rush termed rehabilitation the 'third phase of medicine'.

As the active treatment measures in the psychiatric hospitals began to absorb psychotherapeutic approaches deriving from the theories of Adolph Meyer, Sigmund Freud and his followers, and others of dynamic psychotherapy orientation, a step was made towards blurring the distinction between rehabilitation and treatment. For the first time, treatment was linked to an attempt to understand the patient in his total life situation as well as to understand the bio-physical character of his symptoms. It was considered that only through such an understanding, and through helping the patient to revise his own perceptions of these things, could lasting benefit be achieved. This was in sharp contrast to the tendencies in prior forms of treatment to work toward the removal of symptoms. Moreover, the substance of psychotherapy (which came to mean all methods 'which rely for their effect on an exchange of ideas between patient and doctor'[31] rather than all methods designed to treat the mind) was the interchange of words, ideas, gestures—the stuff of interpersonal relationships generally, the stuff of rehabilitation. However, the psychoanalytic method is time-con-suming, expensive, and in scarce supply (in addition to the limitations on its applicability). While all psychotherapy aimed at improving the individual's personality integration, there were differences in the degree of change to which psychotherapists aspired. A distinction grew up between 'supportive' and 'uncovering' psychotherapy. The former aimed to 'alter the patient's circumstances or his immediate feeling about them so that they will be more bearable to him', while the second attempted to 'alter the patient's innate capacities for dealing with any circumstances'.[32] Both were considered 'treatment' and controlled by physicians when practised in the hospital context. This definition of 'supportive psychotherapy' sounds very much like some definitions of rehabilitation.

With the advent of the 'third revolution' in psychiatry, we see the final tendencies to blur the distinction between treatment and rehabili-tation.

The idea of a psychiatric institution as a therapeutic community has come into vogue in the middle of this century. Whatever its specific treatment methods, there is a tendency for hospitals to provide the kind of environment that will effectively supplement the other kinds of treatment. This movement, resting on an emphasis on group dynamics, has been termed by Moreno and Dreikurs the 'third revolu-tion' in psychiatry. Like the earlier emphasis on 'moral treatment', it stresses the importance of providing favourable environmental condi-tions for the patient—aside from the specifically treatment transactions, whatever they might be. And, like the moral treatment movement, the therapeutic community idea is used as either figure or ground according to the persuasion of the particular practitioner. There are, however, a number of crucial differences between the two approaches, even aside from the sheer presence of theoretical rationales for the contemporary methods.

The contemporary trend has developed partly in reaction to the undesirable qualities of the custodial system,[33] partly under the influ-ence of social science ideas,[34] partly through the application of psycho-analytic ideas to new situations like hospitals[35] or homes for delinquent children,[36] partly in response to the exigencies of war.[37] Other con-tributing influences were the renewed awareness of the capacity of certain colonies like Gheel in Belgium[38] to continue their own psychotics, and in general, a trend towards assuming more large-scale social responsibility for the mentally ill, a task that was becoming more feasible as effective drugs were being developed. As public health medicine triumphed over one mass disease after another, energies were freed to turn to mental disorder, which remains the most complex and intractable of man's pervasive ills.

As the 'third revolution' has taken form and flourished in the psychiatric world, its emphases have been changing from an earlier conception of the patient as a more passive recipient of the milieu therapy methods to a more active participant in the entire programme.[39] Vitale sees the shift from restraint to self-regulation as a core aspect of the development of therapeutic communities. Stainbrook has coined the apt expression 'organization studying organization' to characterize a modern social psychiatric establishment,[40] with the patients as well as staff as the participants.

With regard to the actual carrying through of these ideals, the participants in the trend vary considerably among themselves. Morris Schwartz, in summing up the kinds of things that are thought to be therapeutic in an institutional milieu, noted the following:[41]

A milieu to be therapeutic would be constituted so as 'to provide the contexts and facilities for the kinds of social processes and interpersonal relations that will bring about the following effects in patients:

1. provide the patient with experiences that will minimize his distortions of reality;
2. facilitate his realistic and meaningful communicative exchange with others;
3. facilitate his participation with others so that he derives greater satisfaction and security therefrom;
4. reduce his anxiety and increase his comfort;
5. increase his self-esteem;
6. provide him with insight into the causes and manifestations of his mental illness;
7. mobilize his initiative and motivate him to realize more fully his potentialities for creativity and productivity.'

Schwartz notes that these generalizations embody many diverse ideas of varying consensus among psychiatrists, and our present state is one of exploration and discovery, rather than one in which definite pronouncements can be made.

The goals of the therapeutic milieu as a treatment method are obviously similar to the general goals of psychotherapy. Schwartz observes that the implementation of these goals in hospitals may be (1) the global (i.e., relating to the overall social structure—e.g., as 'democratic' in preference to authoritarian; treatment-oriented as contrasted with custodial; humanitarian as opposed to oppressive; and flexible as opposed to rigid); (2) the level of interpersonal relations (i.e., relating to preferred modes of interaction—e.g., understanding and personal rather than stereotyped and routine; sympathetic and kindly rather than hostile, cruel, or contemptuous; interested rather than unconcerned); and finally (3), the level of attempted effects on patients (e.g., accepting illness rather than projecting it or denying it; correcting distortions rather than continuing in an unrealistic interpretation of expectations).

Obviously these orientations leave a great deal of flexibility in the actual kinds of measures to be adopted, and their relative emphasis within the régime of any particular hospital aspiring to become a therapeutic community.

In general, the socio-environmentally oriented psychiatrists take what Marvin Opler has termed a 'field theoretical' approach, in contrast to the 'class theoretical' approach which sees the locus of the individual's disorder in his psycho-biological make-up.[42]

One approach to the therapeutic implications of socio-environmental conditions within psychiatric hospitals is sometimes called 'administrative psychiatry'. Stanton and Schwartz note:

'Psychotherapy is a technique now widely practised and studied and one held in high prestige. In contrast, administrative psychiatry, the influencing of "the other twenty-three hours" of treatment, is more widely practised but is little studied and is of relatively low prestige.'[43]

Administrative psychiatry attempts to integrate patients' hospital lives outside the specific therapy sessions with the overall goals of treatment and rehabilitation.

A great many techniques for this have been put forward with claims from their enthusiasts for positive results. The plethora of these has caused some professional workers to observe that 'almost anything at one time or another has been of benefit in the treatment of schizophrenia'.[44]

The viewpoint that has come to be called the therapeutic community approach has many variants. However, there seem to be certain common elements or core features that bind them all together. The basic set of beliefs includes:

a. The total social organization in which the patient is involved—and not only the relationship with the doctor—is seen as affecting the therapeutic outcome.

b. The social organization is not regarded as a routinized background to treatment, but as a vital force, useful for creating a milieu that will maximize therapeutic effects.

c. The core element in such an institutional context is the provision of opportunities for patients to take an active part in the affairs of the institution. This trend is sometimes called 'democratization', and it takes a variety of forms. Some attempts at 'democratizing' the hospital system limit themselves to providing meetings for patients in which they can form opinions that will be communicated to the staff, though it is understood that the staff has ultimate authority and responsibility whether or not to implement these opinions.[45] Another type of 'democratization' gives more emphasis to forming all decisions in a group context by consensus of staff and patients.

d. All relationships within the hospital—those of patients among themselves as well as patients with staff—are regarded as potentially therapeutic. Some way is provided to make use of therapeutic potentialities in other kinds of relationships beside the doctor-patient relationship. The extent and type of relationships that any particular institution actively engaged in varies considerably. Sometimes social workers, nurses, occupational therapists, and patients are included, sometimes not.

e. Aside from formal characteristics of structuring relationships, the *qualitative* atmosphere of the social environment is itself considered important therapeutically. This general orientation has reference to what is sometimes called the 'emotional climate' of the institution. While warmth and acceptance are generally regarded as 'good', there are varying views on the optimal degree and condition for tolerating disturbance and disruptive activity.

f. A high value is placed on communication *per se*. One basis for this value is an administrative one. It is considered valuable for people in one part of the organization to know what people in other parts are doing, thinking, and feeling. Furthermore, the act of communicating is thought to have an important morale and therapeutic effect for staff as well as patients. The content of communication is also considered valuable for treatment by making available, through a variety of channels, data supplementing the limited information that emerges in the doctor-patient relationship.

Particular hospitals that exemplify the therapeutic community approach vary in the way they implement these viewpoints and in the specific combination of elements they use. The form that each institution takes is the result of the particular history of that institution, the personality of its leader, the institutional setting within which it occurs (for example, the National Health Service in England as against private, state, or federal hospitals in America), the attitudes of the population at large, the treatment ideology of the staff, and the type and severity of the disorders being treated. Hospitals that have any conviction at all that there is anything in the social psychiatric approach tend to favour, minimally, a 'therapeutic milieu',[46] even though they do not go so far as to institute a 'therapeutic community' as a focal and explicit treatment instrument.

Differences among therapeutic communities may be exemplified by the following:

In one hospital the staff might feel that patients should be allowed to regress in treatment. They might allow patients to go to bed and be treated like sick children more readily than in a hospital where the staff favoured active participation in hospital life and no indulgence of neurotic tendencies. Under the latter conditions, pressures might be exerted on the patient to get up and be active in the regular round of therapeutic community life.

Another kind of variation might be seen in the question of how much expression of aggression should be allowed. To the extent that the staff emphasizes the value of individual patients controlling their aggressive impulses and verbalizing them privately in a doctor-patient interview, they would attempt to discourage or provide restraints against overt aggression. To the extent that the staff value having patients express overt aggression as a diagnostic and therapeutic element, they might be more permissive of such behaviour.

Another example might be seen in the question of occupational therapy. To the extent that the staff feels that work in itself is diagnostically and therapeutically valuable, they would place great emphasis on patients' participation in the work programme. On the other hand, to the extent that they feel the focus of therapy lies in other kinds of relationships and transactions, they would favour work, if at all, only as a diversionary or reality-testing kind of activity.[47]

Similar kinds of variation can be seen about the questions of social mixing; specialization of staff roles; the organization of status hierarchies within the staff; the question of what elements in the patient's experience are relevant for therapy; the problem of which personnel may legitimately administer therapy; the question of degree and type of firmness and discipline to be used in implementing a régime, and so on. These provide the areas of controversy and uncertainty around which different hospitals can organize their treatment programme in quite different ways, and yet adhere essentially to the core set of orientations that characterize the therapeutic community approach.

ORIENTATION TO THE CONCEPTS 'TREATMENT' AND 'REHABILITATION'

It seems, from what we have noted about the trends in social psychiatry, that the *avant-garde* approach tends not to distinguish between the aims, personnel, techniques, or processes of rehabilitation and those of treatment. The definition of social psychiatry proposed by Rennie indicates how social psychiatrists view the two aims of personality change (treatment) and social adaptation (rehabilitation) as of a piece:[48]

'Social psychiatry, by our definition, seeks to determine the significant facts in family and society which affect adaptation (or which can be clearly defined as of aetiological importance). . . . It concerns itself not only with the mentally ill but with the problems of adjustment of all persons in society toward a better understanding of how people adapt and what forces tend to damage or enhance their adaptive capacities. . . . Social psychiatry is therefore the study of aetiology and dynamics of persons seen in their total environmental setting.'

Rennie's emphasis is on *process*, and since his focus is on adaptive processes, treatment of individuals implies their rehabilitation. Maxwell Jones and others view the most meaningful aspect of treatment to be those measures aimed at equipping an individual for performance in the best possible set of roles in society (in contrast to being kept in custodial care). He thus maintains that all psychiatric treatment is 'rehabilitation'.[49] He notes, however, that Tait and Rodger, in their unpublished report on rehabilitation, consider it 'illogical' to reverse the statement and regard all rehabilitation as treatment; though they consider the relationship to be 'very close'. Jones himself prefers a broader view according to which rehabilitation is used to describe 'any treatment situation in which psychological, sociological and anthropological techniques can be applied with advantage to the individual, whether he be recovering from an illness, has reached a static state of disability, be deteriorating or simply maladjusted to a degree which would not commonly be designated "illness".'

Here we have a stress on techniques used as well as goals. There is no mention of process, but the idea of levels seems implicit in his thinking —with 'rehabilitation' implying the conceptualization of goals on the most all-encompassing level.

Several kinds of problems are intermingled here. Separating them out may assist us to develop useful variables in understanding the situation.

First, we have different stages of medical activity—Rusk's three of diagnosis, treatment, and rehabilitation, to which could be added a fourth suggested by Williams, prevention. In each of these, the focus of interest may be on any of three levels—the bio-physiological, the psychological, or the socio-cultural. Conventionally, medicine dealt almost exclusively with the bio-physiological—seeking its aetiological traces, its diagnostic signs, and its therapeutic techniques on this level alone, assuming the others would follow more or less 'automatically'. That is to say, the physician who treated malaria well, found its symptoms on the bio-physical level, administered chemical therapies, and assumed that with good care the patient would recover not only his physiological well-being, but his state of psychic health and his usual level of social adjustment. As it became clear that this did not always work out in medicine generally, 'adjunctive' measures were added, for example, to assist an amputee with the psychological adjustments and vocational retraining that might be necessary for him to return to ordinary society.[50] Gradually all 'good' treatments included rehabilitative considerations, but the order of priority in levels was from the biological 'upward' to the psychological and social. Working with a patient only psychologically would not come to grips with a physical disease. The intervention had to start on the biological level.

In psychiatry the situation is more complex. A patient may have a disorder on the physical level that *can* be affected by intervention at the psychological level—e.g., with the psychoanalysis of an ulcer patient. Here again, the *focus* is on the psychological level of intervention, the aim to reorder the personality, but to achieve an effect on the biological level as well. Effects on the socio-cultural level, if considered at all, are assumed to follow more or less automatically. In general, psychological therapy, of which 'classical' psychoanalysis is the archetype, assumes that sociocultural adjustment will follow on good treatment—i.e., a mature individual will select social situations in which he can function adequately. In psychoanalysis, the treatment situation is explicitly *unlike* ordinary situations. Regression is permitted, even required, and boundaries between the analytic world and the outside world kept as free of 'leakage' (through 'acting out') as possible. In the end, with the resolution of the transference, a modicum of 'normality' is restored to the analyst-patient relationship.

The post-analytic social adjustment of analysands is a much discussed but little studied phenomenon, so it is not possible to say to what extent and in what way social adjustment is affected by a treatment so focused on achieving individual personality integration.

The growth of group methods[51] and ultimately the social psychiatric movement and therapeutic communities brought the socio-cultural level pervasively into focus. Aetiological theories (socio-environmental stresses),[52] diagnosis (interpersonal relationship patterns), treatment (milieu therapy), rehabilitation (adjustment to social roles), and even prevention (e.g., consultation with mental health 'caretakers' in the community)[53] have been conceptualized in socio-cultural terms.

The correlates of therapy addressed to different levels is summarized in *Figure 1*.

The tendency heretofore was to assume that interventions at the lower (biological) level produced results in the higher levels dependably and automatically, while similar processes in the opposite direction did not hold. There are obvious limitations to the extent to which the reverse processes may be said to function (e.g., psychological intervention producing bio-physiological changes; socio-cultural intervention producing psychological and bio-physiological change). But evidence is accumulating that such processes do occur under some circumstances and their manipulation may become a focal method of treatment.

The idea of 'linked open systems' has recently become prominent. It has been derived from the work of Bertalanffy and applied by

FIGURE 1

Intervention Levels	Aims	Methods	Personnel	Illustrative Processes
Socio-cultural	social adaptation, role performance	groups, milieu administrative therapy, rehabilitation therapies	staff and patient groups, occupational instructors, etc.	behaviour adaptation, role playing, education, adjustment
Psycho-logical	personality re-integration in depth, emotional maturity	psychotherapy (e.g. psycho-analysis)	psycho-therapist	catharsis, transference, regression, insight, ego growth
Biolo-gical	cure, physiological health	'physical' treatments (drugs, electricity, surgery)	physician and aides	bio-physiological homeostasis

Caudill[54] to phenomena relevant here. According to this, physicians interested in working with a bio-physiological phenomenon might prescribe a course of socio-cultural experiences to achieve the physical aim. Similarly, interventions on any of the recognized levels may be used to yield results on other levels. This has always been familiar enough in the prescriptions of rest, pleasures, recreation, etc., to allow 'natural' healing processes to regenerate the organism. However, through modern administrative psychiatry, the potentialities at least for even more powerful leverage would seem to be becoming more available as the linkages among the systems become more understood.

In drawing the distinction we have in mind between treatment and rehabilitation in somewhat more operational terms we would make the discriminating criterion *immediate aim*. This seems useful in the light of the general tendency of therapists to expect that in the long run— long after they themselves may have finished their interventions—the patient will achieve some level of socio-cultural adjustment, and thus, in our general sense, be rehabilitated. However, we restrict our own usages to the shorter run. We use the terms as follows:

'*Treatment*' means here all those measures, by any legitimated personnel (and this can include patients in the therapeutic community) that have as their principal immediate aims the alteration of the individual personality toward better intra-psychic integration;

'*Rehabilitation*', on the other hand, means those measures that have as their immediate aim the fitting of a particular personality to the demands of an ongoing social system.

By 'immediate' we mean within the sphere of professional responsibility and involvement of the person administering the treatment. Thus a surgeon, however interested he might be in the ultimate rehabilitation of his amputee case, might not be directly involved in anything further than the treatment, leaving the rehabilitation, if at all, to other specialists.

The differences between psychiatry and other medical specialities are not only differences in degree of specialization. Differences also exist in scope of interest as defined by professional norms. Psychiatrists are increasingly accepting responsibility for the management of situations outside the hospital and consulting room, and to this extent are becoming directly involved in activities closer to patients' ordinary social contexts. They may simply see this as an extension of their treatment techniques aiming at a change in individual personalities. Their techniques, however, come increasingly to resemble those of rehabilitation specialists. Administrative management and leadership techniques become increasingly focal in importance for the milieu therapist. A working knowledge of family and institutional sociology becomes essential for community psychiatrists.

Another element in the situation is the problem of ascertaining 'residual function' in psychiatry as against physical medicine. When a man has his arm cut off, there is no question of his ever growing another. In psychiatry, on the other hand, if a patient loses some of his ego-functions, he may recover them as a consequence of treatment. There are, however, great areas of uncertainty and controversy about the mutability of different aspects of the personality structure. The 'personality disorders', or psychopathic personalities, for example, have been seen as 'constitutionally defective' (presumably unable to develop greater 'residual' functions than those with which they come to the psychiatrist—viz., a congenitally stunted ego-development). Chornyak, for example, states that 'we must learn to face the fact ... that psychopathy is untreatable'.[55] On the other hand, some psychiatrists, including those of the Unit, view patients with 'psychopathic personalities' as essentially of the same stuff as those with other psychiatric disorders, only involving anomalies of ego-growth at different periods and in different contexts of their development as compared with neurotics on the one hand and psychotics on the other. . . .[56]

Clearly, activities that we would conceptualize as treatment may empirically serve rehabilitation ends and vice versa. But this conceptual distinction and our arbitrary cutting points may help to sort out some of the current confusions that perplex a good many contemporary practitioners in the mental health field.

In this context, it appears that the Belmont Unit's merging of the terms treatment and rehabilitation has reference to aims as well as to methods. Its name, the 'Social Rehabilitation Unit', implies its goals of social *adaptation*. Yet it speaks of its methods as 'treatment', implying optimism about the mutability of patients' personality structures in the course of therapy. According to the Unit view, psychopathic personalities can not only be made to adjust socially through group influences, but can also develop their personality structures in the course of treatment in order to ease their 'built-in' limitations on acceptable social adjustment.

There are, obviously, ambiguities and complexities—'slippages'—in the ways in which these ideas are set forth. It is precisely for this reason that we consider it important to devote a major part of our effort to the clarification of these vexed terms. Basically, we are dealing with two abstracted entities—the personality of the patient, and the socio-cultural system to which he must adjust. The set of techniques used in the Unit aims at preparing the patient for adjustment to his system of social relationships outside the hospital. But the short-term interim system to which adjustment trials are geared is that of the Unit—the 'therapeutic community'. We shall concern ourselves with three key questions: Which measures in the Unit seem to serve treatment aims? Which measures seem to serve rehabilitation aims within the Unit? Which elements in the Unit situation serve the ultimate aims of rehabilitating the patient to the world outside the Unit? These questions are not precisely delineated in the Unit; the tendency is to blur the questions and answers as though they were all one. The Unit staff have tended to assume that treatment in the Unit is accomplished through rehabilitation to the Unit, and rehabilitation in the Unit is a dress rehearsal for rehabilitation to the outside world. Our own proposition, based on the research findings to be set forth here, is that treatment and rehabilitation aims ought to be kept distinct, for while the therapeutic milieu activities that serve each of them may sometimes be congruent and mutually re-enforcing, they are often independent and even conflicting.

Our approach is sociological, and so, we hope, gains in generality what it loses in close linkage to the concrete clinical data. Our general point of departure is that the therapeutic community approach is neither necessarily the harbinger of the 'true gospel', nor is it necessarily to be seen as a transient fad; both viewpoints have some currency in the profession. We shall attempt to clarify what is meant here by the concept therapeutic community, what its actual functioning elements seem to be, what factors seem to contribute to the attainment of its goals and what factors seem to hamper their realization, and finally what lessons and principles of practical significance may be derived from the experimentation of the group at Belmont. Professor Redlich wrote recently, in his foreword to Caudill's book, that many people ask the question 'Why do so many patients in mental hospitals not get well?' He states that he finds the question why so many people *do* get well more profitable. . . .[57] The orientation we shall adopt here is that the two questions ought to be asked simultaneously, and that the total fabric of the hospital should, as far as possible, be investigated for insights into these *linked* questions.

NOTES AND REFERENCES

1. Zilboorg, Gregory, and Henry, George A.: *A History of Medical Psychology.* New York, Norton, 1941.
2. Dreikurs, Rudolf: 'Group psychotherapy and the third revolution in psychiatry.' *Int. J. soc. Psychiat.*, 1: 23–32, 1955.
3. Jones, Maxwell, and Rapoport, Robert N.: 'Administrative and social psychiatry.' *Lancet*, 20 August, 1955, pp. 386–8.—Rennie, Thomas A. C.: 'Social Psychiatry—A definition.' *Int. J. soc. Psychiat.*, 1: 5–13, 1955.—Rioch, David McK., and Stanton, Alfred H.: 'Milieu therapy.' *Psychiatry*, 16: 65–72, 1953.
4. Watson, Goodwin: Introduction to Jones, Maxwell, *et al.*: *The Therapeutic Community.* New York, Basic Books, 1953, p. vii.
5. Jones, Maxwell: 'Group treatment, with particular reference to group projection methods', *Amer. J. of Psychiat.*, 101: No. 3, 292–9, 1944.—'Rehabilitation of forces neurosis patients to civilian life', *Brit. med. J.*, 1946, 1: 533.—'The working of an industrial neurosis unit', *Occup. Ther.*, 26: No. 4, 213–21, 1947.—and J. M. Tanner: 'The clinical characteristics, treatment and rehabilitation of repatriated prisoners of war with neurosis', *J. Neurol Psychiat.*, 11: No. 1, 53–60, 1948.—'Emotional catharsis and re-education in the neuroses with the help of group methods', *The Brit. J. med. Psychol.*, 21: Part 2, 104–10, 1948.—'The problem of

the resettlement of the psychiatric Patient', *J. R. sanit. Inst.*, **69**: No. 5, 643–6, 1949. —*et al. Social Psychiatry*, London, Tavistock Publications, 1952 (published in U.S., as *The Therapeutic Community*, New York, Basic Books, 1953.—Merry, J., and Pomryn, B. A., 'A community method of psychotherapy', *Brit. J. med. Psychol.*, **26**: Parts 3 and 4, 222–44, 1953.—'The treatment of character disorder in a therapeutic community', *World Mental Health*, **6**: 1, 1954.—The treatment of psychopathic personalities', *Proc. R. Soc. Med.*, **47**: 636, 1954.—'The concept of a therapeutic community', *Amer. J. Psychiat.*, **112**: 647, 1956.—and Pomryn, B. A., and Skellern, E., 'Work therapy', *Lancet*, 1956, **1**: 343.—'The Treatment of personality disorders in a therapeutic community', *Psychiatry*, **2**: 3, 211–20, 1957.— 'The industrial rehabilitation of mental patients while still in hospital', *Lancet*, 1956, **2**: 985–6.

6. Galdston, Iago: *The Meaning of Social Medicine*. Cambridge, Mass., Harvard Univ. Press, 1954.—Halliday, James: *Psychosocial Medicine*. New York, Norton, 1948.

7. Paul, Benjamin D.: *Health, Culture and Community*. New York, Russel Sage Fdn., 1955.—Foster, G.: 'Problems in Intercultural Health Programs, Memorandum to Committee on Preventive Medicine and Social Science Research.' Social Science Research Council, 1957 (mimeo.).—Leighton, Alexander, and Leighton, D.: *The Navaho Door*. Cambridge, Mass., Harvard Univ. Press, 1944.

8. Simmons, Leo. W., and Wolff, Harold G.: *Social Science in Medicine*. New York: Russell Sage Fdn., 1954.—Stanton, Alfred, and Schwartz, Morris: *The Mental Hospital*. New York, Basic Books, 1954.—Caudill, William A.: *The Psychiatric Hospital as a Small Society*. Cambridge, Mass., Harvard Univ. Press, 1958.

9. Clausen, John A., and Yarrow, Marion R., eds.: 'The impact of mental illness on the family.' *J. soc. Issues*, **11**: No. 4, 1955.—Leighton, Alexander, *et al.*, eds.: *Explorations in Social Psychiatry*, Part II, New York, Basic Books, 1957.—Spiegel John P.: 'Resolution of role conflict within the family.' *Psychiatry*, **20**: 1–16, 1957. —Ackermann, Nathan W.: *Psychodynamics of Family Life*. New York, Basic Books, 1958.

10. Ruesch, Jurgen, and Bateson, Gregory: *Communications: the Social Matrix of Psychiatry*. New York, Norton, 1951.—McQuown, Norman A.: 'Linguistic transcription and specification of psychiatric interview materials.' *Psychiatry*, **20**: 79–86, 1957.

11. Faris, Robert E., and Dunham, H. Warren: *Mental Disorders in Urban Areas*. Univ. of Chicago Press, 1939.—Lemkow, Paul, Tietze, C., and Cooper, M.: 'A survey of statistical studies in the prevalence and incidence of mental disorders in sample populations.' *U.S.P.H.S. Reprint* No. 2534, **58**: 1909–27, 1943.—Milbank Memorial Fund: *Inter-Relations between the Social Environment and Psychiatric Disorders*. New York, Milbank Memorial Fund, 1953.

12. Gilbert, Doris C., and Levinson, Daniel, J.: 'Ideology, personality and institutional policy in the mental hospital.' *J. abnorm. Soc. Psychol.*, **53**: 263–71, 1956.

13. Hollingshead, August, and Redlich, Fredrick: *Social Class and Mental Illness*. New York, Wiley, 1958.—Mishler, Elliot G., and Tropp, A.: 'Status and interaction in a psychiatric hospital.' *Hum. Relations*, **9**: 187–205, 1956.

14. For patients, cf. Simmons, Ozzie, Davis, James A., and Spencer, Katherine: 'Interpersonal strains in release from a mental hospital.' *Soc. Problems*, **4**: 21-8, 1956.—Also, Goffman, Erving: 'The moral career of the mental patient.' *Psychiatry*, **22**: 123-42, 1959—For professional groups, e.g., physicians, cf. Merton, Robert K., Reader, George, and Kendall, Patricia L.: *The Student-Physician: Introductory Studies in the Sociology of Medical Education*. Cambridge, Mass., Harvard Univ. Press, 1957.

15. Henry, Jules: 'The formal structure of a psychiatric hospital.' *Psychiatry*, **17**: 139-52, 1954.

16. Caudill, William A.: *The Psychiatric Hospital . . ., op. cit.*

17. von Mering, Otto, and King, Stanley: *Remotivating the Mental Patient*. New York, Russell Sage, 1957.

18. Caudill, William A., and Roberts, Bertram H.: 'Pitfalls in the organization of interdisciplinary research.' *Hum. Organiz.*, **10**: 12-15, 1951.—Simmons, Ozzie, and Davis, James: 'Interdisciplinary collaboration in mental illness research.' *Amer. J. Sociol.*, **63**: 297-303, 1957.—Luszki, Margaret B.: *Interdisciplinary Team Research: Methods and Problems*. New York Univ. Press, 1958.—Rapoport, Robert N.: 'Notes on the disparagement of sociologizing in collaborative research.' *Hum. Organiz.*, **16**: 14-15, 1957.

19. E.g., Rose, Arnold, ed.: *Mental Health and Mental Disorder*. New York, Norton: 1955.—Greenblatt, Milton; Levinson, Daniel J.; and Williams, Richard H.: *The Patient and the Mental Hospital*. Glencoe, Ill., The Free Press, 1957.—Leighton, Alexander, *et al.*: *Explorations in Social Psychiatry, op. cit.*

20. Stanton, Alfred, and Schwartz, Morris: *The Mental Hospital, op. cit.*—Caudill, William A.: *The Psychiatric Hospital . . ., op. cit.*—Belknap, Ivan: *Human Problems of a State Mental Hospital*. New York, McGraw-Hill, 1956.

21. Williams, Richard H.: 'Psychiatric rehabilitation in the hospitals.' *Publ. Hlth. Rep., Wash.*, **68**: 1043-51 and 1231-6, 1953.

22. Schwartz, Charlotte: *Rehabilitation of Mental Hospital Patients*. USPHS Monograph No. 17, GPO, 1953, p. 2.

23. Zilboorg, Gregory: *A History of Medical Psychology, op. cit.*

24. Dreikurs, Rudolf: 'Group psychotherapy and the third revolution in psychiatry', *op. cit.*

25. Malamud, W.: 'The History of Psychiatric Therapies' in *One Hundred Years of American Psychiatry*. New York, Columbia Univ. Press, 1944.

26. Brigham, Y.: 'Moral treatment of insanity.' *Amer. J. Insan.*, **6**: 1847.

27. Freud, Sigmund: *The complete psychological works*, (Standard edition). London, Hogarth Press.

28. Fenichel, Otto: *The Psychoanalytic Theory of Neurosis*. New York, Norton, 1945.

29. Glover, Edward: *The Technique of Psychoanalysis*. London, Baillière, Tindall & Cox, 1955.

30. Schwartz, Charlotte: *Rehabilitation of Mental Hospital Patients, op. cit.*

31. Stafford-Clark, D.: *Psychiatry Today*. Harmondsworth, Penguin, 1953, p. 167.

32. *Ibid.*

33. Greenblatt, Milton, York, R., and Brown, E. L.: *From Custodial to Therapeutic Care in Mental Hospitals*. New York, Russell Sage, 1955.

34. Sullivan, Harry S.: *The Inter-Personal Theory of Psychiatry*. New York, Norton, 1953; London: Tavistock Publications.
35. Simmel, Ernst: 'Psychoanalytic treatment in a sanatorium.' *Int. J. Psycho-Anal.*, **10**: 70–89, 1929.
36. Aichhorn, August: *Wayward Youth*. New York, Viking, 1935.
37. Wilson, A. T. M.: 'The serviceman returns.' Pilot Papers, Mental Hospital Series, 1946 (mimeo.).—Jones, Maxwell: *The Therapeutic Community, op. cit.*, Chapter I.—Main, T.: 'The hospital as a therapeutic institution.' *Bull. Menninger Clin.*, **10**: 66–70, 1946.
38. Kilgour, J.: 'Colony Gheel.' *Amer. J. Psychiat.*, **92**: 959–65, 1936.
39. Vitale, J. H.: 'The therapeutic community.' Unpublished ms.
40. Stainbrook, E.: 'The hospital as a therapeutic community.' *Neuropsychiat.*, 1955, 69–87.
41. Schwartz, Morris: 'What is a Therapeutic Milieu?' in Greenblatt, Milton, *et al.*: *The Patient and the Mental Hospital, op. cit.*
42. Opler, Marvin: *Culture, Values and Psychiatry*. New York, Thomas, 1956.
43. Stanton, Alfred, and Schwartz, Morris: *The Mental Hospital, op. cit.*, p. 9.
44. Kasanin: 'Critical evaluation of a total push program for regressed schizophrenics in a state hospital.' *Psychiat. Quart.*, **28**: 650–67, 1954.
45. Examples of this would be the 'patient government' method as instituted by Dr Robert W. Hyde and associates at the Boston Psychopathic Hospital and the patient-personnel council as used by Dr Paul M. Howard at McLean Hospital. Cf. Rosenblatt, Daniel: 'Formal Voluntary Organizations Among Patients in a Psychiatric Hospital.' Ph.D. Dissertation, Harvard University, 1959.
46. Rioch, David McK., and Stanton, Alfred H.: 'Milieu therapy', *op. cit.*—Jones, Maxwell, and Rapoport, Robert N.: 'Administrative and social psychiatry', *op. cit.*—Stanton, Alfred H.: 'Problems in analysis of therapeutic implications of the institutional milieu.' *Symposium on Preventive and Social Psychiatry 15–17 April 1957*, Walter Reed Army Institute of Research, Washington, D.C., pp. 493–502.
47. For an illuminating comparison of the different approaches to occupational therapy in European psychiatric hospitals, cf. Carstairs, G. Morris; Clark, David H.; and O'Connor, N.: 'Occupational treatment of chronic psychotics: observations in Holland, Belgium and France.' *Lancet*, 12 Nov. 1955, pp. 1025–30.—Sivadon, Paul: 'Techniques of Sociotherapy.' *Proceedings of the Symposium on Preventive and Social Psychiatry, April 1957*. Walter Reed Army Institute of Research, Washington, D.C.—Jones, Maxwell: 'Psychiatric Rehabilitation.' Report to the World Health Organization (mimeo).
48. Rennie, Thomas A. C.: 'Social psychiatry—a definition', *op. cit.*
49. Jones, Maxwell: 'Psychiatric Rehabilitation', *op. cit.*
50. Jones, Maxwell, and Rapoport, Robert N.: 'Psychiatric Rehabilitation' in *Yearbook of Education*, London, 1955.
51. Corsini, Raymond: *Methods of Group Psychotherapy*. New York, McGraw Hill, 1957.
52. Leighton, Alexander: 'Psychiatric disorder and social environment.' *Psychiat.*, **18**: 367–83, 1955.—Milbank Memorial Fund: *Social Environment and Mental Disorder*. Milbank Memorial Fund, 1953.

53. Caplan, Gerald: 'Mental Health Consultation in Schools' in Kotinsky, R.: *The Elements of a Community Mental Health Program.* Harvard Univ. Press, 1955.
54. Caudill, William A.: *The Psychiatric Hospital . . ., op. cit.*
55. Chornyak, John: 'Some remarks on the diagnosis of the psychopathic delinquent.' *Amer. J. Psychiat.,* **97**: 1326–40, 1941.
56. For an excellent review of professional viewpoints on psychopathy, see McCord, William and Joan: *Psychopathy and Delinquency.* New York, Grune & Stratton, 1956.
57. Redlich, Frederick: Foreword to Caudill, William A.: *The Psychiatric Hospital . . ., op. cit.*

CHAPTER 2

The Unit's Patients

The Unit is part of a Neurosis Centre that serves all the United Kingdom under the National Health Service. It is not part of the special services for any particular 'catchment area', and patients are mainly voluntary admissions referred through a variety of channels.[1] In this chapter we examine the social and psychiatric characteristics of the Unit's patients. While the Unit sees itself as treating 'working-class psychopaths', there is a certain ambiguity about the extent to which the staff and other proponents of the methods consider their approach to be specifically appropriate to 'personality disorders' (as many of the ideological rationales imply), or whether the methods are generally applicable to psychiatric problems of all kinds.[2]

In this chapter we aim at indicating the social and psychiatric *diversity* of the Unit's patients, and specifying more precisely the kinds of patients actually found in the Unit. The task of assessing the strengths and weaknesses of the Unit's methods of treatment and rehabilitation would seem partly to hinge on distinguishing its effect on patients of different kinds. In a later chapter we shall attempt to relate these types of patient to therapeutic results.

TABLE I   COMPOSITION OF REFERRAL SAMPLE: 1953-5

		Discharge Group		
	1953	1954	1955	Totals
Patients				
Discharged	258	259	300	817
Non-Patients				
Referral Refused	21	85	94	200
Non-Appearance	62	67	80	209
Yearly Totals	341	411	474	1226

WHO SENDS THE PATIENTS?

In a study of all people referred to the Unit during the years 1953-5, Rosow found a steady increase in the demand for the Unit's services (*Table 1*):[3]

By far the greatest number of referrals of patients to the Unit come from members of the medical profession, though some are referred by non-medical personnel such as probation officers.

TABLE 2   REFERRAL SOURCES

Type	Referrer-Institutional Setting	No. of Referrals	% of Cases
Medical	Physician in Medical Setting	1082	89
Mixed	Physician in Non-Medical Setting	60	5
Non-Medical	Layman in Non-Medical Setting	73	6
	Totals	1215	100
	No Information	11	
	Total	1226	

According to these data, 94% of all referrals come from physicians, 89% are purely medical, consisting of 83% from hospitals and clinics and 6% from doctors' private practices. Another 5% are of the 'mixed' type, or from doctors serving courts, social agencies, employment exchanges, and other non-medical institutions. Doctors refer almost half the cases that do come from these agencies, while probation officers, social workers, and other laymen refer the rest.

Rosow's study indicates that several kinds of factors operate to determine whether or not a patient will be sent to the Unit for treatment. From a purely scientific point of view, referral criteria would consist exclusively in matching the Unit's treatment to the patient's therapeutic needs. In any actual referral situation, these criteria only partly determine the action taken. Several other considerations characteristically operate to influence the course of events.

Hospitals placed within urban concentrations close to the Unit, mainly the Greater London area, use it more than other urban hospitals. Urban areas use it more than rural areas. Teaching and research hospitals use it more than other hospitals. Hospitals that have been influenced by actual contact with members of the Unit, by being visited, addressed, or served by Unit staff members, use it more than hospitals without such contact. Use of the Unit is not confined to those who are acquainted in detail with its methods and agree with them. Paradoxically, many doctors use the Unit partly because they do not themselves espouse the Unit's methods, but lacking any local method for handling personality disorders with behavioural problems, they refer them to the Unit in preference to providing no treatment at all. While both poles of Unit enthusiasts and Unit disparagers are to be found among referring physicians, most doctors who use the Unit entertain a tentative attitude towards it as an experimental treatment method that fills a gap in the contemporary scene but has yet to demonstrate its actual therapeutic effectiveness.

The study of referrals suggests a large nation-wide network of professional relationships, with nodes in the urban areas, with the most active interest in and use of at least the Unit's innovating treatment method focused in the teaching institutions. Aside from this, actual personal links between members of the Unit staff and acquaintances among their colleagues elsewhere stimulate an additional flow of referrals. These tendencies are clear apart from any appreciable knowledge of the Unit's methods and the 'rational' application of this knowledge to particular patients' needs.

SOCIAL BACKGROUNDS OF PATIENTS

We made a close study of a sample of 168 patients treated in the Unit during the period of research.[4] One hundred and twenty-two were males and 46 females. Almost 50% of the patients were between 20 and 29 years of age. A further 28% were between 30 and 39 years of age; 13% were under 20; and the remaining 10% were over 40, with only 2% of the total over 50.

About 63% of the patients were single, 27% married, and 10% divorced or separated.

Educationally, 64% of the 168 had finished secondary modern education (that is, left school when they were fourteen or fifteen years old), 25% had completed grammar school (left at age sixteen to eighteen), and only 3% had attended a university. Five per cent had received only an elementary school education.[5]

With reference to their social class position,[6] the Unit's clientele is weighted heavily with members of the lower socio-economic groups. In this series of patients, none was classified in the Registrar General's class I. Nine per cent of the 168 were in class II, 51% in class III, 15% in class IV, 20% in class V.[7] It is to be noted that psychiatric patients tend to inflate or be over-optimistic about their occupational classifications. Thus, a man who states on admission to the hospital that he is a TV producer may actually be an assistant cameraman's helper. Wherever possible, we corrected for these distortions by requesting specific job descriptions, but we recognize that our data are far from satisfactory. There is probably a marked bias towards increasing the status distribution toward the higher end.

In terms of religion, 61% of the 168 patients were at least nominally members of the Church of England, 18% were Roman Catholics, 8% members of Nonconformist Protestant denominations (Methodists, Presbyterians, etc.), 4% were Jews, 7% were atheists or agnostics; one adhered to an Oriental religion.[8]

The patients came to the hospital from varied living accommodations. Of the 168, 20% lived alone at the time of their admission, 20% lived with their spouses, 24% lived with their parental families, 6% lived in complex households with spouse and parental members of one or the other families, and 30% had other kinds of arrangements; for example, living with friends or relatives.

The social history of the total series of patients shows that 'objective' difficulties in ordinary social relationships characterize the majority. For example, 34% had a chronic work problem (that is, during a period of full employment, they were not in school and had held no job lasting at least one year in the last ten). A further 43% had intermittent work problems (that is, while they had been able to hold at least one job for a minimum of one year, they had changed jobs frequently, and had experienced difficulties in work adjustment). Only 24% shows no serious problems in the work area.

Thirty-seven per cent of the sample had formal records of criminal convictions. Another 6%, though not formally convicted, told their doctors of crimes they had committed serious enough to get them into jail had they been apprehended. Fifty-seven per cent of the records showed no evidence of overt criminal activity.

Eighteen per cent of the patients studied had records of alcoholism or addiction.

In terms of their general capacity to sustain social relationships, 27% were judged as having lived in a socially isolated condition (no sustained friendships); 31% had histories of discordant and unstable relationships; 40% gave no indication of pervasive difficulties in their history or relationships with others.

Patients were rated according to pervasiveness or localization of their problems, whether their difficulties affected them in one or more areas of their lives—e.g., in work, family, social life, or only psychologically or physiologically. Most of the patients were seriously impaired in more than one area of their lives. Forty per cent were rated as totally incapacitated; 37% were rated as having major incapacities (i.e., more than one area affected), and 23% presented symptomatology in only one area of life. This picture checks generally with the Unit staff's view that personality disorder (psychopathy) tends, in contrast to neurosis, to be very diffuse and pervasive in its manifestation. The less pervasive social incapacities tended to be found more frequently among the neurotics in the Unit.

The data on sexual relations tend to bear out further the Unit's generalizations about its patients' disorders. With regard to sexual functioning, only 5% of the 168 seemed to have satisfactory 'normal' sexual relationships with their spouses or with other sexual partners. Fifty-five per cent seemed to have patterns of heterosexual relationships that were overtly normal, but reported difficulties or disappointments in the heterosexual sphere. Thirty-one per cent were totally inhibited in their sexual practices. Eight per cent customarily practised perversions.[9]

Sociologically, then, the Unit's patients tend to come from lower socio-economic groups, and many have had a history of social deviation. However, these attributes do not apply to all the patients, and there is impressive diversity in each of the dimensions described.

PATIENTS' PSYCHIATRIC CHARACTERISTICS

The Unit staff tend, in describing their patients, to focus on their problems of interpersonal relationships rather than on their physiological or psychological functioning. They do not, however, define these problems in the same terms as do the patients themselves.

Patients appear at the Unit with many statements of what is wrong with them.

The following are taken at random from patients' records as their own views of what was wrong with them initially on admission to the Unit:

> 'Afraid that I'll kill someone'
> 'Afraid of someone killing me'
> 'Unable to control impulses' (e.g., sexual
>   impulses, stealing, exhibitionism, violence)
> 'Drink'
> 'Tensions'
> 'Can't work'
> 'Lack of self-confidence'
> 'Pain in the back of my head'
> 'Mixed-up'
> 'Can't concentrate'
> 'Trouble with the law'
> 'Nothing wrong with me'
> 'Came here to learn a trade.'

The largest number of presenting complaints on admission have a strong psychological component—i.e., they focus on a subjective sense of inner dissatisfaction by the patient that the doctor cannot assign to a physical disorder. Where the complaint contains an *interpersonal* problem, for example an inability to get along with others, it is often accompanied by another, *psychological* complaint, which may be offered as the presenting symptom. Only in a relatively small proportion of the 168 cases (21%) are social difficulties unaccompanied by subjective discomfort. These are most often patients who have come under pressure from others—e.g., families, social worker, or the courts of law. Patients who present purely physical symptoms fall into the smallest category (7%).

In the Unit, patients' complaints are seen as manifestations of underlying problems of personality organization, and are re-defined in socio-psychiatric terms. The welter of complaints are seen as reflections of an underlying core of personality difficulty, whereby patients are seen as more similar to one another than their superficial differences would suggest.[10] Functional psychiatric disorders are regarded by the Unit staff as manifestations of different degrees of 'ego weakness' and personality disorganization. The most extreme cases of this, the psychotics, are not sought by the Unit (though some borderline cases are admitted). At the other extreme, the Unit staff diagnose as psychoneurotic patients whom they consider to have a strong and relatively well developed ego structure. These individuals usually perform their social roles fairly acceptably, though perhaps they suffer from certain discomforts or limited incapacities. In between these two extremes of neurotics and psychotics, the Unit staff see a meaningful group, termed the 'personality disorders'. It is to this intermediate group that the Unit primarily gears its conceptualization and therapeutic activity. Eighty-one per cent of the patients in our sample were diagnosed by the Unit psychiatrists as personality disorders or under some synonymously used diagnostic label (e.g., psychopathic personality, behaviour disorder, character disorder, immature ego-development).[11] Eight per cent were diagnosed as neurotics (e.g., hysterics, anxiety states, obsessionals), 9% psychotics, and only 2% of indeterminate or organic disorder. Some patients labelled 'personality disorders' in the Unit, might be called something else in other hospitals. Terence Morris found, in a series of cases studied in the Unit in 1956-7, that the Unit's diagnoses of its cases favoured labels in the broad category of 'character (personality) disorder' about three times as frequently as did referral agencies in describing the same cases. Because these diagnostic types are used almost interchangeably in the Unit, we follow their usage in our writing, without necessarily agreeing with their position in the controversy as to whether 'psychopathic personality' is a meaningful clinical entity or what the relationship is between 'psychopaths' and the cases called 'personality disorders'.

We thus see that the largest category of patients in the Unit, characterized by a great variety of complaints and of deviations from social norms, is viewed by the Unit staff as essentially a single clinical group towards which the treatment can be directed without further differentiation.

The staff tend to think metaphorically about this group of patients as comparable in ego development to children aged two and a half. Like children of this age, these patients with weakly developed ego structure tend to be self-centred and demanding, unable to empathize with others in ordinary interaction, unable to delay the gratification of their immediate impulses for the sake of long-term goals, unable to plan or to learn adequately from their experiences, and generally exploitative in the way they form relationships with others. In addition, they typically display an unsatisfactory, often perverse, mode of sexual gratification. Furthermore, such adults can be more destructive than children, both physically and in terms of the scope of their effects on others if they occupy social roles of authority and responsibility. The adult patients are seen as persons whose ego development was stunted or warped through unsatisfactory experiences in early relationships. These experiences are thought to produce a personality structure that makes it difficult to perform acceptably in adult social roles—hence the various patterns of failure and deviation.

While the Unit staff loosely class all such social deviants in the 'personality disorder' group, they in fact indicate that they use implicit distinctions in assessing differences within this large and rather heterogeneous grouping. Both in order to make explicit and systematize the Unit's implicit usages, and because these distinctions are valuable in our later analysis of patients' differential responsiveness to the Unit, we make two further sets of psychological distinctions. In this area there is difficulty in establishing 'objective' standards for making the distinctions—comparable to the standards used for the patients' demographic and sociological differentiation. We therefore rely on the joint judgements of clinicians observing behaviour in the Unit and social scientists analysing case records to establish the classifications.

The first distinction is a relatively minor modification of the Unit's idea of ego-weakness as an indicator of degree of psychiatric disorder. If we consider the patients diagnosed as psychotic as a category of 'weakest ego', and those diagnosed as neurotic as a category of 'strongest ego' (in the patient series), we are left with the large undifferentiated group of personality disorders. These were split into two sub-groups of 'personality disorder, strong' (showing stronger egos on specified criteria) and 'personality disorder, weak'. The classification was made by securing two independent judgements on each patient; one by the social scientist on the basis of the patient's medical records, the second by the charge nurse on the basis of observation of the patient in the hospital. Three criteria were used: (a) reality distortion, (b) impulse control, (c) stability of role performance. Agreement was over 90%. This gave us a grade series of four categories of patients (rather than three) in a continuum based on the dimension of ego-strength. The distribution in our series was 16 psychotics (10%); 83 personality disorder weak (50%); 53 personality disorder strong (32%); and 13 neurotics (8%). Three were organically impaired patients.

Our categories of ego-strength implicitly distinguish people according to the degree of their psychological adequacy in meeting life's problems. We would normally expect those with weaker egos to have greater difficulties in managing, to have less personal resources, to be more likely to break down under stress than others, and consequently to require psychiatric treatment.

This, in fact, seems to be the case. According to our data, the weaker-ego group among patients referred to the Unit are more likely to have a psychiatric history, either as patients in a psychiatric hospital or as out-patients in a psychiatric clinic. The stronger-egos are twice as likely as the weaker to have had *no* previous psychiatric treatment (62% *v.* 33%); the weaker-egos are more than twice as likely as the stronger to have been mental hospital patients (51% *v.* 21%) at some time prior to their Unit treatment. To be sure, such a history of psychiatric treatment may affect the way in which the patient is diagnosed. Whether or not such an influence exists, there is a clear relationship between ego–weakness and previous psychiatric treatment.

Similar relationships are found between degree of ego weakness and capacity for sustaining relationships (including marriage), persistence and performance in the occupational sphere, and in early stability and quality of family relationships. Weaker-ego patients showed more transient and discordant relationships, later marriage, more job instability, and a history of early sustained separation from parents and negative orientation toward them (especially mothers).[12] Such expected patterns lend confidence to our classification of patients.

The second distinction we made was based on patients' behavioural tendencies in reacting to stress situations. These 'behavioural defences' are particularly relevant to the Unit's treatment orientation as the staff lay great stress on *behaviour* and patients' capacity to fit their behaviour to the demands of ordinary social life.

We classified these dominant behavioural tendencies into five groups —'aggression', 'emotional insulation', 'conformity', 'illness', and 'physical withdrawal'. By 'aggression' we mean actual physical activity *against* the environment; by 'emotional insulation' we mean a separation between feeling and behaviour, with affective disengagement— e.g. 'intellectualization' as a defence—where participation is sustained with considerable activity (often with covert aggression, sometimes directed against the self, as with some addicts); under 'conformity' we have in mind the type of defence against stress in which the person 'appeals' to the authority figures by being 'good'. Where this conformism is relatively transient and labile we have the familiar 'chameleon' type of reaction, where conformity reflects not a set of internalized standards but expectations in the immediate social situation; by 'illness' (or 'invalidism') we mean the type of defence where the person under stress increases demands for being taken care of, taking to bed with aches and pains, and so on; by 'physical withdrawal' we mean actually leaving the stressful situation altogether.

These classifications are not mutually exclusive. Judgements were made on the basis of typical dominant behavioural defences against stressful situations that have characterized the patient throughout his life. The following excerpts from psychiatrists' case notes will illustrate the types:

Aggression: (male patient, aged 21, home London, unmarried)

Discharged from army after seven months; says he didn't like discipline. Took lorry driving job. Likes this since it keeps him on the move, but he has changed jobs many times. Last Christmas he was accused by police for being involved in a smash and grab raid, and was found guilty. Also found guilty of driving while drunk. . . . Lots of friends, but no one in particular. . . . Got into frequent fights often with parents. Police have had to be called. He sought adventure in the West End to escape parents. He was kept by various older women, and had homosexual advances made to him by a movie producer. Does not trust women . . . usually acts very tense, fed up, belligerent. In the Unit went around with rough crowd—drinking, got into fights, smashed windows. Got some insight into his underlying feelings of inadequacy, but couldn't give up gratifications of being a 'tough guy'. Requested physical treatment.

Emotional Insulation: (male patient, aged 37, London home, unmarried)

Glib and unrealistic person. Tends to say that everything is O.K., and only present in the Unit because of recent court incident in which he was found guilty of stealing a bottle of wine from a carnival shop. He has, in the past, used a good deal of drugs as well as alcohol, and still resorts to them though denying that he does so. Verbalizes well, difficult to pin down . . . understands the principles of the Unit but has the utmost difficulty in applying them to himself . . . has drifted along . . . felt inadequate in relation to women . . . has façade of charming bonhomie, often plays clown role in his relationships, but uses this to keep from looking at his own deeper sense of failure and inadequacy....

Conformity: (female, age 20, Cornwall, unmarried)

Evacuated during war; mother divorced and remarried. Stepfather not interested.... Got on all right at school, but didn't mix well. Played games but not well ... went to school to become children's nurse, and has been looking after children. Never had a boy friend, no special interests. Suffers from slight dissociative states especially in the evenings. These became worse when child she was tending died. In Unit she made a relationship with the instructor of the home group, and this seemed very important to her. She seems to have had a corrective emotional experience—was a good and reliable member of the work group, conformed to the rules, was considered a sensible and intelligent girl.

Illness: (male, aged 37, London, unmarried)

This patient has had many illnesses throughout his life, and has been in observation wards and mental hospital. On admission he proved a poor informant about his problems, wishing only to talk about his physical complaints. He said that he had pains in his legs and face, which started five years ago, and that he had trouble walking in a straight line—tending towards the right. He felt very heavy when he bent down, and had other similar physical problems. ... Although he has had numerous tests that have not revealed anything abnormal physically, he is convinced that something is physically wrong.

During his stay in the Unit he talked only of his physical complaints. He did not like the Unit. He didn't like the groups, and the discussions in the doctor's groups seem to have stirred up his anxieties. It is difficult to know how disturbed he is underneath because his defences do not allow anyone to get very close to him, but a diagnosis of depressive hypochondriasis in an inadequate personality was given.

Withdrawal: (male, aged 22, London, unmarried)

Brought up in an orphanage with his two brothers ... went from job to job—baker's assistant, projectionist's assistant, page boy in hotel, etc. Got into trouble for stealing. Went to jail and put on probation. Got into more trouble . . . several subsequent convictions for stealing, finally sent to Unit. During his stay he was rather passive, attached himself to several women, one after another in a dependent way—idealized them, and then left them feeling upset and disappointed, usually drinking heavily or taking drugs. When he was brought up in groups—which he often missed or came late to, he just looked like a hunted animal and however much the group would try he couldn't use it. Overwhelmed by his primitive feelings, and could only use one relationship at a time but never stuck. . . . Besides arousing the initial 'poor Johnnie' reaction, he couldn't make positive relationships—always backing away, finally left.

While these descriptive categories were not developed with such a conception in mind, it seems that they describe a continuum from activity at the 'aggression' end, through a mid-point of 'conformity' that approximates to social normality, to 'withdrawal' at the other extreme of passive or disengaging kinds of reaction.

The relative ego strengths of patients with these defensive reactions appear in *Table 3*.

TABLE 3 DIAGNOSIS OF BEHAVIOURAL-DEFENCE TYPES

Ego-Strength	Aggression N	%	Emotional Insulation N	%	Conformity N	%	Illness N	%	Physical Withdrawal N	%
Weaker (Psychotic) (PD Weak)	19	76	29	56	8	27	11	52	32	86
Stronger (Neurotic) (PD Strong)	6	24	23	44	22	73	10	48	5	14
Totals:	(25)	100	(52)	100	(30)	100	(21)	100	(37)	100

These patterns are as unequivocal as one could hope for, even with such small numbers of cases. The most socially approved form of behavioural-defence in this array is by definition, conformity, and among the conformists the stronger egos outnumber the weaker by about three to one. This ratio is completely reversed for the most socially disapproved modes of defence at the extremes of the range—the aggressives and the withdrawers. Among these two groups, the weaker egos outnumber the stronger by more than three to one. Among the defence types in an intermediate position of social acceptability, illness, and emotional insulation, the weak and strong egos reach a rough balance. Thus, we find that the stronger egos are relatively conspicuous in the most socially acceptable adjustment, while those with weaker egos become progressively more prominent in the less acceptable patterns of defence. The pattern is clear if we trace the incidence of stronger egos across our five groups: 24%, 44%, 73%, 48% and 14%. This describes a sharply rising, then falling, profile, in which the difference between adjacent groups is substantial.

We have indicated above that the patients' psychological characteristics seem to be related to their social histories in several ways, with weaker-ego patients having had more unstable, deviant, discordant social histories, and more prior psychiatric treatment by the time they reach the Unit. These relationships also hold up in the different 'behavioural defence' patterns. The two deviant extremes show significantly more disturbed backgrounds than the centre group of 'conformative' types.

In other respects, there is no patterned relationship between our independent variables of ego-strength and behavioural-defence and such behaviour disorders as alcoholism or criminal activity. Alcoholism is randomly distributed among our diagnostic groups. Among our behavioural-defence groups, alcoholism increases as a problem at the socially unacceptable extremes, but considering the extent to which the symptoms of alcoholism are likely to correspond to the criteria for judging the behavioural defence types, there is little patterned variation. All this seems to point to the complexity of alcoholism, which probably cannot be regarded as associated with a single psychiatric condition.

In a similar way, and probably for similar reasons, ego-strength bears little relationship to criminal activity, although the weaker-egos are somewhat more prone than the stronger to criminality. Criminal tendencies appear rather more conspicuously among the two diagnostic groups of the personality disorders than among the neurotics and psychotics. But there is no systematic variation according to ego-strength. Among the behavioural-defence groups, two vary from the criminal average about as we might expect (*Table 4*), the Aggressives with an excess of criminal activity, and the Invalids with a deficiency.

TABLE 4   CRIMINALITY OF BEHAVIOURAL-DEFENCE GROUPS

	Behavioural-Defences								
	Emotional								
	Aggression		Insulation		Conformity		Illness		Withdrawal	
	N	%	N	%	N	%	N	%	N	%
Criminal	16	64	21	40	14	44	4	18	17	46
No Crime	9	36	31	60	18	56	18	82	20	54
Totals:	(25)	100	(52)	100	(32)	100	(22)	100	(37)	100

In the sample as a whole, slightly more than two patients in every five (42%) admitted to some kind of criminal action, whether they got into trouble with the law or not. But among the aggressives the proportion that admitted criminal action was close to two-thirds, and it is likely that their *rate* of crime deviated even more than that from the sample mean. Conversely, among the illness group, less than one-fifth admitted any criminal activity. This is only to be expected in this category as the illness behavioural defence group represents the most passive form of response to stress. These people typically react to difficulties in their life situations by invalidism. Where aggressives attempt to deal with their environment by direct action *against* it, the invalids try to control the environment by making themselves extremely dependent upon others.

Because we are here concerned with anti-social behaviour, it seems warranted to deal directly with the raw behaviour, as we have done, in classifying action as intrinsically criminal or not. We have here ignored the person's legal status and his legal responsibility. On the face of it, the percentage—over 40%—of our patients that have admitted criminal behaviour may seem high. But we do not really know how much higher this might be than that for comparable behaviour in the population as a whole. It is axiomatic in criminology that official crime rates seriously understate the actual number of criminal offences. While we may assume that our patient group is higher than the population as a whole, we do not know how much higher it is.

SUMMARY

In summary, then, the patients treated by the Unit are what might be called a 'mixed bag'. They tend to be drawn disproportionately from lower-class, urban backgrounds and to have histories of social discord and instability, but these characteristics do not apply to all Unit patients. A sizeable proportion represent the solid middle and working-class segments of the population and have relatively well-adjusted histories in many areas of life.

While the Unit's patients are mostly diagnosed as 'personality disorders' by its staff, there are sizeable proportions of neurotics and psychotics always present in the Unit, and the group dubbed 'personality disorders' is so broad and heterogeneous that within it fall a great variety of patient types. In order to discriminate further among the types of patients being treated we ranked them on a scale of ego-weakness, using this concept to form two sub-groups of personality disorders—one closer to the psychoses at the weaker end of the continuum and one closer to the neuroses at the stronger.

Another way of classifying patients into meaningful categories, to some extent independently of ego-strength, is that based on characteristic behavioural reactions to stressful life circumstances. Five categories were developed, ranging from socially acceptable conformity in the centre to disapproved aggression and withdrawal at the extremes.

Fairly systematic relationships were found between these psychological types and various social circumstances such as parental situation in childhood, work history, social relationship patterns, and psychiatric history. Anti-social behaviour associated with criminality and alcoholism were less closely associated with these personality types, pointing to the clinical heterogeneity of these forms of social deviance.

While these actual diversities are apparent among the Unit's patients, the Unit staff prefer to conceptualize and organize their treatment programme around an ideal-typical conception of patients, where such differences are minimized as symptomatic variations on a unitary theme.

The ideal-typical Unit patient is a personality disorder, and the apparent variations among actual patients are seen essentially as variations on a single theme of personality anomaly and malformation. To deal therapeutically with this single clinical entity, the Unit has developed an ideology of treatment, constructed a regimen of organized activities and a system of role relationships.

We shall examine these three aspects of Unit social structure in the next three chapters before reporting on the patients' responses to the Unit. We shall then be in a position to attempt to relate the treatment exerted to results for particular types of patient.

NOTES AND REFERENCES

1. A varying proportion, usually under 10% during the period under study, were admitted under court order.

2. Cf. Jones Maxwell: 'The treatment of personality disorders in a therapeutic community.' *Psychiatry*, **20**: 211–20, 1957, and Jones, Maxwell, and Mathews, R.: 'The application of the therapeutic community principle to a state mental health programme.' *Br. J. med. Psychol.*, **29**: 57–62, 1954.—Also cf. Wilmer, Harry A.: *Social Psychiatry in Action: A Therapeutic Community.* New York, Charles C. Thomas, 1958.

3. Rosow, Irving: 'A study of referrals to an innovating psychiatric hospital.' Unpublished ms.

4. Except where explicitly noted otherwise, statistics cited in this and subsequent chapters on the characteristics of Unit patients are based on two samples: Series I, a cross-section of 84 patients comprising the total on hand on a chosen day in 1955; and Series II, comprising 84 consecutive admissions in the period immediately afterwards. Except where the differences between these two sub-populations are relevant, we shall treat them as a single sample representing Unit patients in the period of the research.

5. There is no information concerning the education of about 3%.

6. The Registrar General's classification is used. Cf. General Register Office: *Classification of Occupations*, 1950. London, H.M.S.O., 1950. It is based on occupations with Class I signifying roughly the professional and executive occupations; Class II, the managerial; Class III, clerical, white collar, and some skilled occupations; IV, manual and other skilled and semi-skilled occupations; and V, unskilled manual occupations.

7. Five per cent were not classified.

8. For one we have no information.

9. The sexual adjustment of two patients is not known.

10. The Unit admits a few organically disordered patients—e.g., epileptics—but does not direct its treatment towards 'curing' the physical disorder. It aims, rather, at treating the associated personal and social problems which the individual experiences.

11. Distinctions among these diagnostic types might be made in some psychiatric hospitals. For a good discussion of this problem see McCord, William and Joan: *Psychopathy and Delinquency.* New York, Grune & Stratton, 1956.

12. Cf. Appendix B for statistical documentation and elaboration of these points.

CHAPTER 3

Unit Ideology

The Unit, like any social system, functions according to a more or less explicit and articulated set of ideas about how it ought to be organized to achieve its purposes. As with most contemporary psychiatric innovators, its postulates are controversial and based on convictions as yet untested by thorough-going evaluative procedures. Yet, though backed by a commitment that is not entirely rational,[1] the staff's ideas are still held to some degree tentatively and thus open to the critical analysis of objective observers.

In the present chapter we shall attempt to set forth the Unit's principal ideological tenets about the organization of a therapeutic community, and to indicate how we think they bear on the central problem of the treatment and rehabilitation of the patients who come to the Unit. We shall begin some very general ideas that the Unit staff hold, and then report more specifically on four major 'themes'[2] of thought that seem to underlie many of their concrete policies. As we describe and illustrate each theme, we shall give the rationales that are regularly used by the Unit staff to justify the use of measures subsumed under the theme. We shall indicate some dilemmas which their adoption of Unit ideology poses to staff members. In a later chapter we shall indicate some of the implications for patients of acceptance of Unit ideology.

The Unit staff consider their system of ideas on the organization of a therapeutic community as simultaneously serving the aims of treatment and rehabilitation. On detailed examination, it seems, however, that some of the rationales are closely geared to a programme of rehabilitation aims and others to treatment aims, as we have defined these terms. We shall indicate these affinities in this chapter. In later chapters when we describe how decisions are actually made with respect to the treatment and rehabilitation of patients, we shall attempt to show how the ideological themes serve as one set of determinants, in a field of forces where other determinants also influence the choice of alternatives in any given situation. Other pressures, like those of hospital administration and relations with the community at large, may enter into any particular decision.[3] Clearly, it is valuable to make all the determinants of these decisions as explicit as possible. Decisions will always be influenced by a variety of non-rational as well as rational factors, but to the extent that increasing the rational mastery of the sphere of decision-making is a goal, a refinement of our awareness of what these elements are and how they fit together is essential. The distinction between the measures aimed at treatment and those aimed at rehabilitation is proposed as one such refinement. Demonstrating the utility of keeping alert to the distinction rather than blurring it, despite the major areas of overlap, is our major task.

What, then, are the essential elements of a therapeutic community approach as the staff see it? In the most global terms the staff's conception of the fundamental character of a therapeutic community is based on three general propositions:

'*Everything is treatment*';

'*All treatment is rehabilitation*'; and

'*All patients (once admitted) should get the same treatment.*'

The Unit staff often contend that 'everything (every activity, every relationship) in the Unit is treatment'. New patients in the Unit see signs on the walls with cartoon portrayals of patients at workshops, at play, dancing in socials, or talking in groups, and under each picture is the caption, 'This is treatment'.

When asked a general question, 'What does the term "therapeutic community" mean to you?' the staff tend to answer in a way that indicates that this all-inclusive approach is, in some form, an essential element in their thinking. While some staff members answer in terms of general goals ('a place where people are helped to learn to lead a happier life'; 'a community constructed to develop a sense of belonging and roots in society'), by far the majority of answers are in terms of the all-inclusive aspect of the Unit's approach.

Typical of these answers are the following: 'A place where *everyone*, staff and patients, is to help sorting out current problems'; 'Everyone's contributions are harnessed'; 'All activities are structured for their therapeutic potential, and all used for treatment'; 'A place where the potentials of each member are used as far as possible in relation to (treating) the entire population.'

One member of the staff, a workshop instructor, put his view of the nature of a therapeutic community not in the holistic framework, but in such a way as to emphasize the other core element in Unit thinking about treatment and rehabilitation—viz., that good treatment entails rehabilitation. His conception of a therapeutic community was 'a place where one shares one's experience with patients, so that we can teach them the pitfalls of their behaviour in job situations'.

While the Unit's primary focus, in general discussions, is on *treatment*, they mean a kind of treatment that will be rehabilitative. The staff are interested not merely or primarily in alleviating a particular symptom; nor in improving psychic comfort or increasing happiness; but in improving the capacities and incentives of patients for constructive interpersonal relationships in ordinary social life. They are thus committed to some degree of personality reorganization as a goal. The personality changes, ideally, are to be achieved by learning to adjust to the Unit's social system, and this experience is meant to carry over into ordinary life, hence the title 'Social Rehabilitation Unit' within a neurosis centre; hence Dr Jones' stricture, 'all treatment is rehabilitation'.

Finally an important global aspect of the Unit's treatment ideology assumes that the theories and the organization of the therapeutic programme are generally applicable to *all* the patients admitted. Patients who are 'too sick' to take the treatment are, as far as possible, screened out prior to admission, though this diagnostic observation often takes the form of an *ad hoc* rationalization for patient's unresponsiveness to therapy. Those who are 'suitable' for the treatment tend to be seen, as we have noted in the preceding chapter, in ideal-typical terms as having similar personality disorders, despite their overt differences of social behaviour and personal symptomatology. One social structure is, therefore, set up to treat *all* impartially.

Our view is that important qualifications must be attached to each of these key elements in Unit conceptions of a therapeutic community (i.e. that everything is treatment, all treatment is rehabilitation, and all patients should get the same treatment) if the ultimate interests of the patients are to be kept in the foreground. The Unit staff themselves, if we take a full range of their comments into account rather than the most general and idealized slogans only, do not really believe that literally 'everything is treatment'. They frequently state opinions that indicate how they hold some principles to be therapeutically superior to others. But regardless of their own implicit and explicit qualifications of the general statement, there are further problematic issues in their ideals of treatment method that help to clarify and refine Unit ideas still further. Foremost among these is the consistent blurring of the distinctions between treatment and rehabilitation aims. We believe that these ambiguities may not operate in the best interests of patients. In later chapters we shall attempt to indicate how making the distinctions sharper and more explicit may be of critical importance in therapy.

THE THEMES OF THERAPY

Observation of the Unit in action, discussions and interviews with staff members, have yielded a somewhat more differentiated picture of Unit beliefs as to desirable conditions for treatment and rehabilitation. We have, on the basis of these data, abstracted four principal themes that subsume many of the beliefs that the Unit staff seem to share. We further documented the character of these themes in staff belief through the administration of a value questionnaire.[4]

The four themes which broadly encompass the distinctive elements of the Unit's ideology are:

(a) 'democratization'
(b) 'permissiveness'
(c) 'communalism'
(d) 'reality confrontation'

All these refer to conditions of the social system that the Unit staff feel must prevail if treatment and rehabilitation are to occur.

Some of the themes have sub-themes and each has more than one rationale. There appears to be no hierarchy of themes according to which the ideology automatically values one course of action over another. The choice in any situation of conflict is determined in the situation, not on any *a priori* principle. Further, the principles themselves are flexible enough to provide rationales for various courses of action.

Another feature of the themes is that they have vague and elastic boundaries. When a staff member enunciates one of the slogans that fits one of our themes, he tends to use the shorthand form, omitting qualifications, not indicating limits and boundaries. By doing so, there is a gain in clarity, simplicity and dramatic impact. For example, it is far more viable in the situation to state that the aim of a therapeutic community is to 'free communications', than to state that the policy is to allow a good deal more communication in prescribed situations than is ordinarily allowed in comparable situations outside the Unit. However, while gaining in clarity and impact through the use of these slogans, the Unit staff loses some effectiveness through the generation of certain problems, which will be discussed later in this chapter.

In discussing each theme, we shall indicate its general meaning, illustrate its applicability, and demonstrate the staff's adherence to the principal by reporting on their responses to the values questionnaire. We shall indicate some of their rationales for holding the belief, and then consider the relationship between the Unit staff's rationales and their aims of treatment and/or rehabilitation.

(a) '*Democratization*' refers to the Unit's view that each member of the community should share equally in the exercise of power in decision-making about community affairs—both therapeutic and administrative. They believe that the conventional hospital status hierarchies should be 'flattened' to produce a more equalitarian form of participation. 'Everyone has just one say' is an expression frequently heard in the Unit, and it is meant to convey the sense of joint patient-staff decision-making that is most highly valued.

While the slogan suggests an equalitarian state of affairs, the Unit staff indicated partial agreement with the proposition, '*It is important in running a hospital that orders should be obeyed promptly and without question*'. The majority of the staff chose 'partly agree'. Perhaps their failure to disagree strongly reflected their awareness of their formal responsibility, the need to use their authority under some circumstances, or the recognition that the Unit is deviant in this regard and that for hospitals generally the norm lies more in the direction of agreement with the proposition. Even within the Unit, and apart from the regular situations, when medical affairs warrant surgery or some such procedure that is more along conventional lines, prompt and unquestioning response to orders *is* sometimes required.

A more focal 'democratization' items in the questionnaire, this time phrased in 'pro-Unit' form, is the following: '*Patients should help to decide how their fellow patients should be treated.*' In response to this, the majority of the staff answered *strongly agree*. The proposition, '*Patients should take a good deal of the responsibility for treating other patients,'* also yielded a majority choice for *strongly agree.*

The Unit staff quite clearly feel that patients should participate in decision-making, and that they should be made to feel responsible for these activities—i.e., that these are not merely play-acting or diversionary in nature, but important decisions affecting the lives of individuals.

The rationales for these beliefs in the value of 'democratization' include the following:

Unit staff believe that their patients have negative feelings towards authority figures, based on early unsatisfactory relationships with parental figures. To the extent that they transfer these feelings onto persons in authoritative roles (or who act autocratically), attitudes are established that work against therapy. In extreme cases, patients of this type will leave the hospital and withdraw from treatment, or they may stay but resist forming the kind of relationship that is required for therapeutic influence.

Diffusing the locus of authority is considered valuable not only to remove an immediate target for negative patient reaction, but in general allows for more effective examination of patients' stabilized misconceptions about authority figures. This is enhanced, theoretically, by removing all possible 'reality' bases for their stereotyped use of authorities as loci of hate and blame. The source of their difficulty can then, it is reasoned, be more clearly established as inhering in themselves, rather than in the wicked authorities in a hostile environment.

This set of rationales would seem to be most directly aimed at establishing and sustaining a treatment relationship. The immediate aim is to change patients' basic orientations towards authority figures. While this is of course relevant to the goal of rehabilitation, it is only indirectly so. Individuals like the Unit's patients are not likely to encounter organizations outside the hospital that are 'democratic' in the sense advocated by the Unit staff. Many real life situations, e.g. at work, are organized according to definite hierarchical principles; the powers of decision-making and the lines of responsibility are generally much less diffuse than in the Unit. The Unit's system, to the extent that it is adopted, might actually tend to 'unfit' a patient for such real-life situations outside the hospital (except insofar as the new attitudes that are incorporated make possible positive relationships with *less* benign authority figures than those in the Unit).

Another rationale for the democratization theme is that the legitimation of patient participation in therapy helps to improve communication and keep alive relevant social norms outside the hospital. Staff tend to be of middle-class backgrounds, while patients in the Unit tend to be of working- and lower-class backgrounds. Differences in dialect, and especially in norms, are thought to make for communication barriers that interrupt the work of psychotherapy.[5] There is also a rehabilitation component to this rationale in the recognition of the possibility that staff middle-class values will inadvertently be put forth as 'reality', and thereby hamper rather than promote patients' adjustment after discharge.

Another rationale for democratization is that many patients, though negatively oriented towards authority figures, are observed to be positively influenced by their peers. To the extent that therapy is thought of as a process involving inter-personal influences in which there is an attempt to get patients to give up one set of lifeways for another, the task of the staff is seen as working with whatever channels of influence will be most effective. The Unit staff believe that the democratization measures help to 'beam' therapeutic influences through the collateral channels of patient-patient relationships by encouraging 'constructive' patients to function as effective surrogates of the staff.

From our point of view, this rationale has both treatment and re-habilitation aspects strongly represented. On the one hand, this aspect of the policy is geared to influence patients effectively to make changes in their personalities, with no implication that such peer-centred management typifies any relationships in the 'real world' outside. On the other hand, to the extent that patients are able actually to take responsibility for participating in one another's treatment, the learning experience in the assumption of responsibility *per se* may be said to have rehabilitative effects in that this quality of behaviour is required to some degree in most ordinary social situations.

Another rationale for the adoption of a 'democratization' orientation is that the staff consider it valuable in cultivating latent talents among the patients. When 'treatment' is left only to trained members of the staff, with patients exclusively at the receiving end, there is no development and use of patients' potentials for therapy. Patients are considered to be valuable participants in giving therapy by perceiving one another's difficulties, helping one another to understand them, handling group discussions, grasping the issues in decision-making, representing sub-groups of opinion within the Unit and making the opinion articulate, but these skills are traditionally not exploited. When fully exploited, the staff consider the benefit to lie not only in helping the over-all organization to function more effectively in fulfilling its therapeutic aims, but as valuable as well in making individual patients feel a greater sense of self-respect in contributing to the actual personal assistance of other individuals.

While there may be some instances in which the actual skills culti-vated in this process are directly applicable to the patient's post-hospital situation, in most cases the relevance is indirect. There is one story, frequently repeated in the Unit, of an ex-patient who started group therapy sessions for employees in the basement of the large public institution in London where he worked as a watchman. In other instances the Unit's form of group discussions has been said to have had direct value in solving family problems. However, the Unit does not aim at training its patients for therapeutic roles outside the Unit (as is the usual aim, for example, in a didactic psychoanalysis). It rather stresses the aims of social adjustment, which may be hampered by the kinds of analytic practices that are 'normal' in the Unit.

(b) 'Permissiveness' refers to the Unit's belief that it should function with all its members tolerating from one another a wide degree of behaviour that might be distressing or seem deviant according to 'ordinary' norms. Ideally, this should allow both for individuals freely to expose their behavioural difficulties, and for others to react freely to this so that the bases for both sides of social relationship patterns can be examined.

The staff's view is clearly embodied in the proposition: '*If a patient is very abusive or destructive in hospital, it is better to discuss it with him than to discipline him.*' In response to this the majority of the Unit staff chose *strongly agree.*

Aside from the direct treatment and rehabilitation implications of this position, the staff have a data-gathering and diagnostic rationale for this belief. Patients come to the Unit with a variety of diagnostic labels, are sent for a variety of purposes, and present themselves with a variety of complaints. The way in which the Unit staff reduce this welter of signs and symbols to their own terms is to expose the patients to a fairly unstructured situation (i.e., few explicit rules and regulations) and to observe their reactions. To the extent that patients of this type 'act out' their difficulties, their problems can be seen in their behaviour in these situations. To the extent that the hospital provides a round of activities simulating regular life situations, the 'problems' exposed are assumed to be representative of those the patient experiences outside.

Permissiveness, in the Unit view, consists not only in lightening negative sanctions in the interests of 'understanding', but it also implies a general diminution of bureaucratic institutional restrictions. Thus, the staff's response to the proposition, '*Hospitals should be organized according to a regular set of rules that cover most situations so that each person can know what is expected*', was probably somewhat atypical for hospital personnel. While almost equal numbers of the staff chose *partly agree* and *disagree* (the anticipated position was 'disagree'), members of the core staff (doctors, senior nurses, psychiatric social worker, and psychologist) did choose the disagree position most frequently. Newer, junior staff, presumably feeling a greater personal need for orientation in the situation, responded to the 'expectations' phrase in the proposition and tended to choose *partly agree*. The eschewing of definite expectations is also supported by the 'democratization' theme, which stresses the importance of group decision-making in defining Unit norms and standards.

One consequence of permissiveness in a setting where so many of the participants are disruptive is that a large amount of tension may be generated by the free show of symptoms and the communication of materials ordinarily taboo. This tension, within limits, is regarded by the staff not only as an inevitable burden to be borne in a permissive régime, but of potential treatment value. Anxiety may provide motivation for 'coming into treatment'. The resolution of intra- and interpersonal tensions may entail 'movement' in the individual personalities of the participants.[6]

The staff's view in this matter is illustrated in their tendency to discourage the use of sedatives or other medicaments to allay anxiety. The following two propositions bearing on this position were both marked by staff majorities of '*disagree*': '*Every effort should be made to keep patients from feeling tense or anxious while in hospital*' and '*A restful night is very important for treatment and should be assured if necessary by giving sedatives.*' These apparently humane dictates bear, for the Unit staff, the hallmarks of custodial, anti-therapeutic régimes in psychiatry.

The Unit staff's rationales for taking a permissive orientation are similar, in general outline, to those of the psychoanalysts, with certain extensions to the hospital situation and the particular group of patients being treated. Permissiveness, it is thought, facilitates the expression of ordinarily inhibited materials—in this case behaviourly as well as verbally—that provide problems for analysis. The sheer expression sometimes has value for its cathartic effect. More usually, enduring effects are thought to be contingent on analysis and insight—i.e., interpretations made to the patient about the original sources for the materials expressed, and the patient achieving an awareness of the existence and causes of displacements.

Patients who 'act their disorders out', like children, are thought to need even more latitude than the private consulting room or conventional hospital administration provide. To meet this need, the Unit staff feel that the hospital system should be reorganized to remove excessive emphasis from regulations, neatness, and orderliness, so that opportunities can be provided for application of the therapeutic principles. When this rationale for permissiveness is used it would seem that rehabilitative goals are somewhat more in the background. There is little likelihood that the patient will ever again encounter people who persistently and flexibly attempt to 'understand' him, rather than to react with customary sanctions. His adaptation to this situation, then, must be a transitional one, to be given up before successful rehabilitation can be expected.

Another kind of rationale for encouraging permissiveness is that some kinds of patients show their disorders precisely in their intolerance of others' characteristics. It is considered valuable for such patients to analyse why they become so disturbed at certain kinds of behaviour in others. On the one hand, this rationale directly serves treatment goals in that patients may thus achieve new insight into their own personality problems by analysing reactions that may have passed in the outside world as unproblematic. (E.g., a great sensitivity and negative reactions toward homosexuality might, outside, have passed unmarked as 'normal', while in the Unit it might be interpreted as indicating a latent problem of the patient.) The aim and consequences of this interpretation may include personality changes. On the other hand, whether or not this aim is operative, the Unit does intend, through this rationale, to teach individuals to control their reactions so as to be more tolerant of others, developing a habit of thought that helps the individual to adjust to ordinary social interaction.

Another rationale for permissiveness is to give individuals an opportunity to try out new patterns of behaviour as their old ones become unsatisfactory to them. This involves, on the one hand, what the psychoanalysts call 'working through'. In this context it is part of reorganization processes in the personality as the individual reorganizes his perceptions. On the other hand, it may also involve what sociologists refer to as 'role rehearsals'. In this context it is rehabilitative in its immediate aim.[7]

These permissiveness themes inevitably have rationales that overlap with those of the democratization theme because it is the staff, as formally responsible authorities, who must regulate the boundaries of tolerable behaviour. To the extent that the staff can avoid drawing boundaries in ordinary Unit functioning, or get patients to draw boundaries jointly with them, overtly authoritative behaviour can be avoided. But, if permissiveness limits are strained by extreme acting out, or if patients are not drawing limits as staff feel they 'constructively' should, authoritative interventions are sometimes inevitable. These problems will be elaborated in a later section on 'oscillations' in maintaining equilibrium of the total social organization and social process.

(c) 'Communalism' refers to the Unit's belief that its functioning should be characterized by tight-knit, inter-communicative and intimate sets of relationships. Sharing of amenities, informality (e.g. use of first names), and 'freeing' communication are prescribed.

With regard to the ideal of sharing, for example, the majority of staff 'partly agreed' with the proposition, 'If it were possible, staff and patients should share all facilities and activities in common—cafeterias, work-shops, socials, meetings, etc.' Some reservations on total sharing prevail, but the general tendency is clear.

In response to the proposition: 'Everything the patients say and do while in hospital should be used for treatment', the staff majority chose 'strongly agree'. This is, clearly, an extension of the psychoanalytic ideas of psychic determinism and the use of free association—only here everyone is ideally involved in a therapeutic alliance and is expected to 'feed back' materials into therapeutic groups. Even Unit physicians stress the policy of 'no privileged communications', advocating that everyone be included in everything. Only thus, they feel, can people develop a real sense of participation and can all the relevant data be brought into consideration. Accordingly, they 'strongly disagreed' with

the proposition: 'Many things a patient thinks while in hospital are nobody's business but his own and he shouldn't have to talk about them.'

The 'freeing of communication' emphasis, frequently uttered by the
staff, has administrative and therapeutic rationales. From the administrative point of view, the staff consider it valuable because they feel
that decisions affecting patients can often be more wisely taken and
effectively administered if the patients themselves and those closest to
them contribute relevant information. However, the staff's awareness
of the qualifications that ought to be placed on such a policy in a complex social system is indicated by their choice of 'partly agree' for the
proposition: 'If everyone in hospital freely expressed his thoughts and
feelings to everyone else, it would help the running of the hospital.'

The therapeutic rationalizations for the communalism orientation
include the following:

Many patients are thought to have come from discordant early
family situations, from which they developed the type of personality
sometimes referred to as the 'affectionless character', generally characterized by 'lack of a sense of belonging', 'rootlessness', or 'social
alienation'. The view of the Unit is that the provision of an intensely
counteractive environment of the kind the patients missed when
children, can, under suitable conditions, provide a belated 'corrective
emotional experience'.

The treatment aim seems paramount here. Most patients expect to
live in social networks without the tight-knit, interconnected, warm,
and intimate quality of the Unit's ideal system of relationships. To
judge from the staff's presuppositions about why they need such a
community spirit, patients tend, if anything, to be even less endowed
with these qualities than do most people. The Unit seems to aim
at providing a kind of 'emotional hothouse' in which patients will
develop an increased capacity to endure outside impersonality without
reacting in ways that get them into difficulty—e.g. by behaving in a
hostile, over-demanding or over-dependent manner.

The rationales for 'freeing communications', include a cathartic
aspect. Patients are encouraged to express pent-up emotions on the
assumption that this in itself will have beneficial consequences. One
patient insightfully expressed this 'catharsis' angle as follows: 'A
patient is like a dark bottle. In treatment you shake it all out and have a
look at the contents for the first time properly. Then they don't seem
so bad.'

There is also a rationale more closely geared to the rehabilitation goals. Participation, it is reasoned, is necessary to make any community function. Therefore, patients are expected to participate communally, and the responsibility for doing so is placed on them. Then, where the Unit malfunctions, it is easier to see how the behaviour of individual members may contribute to this than is ordinarily possible in life outside.[8] This makes social consequences of the patients' behaviour clearer to them.

To the extent that it is expected that this well-rounded régime will foster habits of multi-faceted social participation valued in mental health, another rehabilitative aim is present in the all-round participation rationale. It is thought that general participation makes manifest the total range of a patient's interpersonal difficulties. This is considered helpful diagnostically in pin-pointing pathology, which may then serve the aims of treatment and rehabilitation.

(d) 'Reality-Confrontation' refers to the Unit's belief that patients should be continuously presented with interpretations of their behaviour as it is seen by most others.[9] This is meant to counteract patients' tendencies to use massive denial, distortion, withdrawal, or other mechanisms that interfere with their capacity to relate to others in the normal world.

The majority of the staff members, for example, chose 'disagree' for the proposition: 'While a patient is in hospital he should try to forget about his outside problems as much as possible.' Similarly, they 'strongly disagreed' with the proposition that 'Psychiatric hospitals should provide a change from ordinary life with emphasis placed on rest, comfort, and escape from stress and strain.' Their emphatic view is that the patient can solve his problems only by facing them squarely.

They believe that the hospital and the community should be closely interrelated, in contrast to the old custodial system. Where circumstances limit the amount of interchange of people and activities between hospital and local community,[10] they work towards making the organization of the hospital as 'real-life-like' as possible. Ideally, they see the hospital as a miniature society, containing a similar round of activities and functioning according to norms similar to those of society at large, but oriented to treatment and so deliberately mitigating the usual kinds of sanctions.

Thus, the majority of the staff 'disagreed' with the proposition: 'Psychiatry is for the treatment of sick people and belongs in hospitals and *doctors' offices, and not in homes, schools, and outside communities.*' Psychiatry, they would say, is concerned with all interaction, and with preventing pathological development in the community if possible. In this sense, their view of social psychiatry makes it part of the larger tradition of social medicine,[11] Psychiatrists generally, they would say, tend to be too much out of touch with the social backgrounds from which their patients come. If they are to treat with the goal of rehabilitation in mind, and certainly if they are to rehabilitate directly or to work at prevention, they need to increase their knowledge of and interaction with the ordinary community from which the patients come.

The staff is thus concerned for treatment purposes with the 'reality' of the social problems and processes in the social network from which the patients come. They are also interested in these data for rehabilitation aims following hospitalization since it is to extra-hospital relationships that patients must adjust.

An example of the latter type of aim would be the attempt to present the patient with realistic perceptions of the nature of his home, his family, and life situation so that he can fit himself into them in a more satisfactory way, regardless of changes in his personality.

Patients are frequently quoted by staff as having said, 'I didn't realize before how much I was harming others.' It is conceivable in an urban, loosely-organized setting, that individuals may be unaware of the disruptive consequences of their behaviour. Transient relationships, a migratory residence pattern, social distance, and so on, all serve to insulate them from such awareness.

Thus, paradoxically, 'reality confrontation', which seems of all the themes to be most clearly geared to rehabilitative aims, may also be geared to treatment aims. To the extent that they can be distinguished in practice, the latter would prevail if the immediate aim were to change the patient's personality in the sense of his *general* modes of perception, defence, etc. The former would prevail if the confrontation were merely aimed at illuminating the dimensions of a *particular* situation of which a patient might not be aware.

UNIT VALUES AND THE GENERAL PUBLIC

Clearly the Unit's views on many of these matters differ from those of some other hospital authorities, other psychiatrists, penal administrators, and many members of the general public. Unit ideology is a specialized set of beliefs nominally adapted to their work task. One prerequisite for receiving treatment in the Unit would, by hypothesis, be the acceptance, in some degree, of its ideas about how a hospital should be organized for treatment. In a therapeutic community of this type, this is not simply something to be endured while the actual therapy is administered, but the assimilation of these beliefs is of the essence of therapy itself.

The relationship between patients holding these values and their experience in the Unit is examined later, in the chapter on improvement. It may be of interest in this section, however, simply to document disparity between the Unit's ideology and the values of outsiders. A series of new patients on their second day after admission to the Unit was given the same values questionnaire as was administered to the staff. At this point, some influence may already have been established. But on the whole these patients, fresh from the outside, tend to give 'uncontaminated' responses of the social population from which they were drawn. To the extent that influence was already at work on the patients' second day in the Unit, we would expect it to *diminish* differences between new patients and staff.

How, then, do the values of unit staff and new patients compare on issues of treatment ideology?

We see in *Figure 2* that the Unit staff are more heavily concentrated

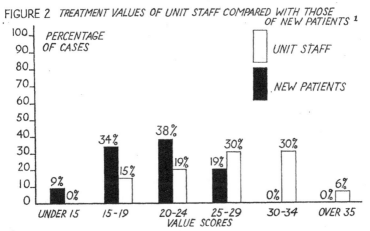

FIGURE 2 *TREATMENT VALUES OF UNIT STAFF COMPARED WITH THOSE OF NEW PATIENTS* [1]

[1] Twenty-six staff and 84 new patients completed the questionnaire. Both sets of scores are represented as percentages of the totals.

at the higher end of the distribution curve. The new patients show a comparable range of variation to the staff, with some overlap in score, but their modal scores are lower than those of the staff members. If a cutting point is set at the score of 25, over three-quarters of newly admitted patients fall below it on initial testing while only a third of the staff do so.

UNIT VALUES

Values occupy a central role in the Unit's conception of treatment. Presumably, patients come in with various problems and defences which distort their perceptions of themselves and the world. Their defences may be reinforced by a commitment to values which differ markedly from those of the Unit's ideology. In general, treatment goals call for a revision of distorted perceptions. The Unit's method of achieving this implies patient's acceptance of Unit values. When this occurs and is manifested in patients' behaviour, they are judged to have successfully 'come into treatment'.

We need not here question the merits of this particular set of assumptions. It is worth while, however, to know how close a correspondence exists between the Unit values and those of the patients when they first enter the Unit and to explore those factors that make for a high correspondence initially. In the later chapter on improvement, we shall examine what variables make for a shift in patients' values to bring them closer to the Unit's position.

Surprisingly, we find through a correlational analysis that no systematic relationship exists between patients' initial values and such demographic factors as age, sex, education, social class or marital status.[12]

Perhaps the greatest anomaly is the lack of relationship between values and class, whether measured by education or occupation. Systematic attitudinal variations are normally to be expected on this variable. Its absence in our sample may reflect the rather special Unit values being tested; it may indicate the vitiation of class determinance of values in the face of psychiatric disturbance; it may represent spurious correspondences masked by the crudeness of the scoring system, or it may reflect a uniform conformity bias in all these groups as a means of coping with anxieties aroused by the Unit. An illustration of this is provided below in our comments on the high 'U' scores of patients who came to the Unit from prison.

There is a very slight and not important connexion between patients' values, on the one hand, and ego-strength (*Table 5*) and types of be-havioural-defence (*Table 6*) on the other. These data suggest slightly higher Unit values among patients with stronger egos or more socially acceptable modes of defence.

TABLE 5   INITIAL VALUES OF DIAGNOSTIC GROUPS

Unit Values	Psychotic N	%	PD Weak N	%	PD Strong N	%	Neurotic N.	%
Low	11	69	57	69	32	60	8	61
High	5	31	26	31	21	40	5	39
Totals:	(16)	100	(83)	100	(53)	100	(13)	100

TABLE 6   INITIAL VALUES OF BEHAVIOURAL DEFENCE TYPES
(TOTAL SAMPLE)

Unit Values	Aggression N	%	Emotional Insulation N	%	Conformity N	%	Illness N	%	Withdrawal N	%
Low	18	72	32	62	14	44	17	77	29	78
High	7	28	20	38	18	56	5	23	8	22
Totals:	(25)	100	(52)	100	(32)	100	(22)	100	(37)	100

The relationships, however, are minor.[13]

The only factor which correlated with the initial agreement with Unit values was the patients' presenting symptoms. And in *Table 7* a slightly lower cutting point is used, which divides patients' initial scores into the lower two and higher four score categories on the six-point values scale. This adjustment of the cutting point highlights the relationship.

The data indicate a greater initial sympathy with Unit ideology among people who arrive with some kind of psychological complaint or a manifest social difficulty rather than with sheer physical symptoms. Those with only physical (often psychosomatic) complaints are less likely to have beliefs which fit in with those of the Unit. The category of 'other presenting symptoms' includes involuntary patients, such as prisoners or persons on probation, who are referred by legal agencies and who arrive at the Unit without symptoms or complaints. The higher value scores of this group may be distorted by a strong compliance bias. Another possible source of this phenomenon might be a spurious agreement which is brought about by criminals and staff members agreeing about the 'levelling' of hierarchies for diametrically opposed reasons. But the small number of cases makes the relationship shown in *Table 7* only suggestive at best.

TABLE 7   INITIAL VALUES ACCORDING TO PRESENTING SYMPTOMS
ON ARRIVAL AT THE UNIT* (SERIES II ONLY)

| Unit Values | *Presenting Symptoms* | | | |
| | *Only Physical* | *Only Psychological* | *Only Social* | *Other (None)* |
	N %	N %	N %	N %
Low	7 87	15 56	15 47	4 29
High	1 13	12 44	17 53	10 71
Totals:	(8) 100	(27) 100	(32) 100	(14) 100

* This table includes only those patients of Series II who report unmixed complaints.

In general, then, there is little firm basis for predicting initial values on arrival at the Unit. Even if the relationship between values and presenting symptoms in *Table 7* were genuine, its meaning would still be quite ambiguous. Hence, the value of even this relationship is moot.

PROBLEMATIC ASPECTS OF UNIT IDEOLOGY

Our observations of the Unit have yielded the patterns of ideological belief and their rationales described above. The ideological themes represent general orientations. At this level of systematization, no *necessary* problems inhere in the ideas themselves. However, there are a great many potential pitfalls and ambiguities between apprehending the ideal principle and applying it most beneficially to the treatment/rehabilitation of patients. The same set of ideas could exist in another setting and be differently applied in practice, since the ideology itself does not specify certain principles of its implementation.

The way the problems of implementation are defined and solved is likely to affect patients' progress in treatment and rehabilitation. It would therefore seem crucial to indicate what problems we consider to be important but not explicitly developed by the Unit staff in articulating the themes logically among themselves, and in applying them to treating problems of patients.

There seems to be four general types of problems of a recurring nature connected with Unit ideology and affecting action. Each individual member of the Unit must work out some *modus vivendi* with these four general problems in the use of Unit ideology before he can become an effectively functioning representative of Unit culture:[14]

A. *Problems of limits.*
B. *Problems of qualifications.*
C. *Problems of hierarchization of themes.*
D. *Problems of resolving treatment-rehabilitation dilemmas.*

A. *Problems of Limits.* Each of the ideals set forth by the Unit staff functions for the benefit of patients only within certain limits.

We can illustrate this for each of the themes:

The doctor who is too autocratic with certain patients with personality disorders might only antagonize them and thus be ineffective in treatment and rehabilitation. On the other hand, a doctor who divests himself too completely of his formal authority and responsibility in the situation might be unable to act authoritatively where it is therapeutically advantageous. The 'abdication' of the responsible exercise of power in situations where it is appropriately required has been shown to be therapeutically harmful.[15]

Similarly, a doctor who is insufficiently permissive with an acting-out patient may lose necessary data on the patient and perhaps even the kind of trusting relationship that is valuable for therapy. On the other hand, over-permissiveness may become negligence.

In the matter of communalism, a staff member who remains aloof from communication and participation networks cannot expect to build up the kinds of relationships that are considered prerequisites for therapy within the Unit. On the other hand, too great communalism may break down staff-patient distinctions altogether and undermine the structure necessary for therapy. These distinctions embody the social reality—viz. that society at large wishes to maintain standards for the responsible administration of therapeutic skills within a permanent and stable institutional structure. The responsibility for maintaining the institutional framework falls to a professional staff. Losing an awareness of the identity of this professional group within the Unit may be both therapeutically damaging for individual patients in the Unit and irresponsible in terms of the Unit's larger social charter.

Reality confrontations, paradoxically, may after a point become 'unrealistic' and therapeutically damaging. While insufficient reality confrontation is undesirable therapeutically because it allows patients to maintain their patterned distortions, too great reality confrontation may be so disturbing to patients with weak defences as actually to work against the patient's progress. The limits, however, are not specified since they are considered to be best applied when tailored to the individual and the situation. The Unit staff do not, however, have a clear and explicit set of principles about how the limits are to be differently defined for different types of cases. Furthermore, they tend to stress the dangers of the 'insufficiency' end of the range—e.g. not being democratic or permissive enough.

B. *Problems of Qualifications.* Each slogan used in the Unit constitutes an expression of at least one of the themes. However, the Unit staff have important implicit qualifications, discovered through observation, of which it is essential to be aware if one is to understand the themes as they actually, rather than ideally, function in the Unit. An appreciation of the actual functions is necessary if a staff member is to perform effectively in his role. Thus, while the staff urge the 'freeing of communications', observations indicate that they in fact favour verbal over non-verbal communications (though the latter may be tolerated and even encouraged at certain stages of treatment and under certain conditions); communications in groups are favoured over communications between individuals in private; communications in groups containing staff members, or at least 'constructive' patients, are favoured over communications in clandestine, hostile, or unsupervised groups. Furthermore, proper communication involves receptivity to others' communications and judgements about the appropriateness of one's own in particular group contexts. The latter may include non-communication.

As we have noted, many of the Unit's slogans, which serve as precepts for Unit neophytes of all kinds and as kinds and as guides to action for the more established members, are simplistic in nature. 'Freeing communications', 'sharing everything', 'making decisions by giving each person one say', are all attractive from the point of view of clarity, simplicity, and emotional impact. They are like the slogans of political parties or religious groups in ordinary life. Yet, in the Unit where there is, alongside the wish to 'win' emotional commitment to therapeutic purposes, the wish to communicate scientific principles of action, these slogans present potential problems. The problems lie partly in the tendency to make the realization of principles embodied in these slogans 'ends in themselves', partly in the tendency for some members to become disillusioned by 'ideal-real discrepancies' when they note that there are a good many implicit qualifications attached to the directives, partly in the inadequacy of these directives for teaching and communication of professional experience.

C. *Hierarchization of Value Themes.* The Unit's view is that all its ideological tenets are valuable in a general way for the organization of a psychiatric institution, and little tendency is shown to regard some as of more import than others. The principles to be applied in any given situation reflect the consensus of the participating group. This view seems to be based on the assumption that arranging a set of principles or regulations in a hierarchical way is a characteristic of bureaucratic and suppressive social systems and may curb the practice of permissiveness and spontaneity.

Study indicates that the *lack* of a clear set of principles for determining which treatment value shall have ascendancy over others at points of intersection leads to recurring dilemmas. These dilemmas tend to be resolved according to various expedients. It seems clear that at some points one treatment value (e.g., 'permissiveness') is more therapeutic for a patient than another in the situation (e.g., 'reality confrontation'); while at another time or for another patient the reverse ranking of the two values might be appropriate. The problem is one of how to resolve dilemmas in a systematic and therapeutically responsible way. It would seem that future developments in the study and formulation of treatment ideologies should concentrate on the principles for articulating the values as well as on the actual delineation of the values themselves.

D. *Treatment-Rehabilitation Dilemmas.* The problem of resolving treatment-rehabilitation dilemmas is one toward the solution of which this entire book is directed. One aspect of the problem entails the degree of replication of the patterns of ordinary life that is desirable within the hospital. The Unit's view is that the hospital community should provide a 'realistic' round of experiences and relationships for the patient—a replica of his outside life—in order to diagnose his recurring difficulties and to work out new socially adaptive patterns. This view, stemming from the feeling that patients' adjustment to the artificial and suppressive organization of custodial mental hospitals fits them only for sheltered institutional life, suggests a continual strain towards making the hospital as much as possible a miniature version of society outside.

On the other hand, it is clear that hospitals as at present constituted *cannot* reproduce identical patterns of relationships—e.g., family life. Furthermore, study reinforces the view that 'too realistic' a confrontation of some patients with the characteristic problems and processes of ordinary life only exacerbates the difficulties initially stimulated outside the hospital. Patients, as casualties of the social processes in the world outside the hospital, may need *different* conditions in which to recover or to nurture their capacity to live with psychological or sociological comfort in ordinary society. Thus, to some extent, the Unit recognizes that its organization is not and should not be a true microcosm—but one that is more permissive, more analytical, more aimed at discovering underlying personality problems and correcting them.

To the extent that the microcosmic emphasis is fostered, rehabilitation goals take precedence. To the extent that the special treatment milieu is developed, treatment goals are in ascendancy. In making any particular decision—for example, the institution of a new kind of group, the selection of a new staff member, the creation of a new staff role, or the scheduling of activities—different choices become 'rational' if one is oriented to rehabilitation via the microcosm conception from those that would be so if aiming at personality change via the special therapeutic milieu conception. If the treatment choice is made, rehabilitation goals can be fostered only by providing pathways (e.g., stages of experience representing 'graded strains') in the direction of the kind of social milieu the patient will have to adjust to following discharge.

Aside from the four general problems stated above, each of the themes seems to have problematic features uniquely associated with it.

With regard to *democratization*, the problematic elements have to do with the diffusion of authority and responsibility. It must be noted that the term 'democracy', as applied here, is employed in a way radically different from its ordinary usage. Politically, democracy implies the delegation of power to a few individuals elected by the majority, with the latter themselves holding ultimate power. In the Unit, the authority, or legitimated power, is formally assigned to the staff, who also hold formal responsibility. The staff is a numerical minority which informally shares its authority and responsibility with others in the Unit because of its ideology of democratization.

One major problem here is that authority and responsibility tend to be diffused differentially. Many people are eager to accept authority without being willing to take the responsibility that may go with it. Since in the Unit both attributes remain formally with the staff, they are left with the problem of having frequently to accept responsibility for the disruptive use of power which they have informally vested in the patients. The balancing of these variables is a perpetual source of concern to the staff in the matter of the realization of the democracy theme.[16]

The problems associated with 'permissiveness' are linked with those of 'democratization' in that limits which the staff set on permissiveness are partly determined by the formal responsibilities they bear. Since the staff are, in fact, responsible for the property, supplies, equipment, organization, and general conduct of the treatment programme, they cannot be so permissive as to be judged irresponsible by the higher administrative authority of the health system, the medical profession, or the external social system of law and government. Their steps to curb behaviour that threatens these responsibilities may take the form of autocratic action.

There are, of course, other reasons for curbing permissiveness— e.g., where its exercise would harm the patients or would allow the patients to harm others, and so on. Illustrations of these instances will be given in the section on 'social processes'. We mean here only to point out that this ideological principle has a complex boundary problem, and because of this a special problem in that the staff must be continually sacrificing *constancy* of permissiveness in order to satisfy other requirements in the situation. This may expose them to feelings of guilt at not being as permissive as they would like; and the patients may feel that the staff are hypocritical. In permissiveness, perhaps more than in the other themes, one can see how the problem of boundaries and hierarchies in themes creates recurring and troublesome dilemmas.[17] It is obviously best not to be permissive with a patient about to commit suicide; on the other hand, the majority of problems in the Unit are more subtle and difficult to assess. For example, if two patients become involved in a sexual affair which represents a 'progressive' maturation experience for one and a 'regressive' exacerbation of symptoms for the other, how much permissiveness is to be granted and how is the situation to be managed if the pair persist even after interpretations make its pitfalls manifest? It is in the resolution of these more subtle dilemmas that refinement in thinking about these themes is most needed.

With 'communalism', the problem that seems especially highlighted is the degree of personal involvement the staff should entertain in their relationships with patients. Free communications, joint participation, and warmth of relationships are prescribed—for treatment and rehabilitation rationales, as we have described above. On the other hand, there is a constant source of difficulty in attempting to reconcile these with the technical necessity for staff to preserve a certain degree of social distance and non-involvement with patients at a personal level. One reason for this social distance requirement is that too strong an attachment between any particular pair of patients tends to undermine participation in the larger group which is the heart of treatment. Another reason is that such alliances may arouse feelings of jealousy and rivalry among other patients that work against therapy. When patients' feelings of jealousy have little basis in objective reality, they can be related aetiologically to an earlier situation and dealt with therapeutically. But this is more difficult to do when there is a 'reality basis' for the jealousy feelings. Staff roles require impartial behaviour toward patients, and favouritism would therefore be a ground for realistic resentment.

Again, if staff members 'fall in love' with patients, it is felt that both may not only be distracted from their obligations to the treatment situation, but that here too, the feelings occurring within the treatment situation may not be the most enduring in the long run. In the immediate situation, it is thought important to analyse feelings that interfere with present conduct but are archaic vestiges of past relationships. This is thought to be made easier if the present relationships do not warrant the highly charged type of feeling. The more impersonal types of professional role relationships allow this neutrality, but more personal relationships do not. Also, to the extent that the feelings of the pair do not belong to the situation, but to other relationships in the past, they are not likely to 'stick' in the kind of way that would make for a good enduring relationship.

Thus, there are elements that specifically complicate the realization of communalism ideals. These elements bear on the particular patient's treatment, other patients' treatment in the immediate situation, the conduct of treatment in the long run (i.e., the maintenance of the treatment structure), and the personal well-being of the staff member.

With regard to 'reality confrontation', we have already mentioned that the confrontation may not only not be *necessary* in some situations, but it may not be *best* for the patient, in that his defences may actually be so weak against assimilating a bit of information that harm rather than benefit will ensue if it is communicated. The idea often heard in the Unit that 'You've got to get worse before you can get better' implies that 'insight' leads to temporary disorganization and distress, but often to subsequent reorganization and improved personality integration. Comparatively little attention is given to the difficult technical problem of defining the situations that ensure the second, reintegrating phase so that they may be fostered; and defining situations that do not ensure it, so that they may be avoided.

A major problem bearing on the interpretation of the 'reality confrontation' theme is that of assessing 'reality'. Democratization is meant to overcome some of the recognized limitations of the middle-class world view of many staff members, but even with the enlarged base of participation, the problem of assessing 'reality' is not automatically solved. Any particular group that is attempting to bring a reality picture to the attention of a patient is hampered by two kinds of problems. The first is the inaccessibility of much clinically relevant material. Even if the group can supplement the patient's own account of his life situation by bringing in families and visiting the patients' homes, there remain serious problems of evaluating conflicting evidence based on retrospection and mediated by individuals with personality problems.

The second is that, even given the degree of valid material with which the group can work to construct an objective picture of a patient's real life situation, groups as wholes are subject to distortions of perception and judgement that can lead to very 'unrealistic' consensus. To some extent, a group acting in concert has some properties similar to those of an individual in this regard. The group may collusively deny, become anxious, punitive, guilty, etc., and behave in ways that are not desirable for the patient's treatment or rehabilitation.[18]

In general, then, any practitioner of the Unit's methods of treatment and rehabilitation will have to work out for himself means of qualifying and limiting the application of the principles. He will have to learn to resolve treatment-rehabilitation dilemmas where they exist, and in general to develop principles for articulating and hierarchizing these values where they meet or come into conflict if he is to function adequately within the framework. Unless these problems are given explicit attention, the innovator is likely to be faced not only with recurring dilemmas that are difficult to resolve in this framework, but also the situation where a variety of expedient resolutions can be used with facile application of broad ideological rationales. The latter kind of problem can promote social discord as well as blurring issues of therapeutic method.

In working out systematic solutions to these problems the dual considerations of individual needs for treatment and rehabilitation on the one hand, and social functioning of the hospital social system on the other, must constantly be kept in mind. The former suggests individualizing treatment and rehabilitation relationships and programmes; the latter suggests functioning according to some jointly held, standardized, and cooperatively executed programmes. The latter approach, working on the basis of a lowest common denominator conception of some kind, obviously has its strengths and weaknesses, its facilitating and complicating aspects. We have tried in this chapter to bring out some of those that are implied in the ideological system itself.

It would seem that those problems intrinsic to applying the ideology reflect several aspects of the Unit's situation—e.g. the attempt to innovate a familistic-communalistic system within a larger structure that is universalistic-bureaucratic in nature; the diversity of sources for the ideas used and the avowedly eclectic approach pending their empirical evaluation. These same problematic aspects of the Unit situation are reflected in the overall organization of activities, the definition of social roles, the patterning of dilemmas in the performance of staff roles, and, ultimately, the outcome of patients' therapeutic careers. These areas of Unit functioning will be examined in the chapters that follow.

NOTES AND REFERENCES

1. Mannheim, Karl: *Ideology and Utopia*. London, Routledge; and New York, Harcourt Brace, 1940.

2. Opler, Morris: 'Themes as dynamic forces in culture.' *Amer. J. Sociol.*, **51**: 198–206, 1945.

3. Stanton, Alfred, and Schwartz, Morris: 'Medical opinion and the social context in the mental hospital.' *Psychiatry*, **12**: 243–9, 1949.

4. As a technique to determine the degree to which people held the ideological tenets we had attributed to the Unit's staff through participant observation, we constructed a questionnaire giving specific items of policy which would elicit attitudes of agreement or disagreement in the respondent according to where he stood on the issue involved. In some of the questions, agreement signified a pro-Unit-ideology view (hereinafter referred to as 'U'); in some questions the same view was indicated by disagreement with the proposition. In response to other questions agreement would signify the 'non-U' view. In each case we scored the answers on a four-point scale. If the respondent answered either at the extreme of a 'strongly agree' or 'strongly disagree', depending on the end of the continuum at which we hypothesized the Unit's views to lie, he received the highest score. Correspondingly lower scores were assigned as individuals chose one of the other responses. The set of four were: strongly agree, partly agree, disagree, strongly disagree. In the end, the highest scores we took to indicate the most extreme 'U' views; the lowest scores, the most 'non-U'.

5. Hollingshead, August, and Redlich, Fredrick: *Social Class and Mental Illness.* New York, Wiley, 1958.

6. Rapoport, Robert, and Skellern, Eileen: 'Therapeutic functions of administrative disturbance.' *Admin. Sci. Quart.*, **2**: 82–96, 1957.

7. Parker, Seymour: 'Role theory and the treatment of anti-social acting-out disorders.' *Brit. J. Delinq.*, **7**: 285–300, 1957.

8. There is a problem here about the validity and consequences of the Unit's assumptions about the ways in which patients' behaviour determines the overall state of Unit organization. This will be discussed in Chapter 6.

9. There is a problem here in distinguishing between consensus in the Unit and norms of people outside. This will be discussed in Chapter 7.

10. During the war years, when the Unit treated service-men, the interaction between hospital and community was at a peak which it has not been possible to sustain in post-war years because of a different type of patient population and changed public attitudes.

11. Galdston, Iago: *The Meaning of Social Medicine.* Cambridge, Mass., Harvard Univ. Press, 1954.

12. The only group worth special mention are the patients who have been divorced or separated, and they average even lower value scores than the others.

13. It is noteworthy that the relationship is even less discernible on admission. There seems to be some tendency for the Unit ideology to filter through slightly better to most patients of the stronger ego groups than to those with weaker egos. This will be mentioned again in Chapter 7.

14. Jones, Maxwell, and Rapoport, Robert: 'The Absorption of New Doctors into a Therapeutic Community' in Greenblatt, M.; Levinson, D. J.; and Williams, R. H.: *The Patient and the Mental Hospital.* Glencoe, Ill., The Free Press, 1957.

15. Stanton, Alfred, and Schwartz, Morris: *The Mental Hospital.* New York, Basic Books, 1954, p. 274 ff.
16. Rapoport, Robert and Rhona: 'Democratization and authority in a therapeutic community.' *Behavioral Science,* 2: 128–33, 1957.
17. Rapoport, Robert and Rhona: 'Permissiveness and treatment in a therapeutic community.' *Psychiatry,* 1959.
18. Some of these problems will be further discussed in Chapter 6 under 'oscillatory' processes.

CHAPTER 4

The Organization of Activities

The Unit staff attempt to implement their ideology through a system of organized activities. Each kind of activity can be seen in terms of its function with reference to the ideology of treatment and rehabilitation. Viewed atomistically, each also has a separate history in the Unit and in the profession as a whole. The general tendency among the Unit staff, however, is to view the programme of activities as an organic whole in which each of the parts derives its principal meaning from its place in the total pattern. Unit staff make statements like the following:

> 'The Unit treatment is like a symphony; each person's contribution, singly or in groups, is like the contribution to music made by the parts of a symphony orchestra.'

The Unit staff attempt to apply their ideological principles and rationales pervasively to every aspect of Unit life. Their therapeutic rationalizations for every aspect of Unit life can be illustrated by their attitudes toward the physical plant. The building is an old-fashioned, poorly constructed (originally a workhouse, not a hospital), bomb-damaged, structure in which patients are housed in very large wards which tend to be rather poorly heated and generally uncomfortable. The Unit sees these as favourable conditions for the patients they are treating in that the poverty of the surroundings provides a realistic background for treatment, similar to the working-class neighbourhoods to which patients will have to return. In addition, the shabbiness of the amenities is seen as an advantage for the occupational therapies in that there is a great deal of work to be done by way of decorating, furniture repair, etc., that constitutes a tangible and really needed contribution— not just 'make-work'.

Technically, the Unit staff's holistic approach may be seen as an attempt by them to view the entire social structure as a treatment instrument constructed in such a way as to maximize the institution's therapeutic effectiveness. In this chapter we are concerned with that aspect of the instrument that consists of the organization of activities. We shall look first at the overall pattern of the organization, indicating how its characteristics fit the Unit aims of treatment and rehabilitation. We shall then look at component elements in the organization of activities to attempt to understand each one's contribution.

With regard to the overall pattern, *Figure 3* gives its components and rough time patterning:

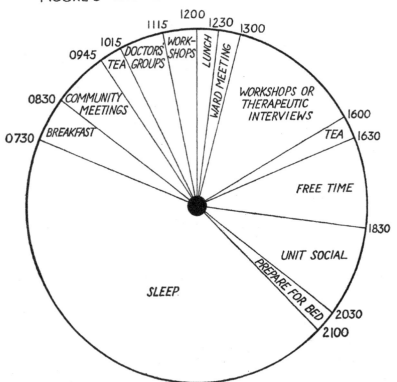

FIGURE 3 *DAILY ROUND OF ORGANISED ACTIVITY*

Treatment potentials are seen in every aspect of this pattern, and the ideologies of treatment and rehabilitation are meant to apply pervasively

throughout. In any particular kind of activity, be it doctor's therapeutic group, furniture repair shop, or evening social, all members of
the Unit are meant to be 'permissive', 'democratic', 'communal', and
'reality-oriented'. The participants ideally orient their activities in terms
of these values, rather than predominantly in terms of such other
potentially cross-cutting aims as personal gratification, efficiency, or
orderliness.

While in the abstract permissiveness allows patients to participate in
any way they choose, including non-participation, the Unit stresses
two important points of conformity as indicating *minimal* positive
orientation to the treatment as a whole. These are (*a*) attendance at the
8.30 morning meeting, and (*b*) being in the ward in pyjamas at 9.00
p.m. These two points are often mentioned as 'the only two rules in
Unit life'. There are, of course, a great many less explicit norms and
sanctions associated with participation in the Unit's activities. Many of
these will become apparent in the course of our analysis.

The timetable pictured in *Figure 3* indicates the usual daily round of
activities, excluding a variety of special groups, committees, and the
like. The principal rationale for the pattern is that it includes a round of
activities that is to some degree a replica of the social life of individuals
living in the non-hospital community. In many hospitals the actual
treatment and rehabilitation occur in brief focused sessions dedicated
to these purposes, while the rest of the time is taken up in routine care
and diversionary activities. In the Unit, treatment is meant to be all-
pervasive, and the rehabilitative effect of treatment is meant to be
enhanced by creating a pattern of activities that is like that of the average
person outside.

It may be pointed out that the Unit's daily round resembles that of
Mr Everyman only in a few aspects. There are daily workshops, which
are considered essential both to the individual and the system; there are
socials that stress ordinary forms of interaction between the sexes; there
are opportunities for spontaneous and self-selected associations. However, aside from whatever other limitations the workshops may have
as realistic occupational settings, they necessarily occupy a much
shorter part of the patient's day than work outside would. This stems
partly from the Unit's desire to have other treatment-oriented groups.
The socials, unlike those of the ordinary man's life, occur nightly and
often impel a kind of interaction that would not necessarily apply
outside the Unit, and which might actually lead to trouble in

post-hospital adjustment. For example, married men sometimes form heterosexual relationships in this setting that may interfere with their marital relationship. The meaning of the social for a young, inhibited, or inadequate single person is different from the meaning usually given to it by either single people who have no problems about unsociability (for example, alcoholics or 'con' men) or married patients.

Another aspect of the overall patterning of activities can be seen in the structure of group activities in *Figure 4*, which graphically portrays staff-patient interaction versus segregation:

FIGURE 4   *PATTERNS OF STAFF AND PATIENT INTERACTION IN THE DAILY ROUND*

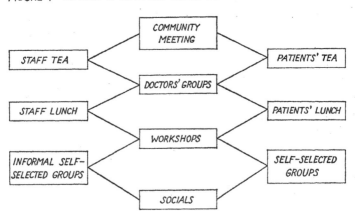

It is clear from this view of the organization that there is a kind of alternation between joint and segregated activities of patients and staff. As far as we can determine, this pattern developed independently of recent social science research on the social structure of mental hospitals. However, it seems to provide admirably for dealing with some of the phenomena behind the so-called 'Stanton-Schwartz effect'. Stanton and Schwartz, in their study of determinants of pathological excitement among patients, concluded that unrecognized disagreements between administrators and therapists were often at the basis of the patient's disturbance.[1] The Unit's pattern of alternating interaction and segregation is often now rationalized in terms of its capacity to avoid such staff splits. The type of patient treated by the Unit is considered especially prone to splitting staff by relating differently to different members and stimulating discord between them. Communalism notwithstanding, frequent staff meetings apart from the patients, are considered valuable for attempting to avoid such splits. This element of the organization of activities seems to enhance the quality of communication by structuring (and thereby curtailing) the degree of actual staff-patient interaction.

One further aspect of the pattern of activities as a whole may be pointed out. This is the progressive fragmentation and reshuffling of groups. This is graphically portrayed in *Figure 5*.

FIGURE 5   USUAL DAILY TIMETABLE SHOWN AS GROUPINGS [1]

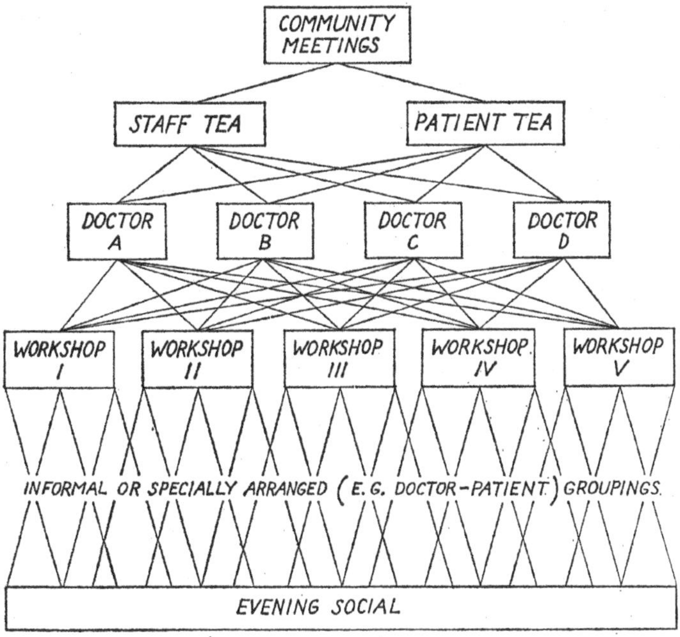

1 EXCLUDING MEALS AND SPECIAL GROUPS.

If we consider that a patient's ward is his 'home', we can see that he leaves home in the morning to go to a community meeting which includes all members of his own home group and all other groups in the Unit. This gathering is meant to be of special value in dealing with problems affecting the Unit as a whole and problems involving individuals from different sub-groups, Following the community meeting and the tea break, patients assemble in their doctors' therapeutic groups.[2] Here they interact with individuals from all the other Unit wards as well as members of their own. Eventually, owing to the cross-cutting membership of each group, and the continual reshuffling of group membership, each member of the Unit interacts with every other member in one group or another.

The explicit advantage of this pattern is expressed as a treatment rationale. Briefly stated, treatment presumably depends on a knowledge of any individual's total pattern of relationships. If in any one group, such as the workshop, a patient sees only other patients who know him in his work role, data from other areas of the patient's life will not be available in discussions of therapeutic importance within that group. For example, it is valuable in a workshop discussion group that individuals who know any given patient's patterns of interaction in his other spheres of activity be present to indicate how his behaviour in the work situation is related to his larger social experience. Thus, in the workshop a patient will have members of his own ward and of all other wards, so that all data about his relationships in the ward setting may be potentially available. He will also have members of his own doctor's group and members of all other doctors' groups where his name may have come up in connexion with someone else's problems. Similarly, in his doctor's group there will be representatives of his ward, his workshop, and all other spheres in his life in the Unit. According to this plan of organization, each patient gets an opportunity to interact closely with all other members of his community, and to have fed back into any particular group information from all of his spheres of activity.

While this is the rationale for the continual reshuffling of groups in the Unit, the actual group composition results from chance rather than deliberate assignment. Thus, at any given time group composition may only very roughly approximate to the valued structure. In the terms of our analysis, the Unit's argument is, essentially, that a much more tightly interconnected network of relations than is prevalent in the world outside the hospital is valuable for providing the 'feedback' of communications considered necessary for treatment.

The overall pattern, as we have described it, thus has some elements which serve patients' rehabilitation and some that are rationalized for treatment aims and may have little direct application to rehabilitation, or even be detrimental to it.

With regard to particular Unit sub-groups, some are more directly geared to one or the other of the Unit's principal goals. The tea-breaks, meals, and spontaneous self-selected associations have in common their apparent diversion from the pressing and pervasive tasks of therapy. The Unit differs from the more conventional hospitals (and this is characteristic of the therapeutic community approach) in attempting to use the transactions of even these informal associations to supplement its work in the formal groups in the interests of therapy. In this, as in its overall pattern of alternations of groups, it anticipated the social science findings of such researchers as Caudill[3] and Belknap[4] on more conventional hospitals, where informal associational materials were ignored to the detriment of therapy. In the Unit, these groupings are considered part of the daily round of 'ordinary' activies and, as such, arenas for the observation and collection of data on patients' interaction patterns as well as for the development of relationships that may facilitate treatment-rehabilitation in other contexts. The ways in which this may occur are legion. Sometimes the effect is an immediate and direct one—e.g., where one patient influences another patient to control his impulses to go out drinking. Sometimes the effect is direct, but not immediate—e.g., where a patient 'pairs off' with another and forms a relationship that is a 'good' one—i.e., that can last and be of benefit to both in their attempts to adjust to the outside world.[5] Sometimes the effects are delayed and indirect, as when a patient learns to trust another, and then in a therapeutic group is influenced by what a doctor says, not so much because it is the doctor saying it, but because his friend is present in the group and seems to concur, casting doubt on his defensive suspiciousness of the doctor's view.

In the therapeutic use of materials from the informal contexts, patients who take active parts in relaying back information and apply-ing Unit ideology in collaboration with the staff are in a complex position. They are acting consistently with Unit staff ideals, thus assist-ing with the therapeutic tasks and acting in their own interests to the extent that the assumption of responsibility and constructive activity are beneficial for them. On the other hand, they may be seen by their peers, particularly in times of staff-patient discord and general Unit disorganization, as 'stool pigeons' who 'rat on' rather than 'help' their fellow patients.[6]

The staff, too, may have a problem with reference to these 'construc-tive' patients. Sometimes patients who are overtly taking the prescribed parts of staff-surrogates may be perceived by the staff as showing their own problems (e.g., sadism, obsessional need to control, manic domin- ance in group interaction) and not contributing to the therapy of themselves or others. Staff interpretations along these lines may com- bine with peer-group resentment to make life in the Unit difficult for patients of this kind who perceive themselves as constructively oriented.[7]

Another set of groups that has a complex relation to the Unit's goals is that primarily concerned with staff problems. Staff meetings and tutorials are concerned in varying degree with teaching, administra- tion, helping staff in emotional problems they may have in their day- to-day work with patients or their relationships among themselves, and coordinating the staff policies and activities in their joint treatment/ rehabilitation enterprise.

There is a problem in the contradiction between the practice of separate staff meetings and the ideal of 'communalism'. This is often noted in the Unit—either by patients who feel acutely their exclusion from these meetings, or by staff who do not value the benefits of staff meetings as much as they value a sustained interaction with patients. This contradiction is sometimes the basis for staff factionalism or alien- ation.

The staff meetings do not take the form of formal presentations and case conferences, but of spontaneous discussion along similar lines to other Unit groups. People are expected to participate as they feel impelled. The need may be role-determined (e.g. director concerned about an admissions or public relations problem; DRO about a job placement problem), or personality-determined (e.g., homesick social therapist). In general the policy is to weave didactic discussions around problems of contemporary involvement, though the senior staff attempt a broad coverage of theory for the social therapists in their tutorials.

To some extent, the patients' committees are a counterpart of the staff meetings. The reception of new patients, the organization of socials, the conduct of certain interest groups (e.g., play-reading) are all patient-run activities. Though the staff, being formally responsible, retain ultimate power to curb or influence the conduct of these com- mittees, patients retain a good deal of autonomy in the actual day-to- day conduct of these groups.

The 'visitors' group', which receives professional visitors to the Unit

once a week, is, similarly, tangential to the core goals of Unit functioning, though indirectly related to them. In visitors' groups, for example,
staff and/or patients may, in the course of presenting viewpoints for the
enlightenment of the visitors, shed new light on their own understanding of the Unit situation or contribute to the working-through
of their own problems of living. These are not, however, the focal
aims of the visitors' group. The Unit staff tend to feel that visitors can
get a more realistic view of how the Unit works by allowing these
groups to function as small community meetings or therapy groups.
But to the extent that this aim transcends and is offered as a substitute
for the aim of a professional discussion with visitors on a technical
level, some visitors are dissatisfied with groups of this type.

The three groups most directly concerned with the task of treatment-
rehabilitation are the doctors' groups, the workshops, and the socials.
The community meeting, a fourth group that might be considered in
this category, will be discussed separately. Each of the three types of
group is meant to help the patient in different ways. The doctors'
group, modelled on general psychiatric principles of group therapy,
derives its main impact through *verbal communication*, and supplements
the pervasive Unit attempt to demonstrate 'here and now' problems of
interactions with analysis of personal motivations, and family-based
aetiological factors. The workshops, on the other hand, are *activity*-
centred. They supplement the general attempt to elucidate contemporary patterns of interpersonal difficulty (in this case, especially in the
work sphere) with opportunities to work out new, more satisfactory
patterns. The standards for conduct that apply here resemble more
closely than any others in the Unit those of ordinary outside activities.
For this reason, the workshop groups are highly valued as arenas for
rehabilitation efforts. The socials, too, approach 'normal' extra-
hospital types of situations—with dancing, small-talk, card-playing,
group games, and entertainment programmes. Their focal medium is
interaction of a more expressive affectual kind—i.e., less emphasis is
placed on what is said or done than on *how* it is said or done.

Each of these groups has, of course, its unique organizational problems, and these bear on the overall therapeutic goals of the Unit.
In the doctors' groups, the problems for the staff members concerned
lie mainly in the technical treatment sphere (i.e., which style and
technique of group therapy to emphasize; how much to supplement
group sessions with individual sessions with particular patients, etc.).

For the patients, the doctors' groups are the closest thing in the Unit to 'treatment' in the conventional sense. Here, at least, is a doctor conducting activities that, unlike most Unit groups, have no outside counterpart. These groups also differ from most Unit groups in their focus of interest. The *individuals'* problems, and not the Unit's problems, are in focus. Also, while everyone participates here, as elsewhere, the doctor's expertise is more clearly in relief.

Although they see group dynamics in terms of each patient's tendency to repeat earlier patterns of relationships in new situations, the doctors vary somewhat in their theoretical orientations and their personal styles of treatment. One doctor gives special emphasis to the interpretation of basic tendencies of the group as though it were an individual, and from this to see each person's part in creating the group tendency.[8] Another doctor has developed a technique that combines the 'leaderless', non-directive approach with 'excitatory', directive elements.[9] One doctor stresses the importance of positive affectual qualities in the therapeutic relationship ('Love *is* enough'), while another stresses the 'tough, masculine' approach as important in resisting attempts to manipulate the therapist and also in providing the kind of role model with which psychopaths might be likely to identify.

With regard to the workshops, the situation is more complex. The attitude of the staff is stated in their recent *Lancet* article:

'We came to realize that the work would become meaningful to the patients only when the tasks met some of their fundamental needs.

'Because we were housed in a neglected bomb-damaged building, there was a real need to redecorate the rooms to make our home more cheerful. The rooms contained many broken-down pieces of furniture which urgently needed attention if we were to have any pride in our surroundings, let alone any comfort... (patients) needed new clothes or at least repair of those they had. Also, their monotonous diet could be varied by growing more vegetables. By forming a home group, we shifted the emphasis from pre-vocational training to work to meet the more urgent needs of the community. Now we have five groups—furniture repair, painting and decorating, gardening, tailoring, and home groups—all engaged on tasks relevant to the needs of the community; and the patients' attitude to work has changed. In observing the social processes within the groups we have been helped by weekly workshop discussions, which were suggested by the patients themselves . . . the subjects of discussion include absenteeism, lateness, difficulties with authority, and relations within the group. Present working problems are related to outside factory problems and this trial period allows the patients to analyse their attitude to work.'[10]

In the workshops we have the clearest case, among Unit groups, of relatively undiluted rehabilitation aims. Even here, however, the aims of treatment are present, though in considerably subordinate form. When patients, for example, request changes in their workshops, the criterion of whether or not the workshop in which they are at the time engaged resembles that of their long-term occupation is not always paramount. More often, the consideration is whether or not the patient might have personality problems that could be analysed in relation to this or any other work situation—presumably with the intention of acting to change the personality. According to this view, any kind of work task provides 'grist for the treatment mill'—a viewpoint similar to that frequently found in psychoanalytic practice. The personality problems, being pervasive throughout the individual's spheres of activity, are considered to be the focus of interest and capable of being worked out, using any of a variety of 'reality' stimuli.

In line with the treatment orientation is the effort to foster identification with the Unit as a whole and its needs. In the staff's view, the most effective way to accomplish this is by setting the patients to work on tasks that have direct relevance to their own interests, which can be realized only in social living. This, too, provides the rationale *against* cash payments despite its 'realistic' reflection of the outside money-wage economy.

In the larger society, it is not so immediately apparent to any particular individual how absenteeism, for example, affects his lot in life. In a small community like the Unit the effect of any individual's behaviour on the whole system is more easily apparent. It becomes 'felt' by any individual to the extent that he identifies with the community as a whole. This identification, the Unit staff hope, will carry over to comparable situations outside. It is also seen as valuable in making patients more receptive to the attempts of staff, as community authorities, to work at changing their personalities while they are within the Unit.

From the point of view of fitting the individual to the kind of social situation to which he might have to adjust outside the hospital, other considerations are worth elaborating. In analysing the 'social reality' of the workshops, it is clear that they differ among themselves in several important characteristics (even aside from the physical differences in plant facilities, and the differences in personality and policy of the instructors). Some workshops tend to be more linked in local cultural definitions with one sex or the other (e.g., furniture repair is more 'masculine', the home group more 'feminine'). While the Unit staff note in the article cited above that many of the patients do not conform to the popular sex-linked occupational patterns, it is also true that many do, and, to the extent that rehabilitative aims are being pursued, it would seem desirable to sort out and match these patients with their appropriate job contexts.

Workshops also vary in tangibility of product (the furniture repair shop produces tangible, permanent products, while the home group cleans the physical plant only to have its work immediately obliterated each day).

The workshops also vary in terms of the social organization required for task completion (the furniture repair shop uses assembly line methods, division of labour, and factory-like hierarchies of worker-foreman-boss; the gardening group employs its individuals in a dispersed pattern of non-interacting, often widely separated tasks).

The groups also differ in terms of external relations and the repercussions of their activities (the effects of the gardening group on diet are rather small, since the hospital provides for the commercial purchase of most of its food, and the actual results of the gardening activities are not highly visible to other members of the Unit; at the other extreme, the cleaning group's activities affect the everyday life of everyone in the Unit and the group may be observed at work by anyone who enters the wards).

All the above variables that distinguish one workshop from another are relevant for treatment and/or rehabilitation. To the extent that rehabilitation ends are immediate, the major factor is the workshop's similarity to a patient's outside work situation. To the extent that treatment aims are relevant, the workshops are appraised in terms of their capacity to gain interest, trust, identification, and other prerequisites for fostering the relationship with therapists that may lead to personality change.

All the workshops may thus be seen as attempts to change individual personalities by fostering identification with the community as a whole, which makes patients more receptive to the larger community's influence on them. They may also be said to be rehabilitative in their general aim to the extent that they are more realistic than the usual hospital occupational therapies. Attempts are continually being made to foster both emphases. For example, during the course of this study the workshops began a policy of 'sacking' patients who did not work well, thereby increasing the similarity of these workshops to those in the outside world. At the same time, innovations that strengthened the treatment potentials of these groups were also made—e.g., by doctors (unlike executives in the outside world) joining work groups, chatting informally and working with patients on the job in order to develop a more spontaneous, intimate relationship, and implementing the staff's ideological tenet of communalism.

Unit staff tend to conceptualize the problem of the place of work-shops as one of striking a balance between making the workshops so 'realistic' that they are not therapeutic, on the one hand, and, at the other extreme, establishing such a therapeutic milieu through permis-siveness and communalism as to be unrealistic in terms of normal work expectations in industry. The awareness of our distinction between treatment and rehabilitation would enable workshops to exemplify in practice various proportions of each, and assign patients to work according to their therapeutic needs.

The socials are rationalized almost entirely in terms of their aim of assisting individuals toward normal patterns of social interaction. By creating a warm sense of communal participation, patients who are timid and distrustful in social situations may develop a sufficient sense of 'safety' and 'belonging' to be able to enter and participate in such situations outside the hospital. The patient committees that organize and run the socials present opportunities to practise social roles, assume responsibility, and carry out complex, cooperative tasks. Many patients who grow up with strong feelings of inadequacy often miss, successfully avoid, or mishandle such simple social relationships as carrying on small talk with members of the opposite sex. Being inept at even these preliminaries, their realization of the potentialities of such relationships tends to remain stunted. By learning how to control their fears and suspicions and to use the ordinary channels for informal social interaction, patients are thought by the Unit staff to be made more capable of carrying on a rewarding social life even with their basic personality difficulties.

In fact, the socials also have many recurrent patterns of interaction that have strong treatment intent and potential, even aside from their provision of data for the doctors' therapeutic groups. The ways in which the staff members present (usually social therapists) handle such recurrent problems as pairing-off, monopolization of the programme by special interest groups (such as jazz fans, old-time waltz enthusiasts, etc.), apathy, or refusal to terminate the social at bedtime, may have a direct intention of changing the particular patient's personality.

On the whole, however, most interaction in the socials has as manifest rehabilitative aims as any other sub-group within the Unit, with the possible exception of the workshops. Under the present form of Unit organization, it would seem that rehabilitative effects probably stem, for some patients, mainly from the workshops, and for other patients mainly from the socials. All patients, however, are exposed to both these activities with little discrimination.

The community-meeting ('the 8.30') is a group that is unique to the Unit. Group therapy, occupational and even work therapy, staff meetings and tutorials, ward meetings, patient committees, socials and so on are common in modern psychiatric hospital practice. The community meeting, however, is a distinctive form that can be understood only in relation to the Unit's history. It has several facets. On the one hand, it resembles group therapy, except for the unconventional size of the group—125 or so, as against the usual size of under a dozen. The intimate, public-confessional aspects of this community meeting, unusual in gatherings larger than the usual therapeutic groups, is often thought by observers to give it the quality sometimes found in congregations of religious sects like the Buchmanites (Oxford Group), Quakers, and others that stress leaderless public-confessionals. The Unit staff use the term 'community therapy' to refer either to a group of this *size* or to the use of the *entire community* with all its activities and relationships for therapy.

'The 8.30', however, is not predominantly seen by either staff or patients as a treatment group in the same sense as the smaller therapy groups. While it is recognized that treatment occurs here, and that there are powerful social forces at the disposal of treatment aims in such a group, the *principal* aims of the community meetings are those of social control. The actual devices of social control are varied. Much of the work of the meeting is taken up in data-gathering—but specifically on cases of deviant behaviour within the Unit's set of normative regulations. Early in the research the 8.30 meeting was divided into two sections, the first of which was given over specifically to naming 'defaulters', and having them discuss their deviant behaviour. Their names were compiled by the social therapists and night staff, and matters dealt with consisted of such social deviations as lateness or absence in the ward, absence from the community meetings, disorderly behaviour in the evening, and so on. In keeping with the general democratization trend, this group was absorbed into the larger 'community' meeting, and instead of being named by staff, the 'defaulters' were incorporated into a regular patients' news bulletin, read by the patient who was chairman of the entertainments committee, which also functions as a 'patient government' group. The patients' entertainments committee consists of elected representatives from each ward. They are important opinion setters, and represent the patients as a group for a variety of transactions with the staff.

Those patients who are especially sensitive to the public exposition of social deviation tend to see the community meeting as a punitive session and compare it with a criminal court. The distinction that the staff emphasize between this group and outside social control agencies is that there is collection of evidence and judgement (about what is 'reality') in the Unit, but not punishment. Patients are confronted with the 'reality' of their deviant behaviour and its effects on other individuals and on the system as a whole (e.g., getting the Unit into trouble with the hospital authorities or the police, and thus endangering its survival), but the intended consequences of this confrontation are not punitive so much as educational. While everyone recognizes that shame functions as a powerful social sanction, the purpose of the discussions is not to arouse feelings of shame or guilt. These feelings, where mobilizable, are seen as sometimes useful in bringing about changes, but it is the change itself that is sought—whether through the use of guilt and shame or through rational consideration, or substitution of new patterns for the old. Patients who see this 'educational' aspect of the community meeting as focal tend to compare its sessions with those of schoolrooms, stressing the amount they have learned in a straight educational sense about 'life' and 'people' in these sessions.

From the staff point of view, the meeting, whatever treatment/

rehabilitation value it may have for patients, is an essential channel of communications. In this group a variety of functions considered necessary for system-maintenance are fulfilled. Only through fulfilling these functions can those who hold formal responsibility gain enough reassurance about the consequences of their policies of democratization and permissiveness to carry on without excessive anxiety. All the Unit's personal resources—those of staff and patients—are, in this group, mustered to account for the deviant behaviour that is prevalent in the Unit. The knowledge of this deviation level gives the staff one 'social barometer' that helps them to judge the advisable limits of permissiveness. The situation is gauged not only by the actual number of deviant episodes brought to light, but by the manner in which they are handled. When the Unit is functioning well and the patients are constructively oriented to the joint enterprise, these meetings are therapeutically productive. Communications are relatively free and frank, attitudes toward the Unit and its work are positive. When the Unit is not functioning harmoniously, apathy and 'non-U' approaches (e.g., punitiveness, moralizing, domination) may characterize both staff and patients in interaction.[11]

This account does not exhaust the range of the Unit's organized groups. There are also weekly ward meetings, which resemble the community meetings, but are smaller, and concern only the affairs of single wards; there are family groups for the purpose of studying family relationships relative to the treatment/rehabilitation enterprise;[12] and there are patient committees of various kinds.[13]

What, then, can be said about the Unit's group organization in general? First, observers are often impressed with the sheer number of groups in the daily round of activities, and to the importance attached to 'groups' as the core treatment approach. 'Groups, groups, groups' is the refrain of the staff and the patients in informal discussion. 'Take it to the group' is the standard referral gambit in problematic staff-patient encounters. Between the '8.30' and afternoon tea at 4.00 P.M., there is constant group activity, with little time off even for lunch. Then the informal groups of the afternoon 'free' time often engage a patient's attention in activities until supper, which is followed by the evening social which draws together the entire Unit patient community for a final set of group activities before bedtime.

This constant collective activity is seen as valuable by the Unit in terms of catching emotional problems as they are 'hot'—'lancing the boil' at the crucial moment—rather than asking patients to contain their feelings until a formal treatment time the following day or week. To delay communication on emotional problems is seen as less effective than dealing with them on the spot, and also as literally impossible with this type of patient, who is distinguished by an incapacity to defer the immediate translation of feelings into activity. The Unit has thus become what one psychoanalyst has called an 'acting-out playground', in which the basic psychoanalytic principle of discouraging acting-out has been modified in dealing with adults with 'acting-out disorders'. However, even those observers who are impressed with the desirability of 'utilizing the other twenty-three hours', and the effectiveness of 'working with the problem while it's hot', still often feel that the pace is one that encourages the defences of manic activity and verbalization-intellectualization to the exclusion of introspective activities. While each group in the Unit functions with a good deal of 'self-determination', this sometimes increases external pressures on any particular patient, with a corresponding decrease of his internal self-determination.

There are patients who are not able to sustain participation in 'democratic' groups—e.g., if a patient so dominates their activities, that either he must be suppressed or the group must give up any idea of functioning in a democratic way. There are some patients who cannot communicate about the requisite personal materials in such a setting at all. Neither type seems best suited for the Unit's mode of treatment, which requires the alternation of active participation with reflection and passive participation. It seems paradoxical that such a preponderance of the Unit's organized activities is of a verbalizing, cognitive-reorientation type. Verbalizing comprises such a comparatively small proportion of the daily life of the ordinary British working-class man that immersion into the Unit's groups constitutes for many a rather severe iolt. The pace and tempo of this kind of psychotherapy makes it seem to patients that they are 'given' problems rather than find them in themselves and in their relationships. This approach to psychotherapy has been found useful in other attempts to speed up the process, but in other situations where the therapy occurred in a two-person relationship, the pace could be geared to the individual. In the Unit, while there is considerable leeway for participation in groups according to one's own, inclination, many patients find it difficult to sustain an involvement, even of vicarious participation, let alone activity in groups.

Another important aspect of the overall group picture is that some groups are associated with doctors or other core professional staff (e.g., doctors' groups), while other groups are associated with others in the staff (for example, the socials are associated with the social therapists, who are the only staff members relied upon to be there night after night). On the whole, the diversified groups associated with the core staff (doctor's groups, community meetings, ward meetings, family group) emphasize cognitive modes of therapy and have a predominantly treatment agenda. The workshops and socials, associated with non-psychiatrically-trained and transient staff respectively, concentrate on behavioural and attitudinal elements in therapy and have a rehabilitative emphasis. Their activities are aimed primarily at fitting an individual to a social context outside the hospital. But it is important to note that while activity rather than verbalizing provides the dominant content of these groups, the interpersonal expressive rather than the instrumental aspects of the activities are stressed. In the workshop, for example, the rehabilitation is oriented towards helping the patient to get on well with his fellows and his boss rather than towards superior technical performance. The assumption seems to be that these individuals are so incapacitated in their interpersonal relationships that no matter how great their technical performance skills in these occupations, they would experience work difficulties. On the other hand, if they could learn to sustain reasonably harmonious interpersonal relationships, they could find a job that would absorb them at whatever rudimentary level of task-performance they could show.

While the staff stress the importance of all groups and all activities in their attempt to 'treat the whole person', both staff and patients feel that some groups are more important than others—*but they do not agree on which groups are important or unimportant.* Staff and patients were asked to rank the three most helpful and three least helpful in the Unit. Their responses are summarized in *Table 8.*

The differences indicated here stem both from differences in staff and patient viewpoint in evaluating the groups, and from differences in their relative knowledge of and participation in the groups. Thus the family group, for example, is apparently more highly thought of by staff than by patients. But this is at least partly an artefact of the situation, in which most staff members know of and have an opinion about the value of the family group whether or not they actually attend it, whereas patients may, if their families do not figure in their treatment, have no special impression of it. The relative paucity of strong opinions about it among patients is probably in part, at least, a reflection of their differential exposure to and use of the group. Thus while the patients tend to feel more positive than negative towards it, the staff give the family group stronger favourable votes than they do to any other group.

TABLE 8 STAFF AND PATIENT EVALUATIONS
OF UNIT GROUPS*

Groups	Most Important		Least Important	
	Staff	Patients	Staff	Patients
	%	%	%	%
Community Meeting	21	10	2	23
Ward Meeting	7	3	7	28
Departure Group	1	1	25	6
Family Group	27	9	1	3
Socials	2	10	4	4
Indiv. Doc-Pat.	1	12	17	3
Indiv. Non-Med-Pat.	2	9	6	6
Doctor's Group	25	27	—	3
Workshop	14	11	1	10
Leisure Groups	—	2	23	9
Other	—	6	14†	5
Totals:	100	100	100	100

* The scores are expressed as percentages of total scores. Scores are computed by awarding three points to each first choice, two to each second, and one to each third. 'Least important' patient views only included two choices. All figures here are, thus, weighted percentages.

† This includes 13 per cent for staff meetings, a choice not available to patients.

The greatest difference of the other type—i.e., where accessibility and use are evenly distributed among staff and patients—focuses on the community meeting. The staff, obviously, regard it as one of their principal groups, while the patients tend to have strong negative feelings towards it. This is consistent with our analysis of the community meeting as primarily concerned with social control, a type of transaction understandably unpopular among *patients* in the Unit, while indispensable to Unit *staff*.

There are other less striking differences worthy of note. Patients tend to value individual doctor-patient relationships more highly than staff, many of whom see them as a handicap to the most desirable kinds of diffuse involvements. A much larger proportion of the patients than of the staff consider the workshops to be unhelpful, while a sizeably larger proportion of the staff than of the patients consider the leisure activities unhelpful.

The high negative score for the patients' evaluation of the ward meetings needs explanation. Interviews with patients indicate that their opinion is based less on the potential than on the actual value of such meetings. The amount of time given them and the tendency for patients to drift in and out because of the meeting's proximity to the lunch hour detract from its efficacy. Patients feel that as the group currently functions it does not do the kind of job that needs to be done, rather than that the job itself is not worth doing.

The departure group, which was eventually discontinued, illustrates a case of negative evaluation of the type of activity *per se*. The institution of a relatively formal, specialists' group to plan patients' discharges was felt by most staff to be going against the trend toward communal decision making and also negated the ideal of consistently thinking ahead towards discharge from the very beginning of treatment.

In general it seems that 'treatment' interactions are most highly valued by both staff and patients, while 'rehabilitation' groups yield differences of opinion. Some groups that are focused on facilitating social adjustment are more highly valued by staff than patients (workshops), others by patients more than by staff (socials). This, too, is not surprising in view of the patients' characteristic problems and the staff's ideology with reference to work therapy.

NOTES AND REFERENCES

1. Stanton, Alfred, and Schwartz, Morris: *The Mental Hospital*. New York, Basic Books, 1954.
2. Some doctors see their patients in two smaller briefer morning sessions rather than in the one large grouping that lasts from morning tea until lunch. In these cases, the patients go to their workshops for the period in which the doctor's group is not in session.
3. Caudill, William A.: *The Psychiatric Hospital as a Small Society*. Cambridge, Mass., Harvard Univ. Press, 1958.
4. Belknap, Ivan: *Human Problems in a State Mental Hospital*. New York, McGraw-Hill, 1956.
5. Examples of this will be mentioned in the section on 'pairing off' in Chapter 6.
6. In the section on patient leadership and clique formation in Chapter 6, some of these problems are discussed.
7. The vicissitudes of 'constructive' *v.* 'destructive' participation will also be discussed in Chapter 6.

8. Bion, W. R.: 'Experiences in groups' (seven-part article). *Hum. Relations*, Vols. 1–3, 1948–50. Also in *Experiences in Groups and Other Papers*. London, Tavistock Publications, 1961.

9. Merry, Julius: 'Excitatory psychotherapy.' *Brit. J. med. Psychol.*

10. Jones, Maxwell, Pomryn, B.A., and Skellern, Eileen: 'Work therapy.' *Lancet*, 31 March, 1956, pp. 343–4.

11. Cf. the section on 'oscillations' in Chapter 6.

12. To be discussed in Chapter 8.

13. The New Patients' Committee will be discussed in Chapter 7.

CHAPTER 5

The System of Social Roles

Each individual who enters the Unit must work out some way of behaving that will satisfy two distinct sets of social role prescriptions. The first is a set peculiar to the Unit (according to which the blueprint for the role system is implied in the treatment ideology). The second is a set deriving from the customs, ethical codes, and statutes of the larger society (according to which the blueprint for the role system is implied in professional canons and in the provisions of the National Health Act). In this chapter we shall indicate some of the cardinal features of each of these sets of role directives, and describe some of the characteristics of the Unit's role system as it takes form under the influence of these diverse forces. We shall then indicate some patterns of role performance that have actually emerged as characteristic of particular roles as their incumbents have sought ways of reconciling dilemmas implied in combining the two sets of role prescriptions. Since the treatment instruments of social psychiatry are to be found in the *actual* rather than the ideal patterns of role performance, it is important to understand the factors that forge the actual social structure and to trace the therapeutic implications from this point rather than from the ideal structure.

According to Unit ideology, everyone, regardless of his social role in the formal organization, should participate in Unit life according to a similar set of principles. These are:

a. Everyone is expected to attend as many groups as possible, including as a minimum, the community meetings, and to participate in discussions (to 'verbalize').

b. Everyone is expected to express his *feelings* in these groups—to 'say what he feels'—spontaneously and fully.

c. Everyone is expected to 'feed back' information about others that might be relevant to the functioning of the Unit or to the others' treatment.

d. Everyone is expected to participate in decision-making on practical or administrative problems affecting the Unit's functioning.

e. Everyone is expected to share a sense of responsibility for the course of events as it is affected by group decision-making.

f. Everyone is expected to receive as well as to give treatment—to 'trust the community'—at least to the extent of listening to others and accepting the consensus of Unit groups as 'reality'.

g. Everyone is expected to respond to group consensus by modifying his behaviour accordingly—i.e., to be responsive to social pressure.

h. Everyone is expected to 'help' others in prescribed ways—i.e., by being permissive, sharing, forming relationships, providing models for socially adaptive behaviour, providing supportive (non-punitive) controls against patients' anti-social 'acting out' while they are in the Unit.

Within this general blanket prescription, the general view of the Unit staff is that 'everyone should find his own role' in the Unit, by which they mean that each individual should find a way of participating that is compatible with his personal needs and that allows maximal expression of his personal capacities. For patients this is meant to provide a framework that would be of direct diagnostic and therapeutic value. Since many of them have experienced difficulty in performing in social roles outside the Unit because of their underlying personality problems, it is reasoned that a regimen of formal prescriptions in the hospital would only obscure the real source of the difficulty by enforcing behavioural uniformity. This was the general picture in prisons or in the old-fashioned mental hospitals. On the other hand, if a rather unstructured social situation were provided, patients' behaviour would be determined more by their underlying personality needs than by external social pressures. Through making the personality determinant of behaviour manifest, those giving treatment could become aware of the underlying problems and those receiving it could be confronted with others' perceptions of them. In this chapter we shall be concerned primarily with staff roles, reserving the analysis of patients' roles for a later chapter.

For the staff, the emphasis on ideologically-based role prescriptions that are meant to apply to everyone in the Unit is thought to have advantages over implementing therapy. In the old-fashioned custodial system, lower echelons of the staff tended to be excluded from the more interesting work (where it did exist) of study and analysis of patients' problems, and to be 'saddled' with the routine jobs of care for the patients. Part of the Unit staff's rationale for the emphasis on universality in role prescriptions is that the diffusion of knowledge about and participation in treatment of patients' problems is valuable for staff morale. Maxwell Jones has maintained in a recent paper with the present author that one possible cause for the nursing shortage in mental hospitals is that conventional roles exclude them from the more interesting kinds of participation in medical discussion.[1]

Aside from the morale that may stem from general participation, the Unit staff consider that the emphasis placed on allowing personality determinants of role performance to come into ascendancy yields increments of therapeutic power. The skills that are necessary for therapy, it is reasoned, are very diverse. Information must be gathered about the patient—and this involves being on hand to observe him and having the kind of relationship with him that will entail his frank and spontaneous communications. Judgements must be made about the nature of the underlying difficulty that recurs in a patterned way in different situations. Strategies must be formed for the exertion of therapeutic influence. The actual influences must be brought to bear on the patient, and anomalies in his response dealt with by constant revision of strategies. Some of these therapeutic requirements, it is reasoned, may best be met by lower echelon staff or by the patients themselves (e.g., observation of a variety of spontaneous interaction situations; communication on frank and spontaneous levels; effective exertion of certain kinds of influence); on the other hand, the senior staff might tend to excel in matters involving specialized training. Since none of the requisite skills is considered the monopoly of any of the participants, and since the staff does not maintain that some skills are necessarily more important than others, the general prescription is for universal participation in all the phases of the therapeutic endeavour, with relevant skills to be encouraged and exploited wherever they turn up in the system.

The Unit's ideology, then, implies a set of role prescriptions that is to be applied universally to all participants in the system. This situation is consistent with the democratic and communal ideological themes, and altogether these ideals may be said to imply a social structure that has the following characteristics:

a. The social structure is, ideally, 'acephalous'—i.e., there is to be no formal, authoritative head to lead or direct any of its groups. Consensus through equalitarian participation is to replace division of authority.

b. If the social structure is considered as a network of social relationships, the ideal Unit structure is one that is tightly interconnected—i.e., each individual is to have as part of his social network every other individual in the Unit, and they are thus to be totally interconnected.

c. The expectations of each individual in the network are to be very broadly defined, and exercised with diminished or muted sanctions in comparison to those prevailing in the world outside the system.

d. All relationships in the system are to be verbally reciprocal—i.e., individuals are to 'hold up a mirror' to others, and to confront them with a verbal reaction that makes clear the effects of their behaviour on others.

e. Role functions are to be interchangeable—i.e., everyone is to give and to receive treatment and everyone may choose the modes of participation that are most suited to him personally. However, 'constructive' participation, in 'U' terms, is the most highly valued mode for both staff and patients.

Aside from these general role prescriptions stemming from Unit ideology, each member of the staff is subject to certain role prescriptions following from his position in the *formal* system of the Health Services. Each staff member technically occupies a formal position *different* from others within a national system for organizing hospitals. Each of these positions incorporates certain expectations, obligations, privileges, and rights that are customary and sometimes enforced by statute or canons of professional ethics. The incumbent of each position has, furthermore, a set of expectations of others in the variety of formal positions with which his own role articulates. Together, these form what Merton has called the 'role set'.[2] Thus, a doctor must not only know what is expected of doctors by the medical profession, by the public, by the National Health Service and by the particular hospital, but he must also know what to expect of persons in other roles which articulate with his own—e.g., social worker, nurse, patient, and so on.

The statutory prescriptions governing the organization of hospitals and associated administrative structures is usually represented in the familiar 'tree' type of organizational chart of *Figure 6*.

Each hospital is staffed according to specifications authorized by its Regional Board but along lines consistent with this basic pattern. Belmont Hospital, though administered by a local Regional Board, receives patients from all over England and not only from the local 'catchment area'. The Unit is authorized, within Belmont Hospital, to have a fixed staff, including a director (with rank of consultant physician psychiatrist), three other physicians of various grades, a charge nurse (sister), two staff nurses, twelve assistant nurses (social therapists), psychiatric social worker, psychologist, four workshop instructors, two Disablement Resettlement Officers (delegated from the Ministry of Labour), and secretarial and domestic staff.

FIGURE 6 *TYPICAL CHART SHOWING ORGANIZATION OF HEALTH SERVICES*

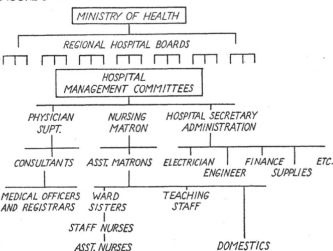

Patients, too, have a formally recognized role, distinct from staff roles generally, and are subject to certain expectations within the hospital system. Patients are admitted to the hospital for 'treatment', and this is bestowed upon them as their *right* as taxpayers under the National Health Service, not simply as paid services or as favours. In their role as 'ill' persons, patients may behave in ways considered deviant outside the hospital, but it is expected that they should *want* to take steps to correct this, to get 'into treatment'. Essential in this is the idea that they should have some desire for therapy. Lacking the wish to change, they are still to be assisted, if medical opinion recognizes potentiality for change, but the prognosis tends to be poorer in such circumstances.

In summary, the structure prescribed by the formal-conventional system is hierarchical rather than flattened; heterogeneous and specialized rather than homogeneous (equalitarian) and generalized (interchangeable functions); impersonal and segmental rather than intimate; diffuse rather than interconnected; orderly and disciplined rather than permissive of deviant personal modes of participation.

EMERGENT STAFF ROLES

All together the expectations associated with any particular role tend to fall on the one hand into a formal set that is fairly coherent and well worked out in custom, generally adhered to in the profession, and embodied in canon and statute; and on the other hand the Unit's ideological directives, which form a new and very different set of prescriptions, which must then be reconciled with the formal set. This reconciliation is mediated by the personality of the role incumbent and the exigencies of the particular situation, forming an emergent pattern of role performance. The new system of roles worked out by the Unit staff members forms the actual social structure of the Unit.

The general picture we get for each social role may be represented schematically as follows:

FIGURE 7   DETERMINANTS OF STAFF ROLES

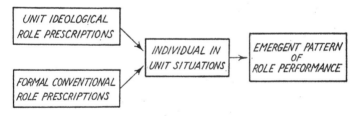

For the Unit as a whole, the emergent structure of the system of roles is, indeed, intermediate between the formal traditional 'tree' type and the Unit's 'flat' homogenized ideal. It may be thought of as comprising, on the staff level, three sub-groups:

a. The 'core staff'—comprising the most highly trained professional psychiatric staff—the doctors, the charge nurse ('sister'), and psychiatric social worker (p.s.w.), and the psychologist.

b. The adjunctive permanent staff—comprising those whose training is not psychiatric but in some special skill that supplements the psychiatric to make up a team capable of conducting 'community therapy'. These include the workshop instructors, the disablement resettlement officers, and the staff nurses (who are medically but not psychiatrically qualified).

c. The transient staff—comprising the 'social therapists', who are untrained in any of the core or adjunctive professional skills, but are employed in the formal position of assistant nurse. In the Unit, unlike elsewhere in the Health system, these girls are not part of the nursing hierarchy, but are transient personnel brought in for six months to a year to implement the Unit's particular approach to treatment rehabilitation. In many cases they have had some university education, usually in social work but they seldom have any nursing training. They do not, however, form part of any definite career line, and go into various occupations after their experience in the Unit.

These groups may be pictured graphically as follows:

FIGURE 8   *THE STRUCTURE OF UNIT STAFF ROLES*

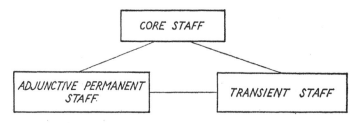

We may describe the general characteristics of each of these groups, and then, through the analysis of role problems and dilemmas of a selected role from each group, show how the Unit's system of social roles bears on the treatment/rehabilitation of patients.

The core staff is made up of four doctors, a p.s.w., a nursing sister, and a clinical psychologist. They are distinguished from other staff members by a good deal of professional training and/or experience. For most purely Unit functions, the division of labour according to differences of formal status is not operative in that core staff may perform many functions interchangeably. Any member of the core staff can conduct a group without arousing particular discomfort. They may substitute for one another. When a doctor is away, the leadership of his therapeutic group may be taken over by another doctor, or may fall to the nursing sister, or psychiatric social worker. Difficulties encountered in this substitution are not usually attributed to status differences, but to differences in personality or to the difficulties inherent in loss of a 'parental figure' and substitution of a new one. Because of their positions in the Unit, each of the core staff members is expected to, and indeed does, participate on a more sophisticated level than members of other staff or patient groups.

Each core staff member has his specialized duties as well as those he performs jointly or interchangeably with others in the core group. The psychiatric social worker, for example, is mainly concerned with relationships to social service agencies and the practical problems of patients' families outside the Unit; the psychologist is the only one in the Unit who administers tests; the nursing sister is more concerned than others with the immediate problems of hygiene, sanitation, care of equipment and supplies, and maintenance of nursing records and rosters; and the physicians are more immediately concerned with medical records, diagnosis, referral and problems of physical illness when they become pressing. Sister, having a more *general* jurisdiction than simply over the more junior nurses (who, in the Unit, are directly responsible to the medical director), actually performs many functions of a liaison and integrative type that are prescribed neither by the formal nursing requirements nor by the Unit ideology. These seem to fall most appropriately to her because of her high status, and partly because of her personality which both attracts persons in need of help to her as a central 'mother' figure and draws her towards integrating discordancies in relationships. Both sister and the psychiatric social worker often function along with male doctors as distaff group leaders in 'doctor's groups'—enhancing the 'familistic' quality of the groups by providing convenient figures for 'mother' as well as 'father' types of relational objects.

The permanent adjunctive staff is made up of individuals trained and experienced in occupations relevant to the therapeutic community venture, but not in psychiatry or other core disciplines associated with conventional psychiatry. The principal value of the workshop instructors and D.R.O.s, for example, is considered to be their long experience with 'real' industry. In order to apply this experience to the therapeutic community context they must be appropriately indoctrinated in the special problems of working with patients with personality disorders, and they must, of course, be of suitable personality. To the extent that they become more involved in interpreting patients' motives beyond what is necessary for them to modify their own approaches to fit the Unit's general approach, instructors are seen as losing some of their special value. Thus if a workshop instructor loses touch with the realistic requirements on jobs outside the Unit, his value to the Unit as an agent of rehabilitation efforts diminishes—regardless of how therapeutic his approach may be in other respects. The workshop instructors vary in their actual practice from those who organize their shops very much like industrial workshops to those who simply provide organized activities for the patients with little resemblance to the occupational structure to which the patients are likely to return.

The staff nurses, while not so directly tied into the rehabilitation effort as are D.R.O.s and workshop instructors, maintain their external links for still other reasons. Their principal task is that of system maintenance with regard to physical medication, records, rosters, and so on. While the Unit emphasizes none of these impedimenta of usual hospital practice, the nurses are expected to sustain the daily records of patient care required by the hospital. Technically, the staff nurses are in a hierarchy between the nursing sister and the assistant nurses (social therapists). The situation in the Unit is such that the nursing sister functions as a member of the core group, partly because of the Unit's ideology, partly because of her special training and personality—leaving most routine formal nursing matters to the staff nurses. The social therapists, on the other hand, are given a special role, directly responsible to the medical director of the Unit and not performing the usual tasks of assistant nurses in hospitals. This situation creates certain problems in the role of staff nurse that will be discussed below.

The D.R.O.s in the Unit at the time of study strikingly exemplify the range of role adjustments to the Unit's dual determinants. There are two D.R.O.s, and one performs in his role primarily according to the *formal* prescriptions, with only minimal concessions to the Unit as a context for the performance of his duty. He is a fine type of British civil servant, impeccably groomed, punctual, reliable, and universally 'correct' in his dealings with everyone. He addresses patients with the use of the title 'Mr', 'Miss', or 'Mrs' and their surname, and is addressed similarly by almost everyone in the Unit. The other D.R.O., on the other hand, equally fulfils her formal responsibilities, but uses the Unit context and ideology to its utmost in enlarging the scope of her role. She attends many more groups than she has to, participates according to the general Unit ideological principles rather than confining her contribution to matters technically concerning the D.R.O., and deals with patients in a more informal and personal way than is customary among her professional colleagues. In keeping with this, she is almost universally addressed by her first name.

The social therapists tend to be unmarried girls between the ages of 20 and 30, who have had some university training, often in social work, and who stay in the Unit from six months to a year. They come for a variety of reasons, are recruited informally (e.g., by ex-therapists, by the director on lecture tours, by referrals from people who know of the Unit's system), and on leaving the Unit go into a variety of occupations. In selecting them, the Unit staff stress the importance of their being relatively healthy emotionally, attractive, intelligent, of responsive temperament and interested in people. These requirements are surprisingly like those of airline hostesses, and many of the Unit therapists at least have fantasies of becoming airline hostesses after leaving the Unit. Scandinavians are thought to be especially suitable for the job of social therapist, not only for their physical attractiveness, but because of their 'democratic' approach. They do not typically relate to patients in terms of formal status differences as is so common among many British nurses. Their lack of nursing training is thought to facilitate this 'equalitarian' approach. Being foreigners, formally un-trained and transient, they are thought to have a lot in common with the patients. When new in the Unit, social therapists may have to look to patients for many items of day-to-day orientation in their new culture, giving the latter feelings of social worth and enhancing the Unit ideal of interchangeability of role functions.

The social therapist, ideally, identifies herself with both staff and patients[3] and serves as an important intermediary. Her regular tutorials with members of the core staff provide 'on the job training' woven around issues of current importance in the Unit's life. The patients get the sustained contact with the social therapists—in wards and other groups, and in socials. The social therapists serve as 'good' female figures, who by accepting patients are thought to stimulate many positive emotions which assist patients to identify with the established order. In most of the patients these feelings were diverted or stunted in their early relationships with unsatisfactory parental figures.

Two characteristics of the therapists' social role make them valuable to the core staff as indicators of the state of patient opinion in the Unit. First, among staff, they have the most sustained, pervasive contact with patients, giving them an unparalleled overview of the situation. This comes by virtue of their participation in *every* organized Unit group. The second factor is, paradoxically, their lack of formal training. This tends to make them more than usually dependent on the permanent trained staff for forming judgements as to the state of affairs. They report what they experience with relatively little bias either from the stylized conventions of traditional hospital nursing routines or from the sophisticated abstractions of enthusiastic but relatively inexperienced junior members of other disciplines. Their 'ordinariness' is seen as their greatest asset, and their role has been described as dealing mainly with socializing aspects of treatment within the Unit.[4] As we shall see below, these critical elements in the social therapists' role contribute to a set of role dilemmas that manifest crucial problems 'built in' to the Unit social structure.

PROBLEMS IN THE RESOLUTION OF ROLE DILEMMAS

As we have seen, the Unit's ideal role prescriptions are at variance with those of the formal system underlying it. This variance poses, for each role incumbent, certain dilemmas that he must resolve in working out his emergent pattern of role performance. The variation between ideal and formal role prescriptions is different for different roles, and this fact will determine the patterns of resolution that may be observed in actual Unit role performance. We shall examine here three roles—one representing each of the major groupings of roles in the Unit—and attempt to analyse the types of dilemmas posed, the patterns of role performance that tend to emerge as resolutions of these dilemmas, and their implications for treatment/rehabilitation of patients. The Unit staff stress the idea that the flexibility provided for personally determined role performance is favourable for treatment/rehabilitation in that it allows each staff member to perform in a 'natural' and sincere way, contributing to the genuineness of his personal relationship with the patient and to the 'realism' of his mode of relating. Ideally this allows for individual satisfaction for the staff member in his role, and effective rehabilitative influence for the patient (cell A in *Figure 9*). This ideal situation is, in fact, exemplified by some of the patterns observed in the Unit. However, other patterns that deviate from the ideal either in personal satisfaction of the incumbent in the face of the flexibility in role resolutional patterns or in the benefits to patients from the treatment/rehabilitation viewpoint are also observable. Essentially we have a 'four-fold' typology which is shown in *Figure 9*.

FIGURE 9   TYPOLOGY OF RESOLUTIONS
                           TO UNIT STAFF ROLE DILEMMAS

| | | *Therapeutic Effects* | |
		Good	*Bad*
	Good	A	B
Personal Satisfaction			
	Bad	C	D

The type represented in cell A is the one most valued in the Unit. Some behaviour of staff (cell B) satisfies personal needs in the conflict situations but entails antitherapeutic consequences for patients. Other behaviour is geared to the therapeutic task but at the cost of personal strains for the staff members (cell C). Finally, some behaviour (cell D) yields negative results for both, the staff member and the patient. To a large extent these patterns are recognized and watched for by Unit staff and dealt with as 'problems' relevant to the therapeutic enterprise as a whole. To some extent they are not explicitly understood nor are they systematically dealt with. In this chapter we shall illustrate how some characteristic dilemmas arise in staff roles and are resolved in a variety of ways encompassed by the categories just described.

The three representative roles that we shall analyse in this way are the role of junior physician, to illustrate some problems of core staff members; the role of staff nurse, to illustrate some problems of permanent adjunctive staff; and the role of social therapist.

THE ROLE OF JUNIOR PSYCHIATRIST

The Unit provides for only two permanent doctors' appointments, with two junior psychiatrists participating on two to four year tenures. This fact, together with the Unit's frequent practice of absorbing visiting doctors for periods of up to six months for didactic purposes, provides a group of doctors with characteristic problems of adjustment in the Unit overlapping with, but somewhat different from, those of the two senior doctors and the other more permanent members of the core group.

Some general points may be made about the doctor's role[5] and about the problems of absorption of new doctors into the Unit.[6]

Doctors are, characteristically, located at the pinnacle of the treatment hierarchy of hospitals. They have authority to carry out their treatment within the institutional structure, and are held responsible in law, canon, and custom for their professional conduct. 'Doctors' orders' tend to be imperatives of the utmost force in the system, and are always considered immediately relevant to health, even to life or death. In any hospital, the physician's group ordinarily comprises the highest concentration of technical training and skills to which all other roles are oriented. This is particularly true in psychiatry, where the technological impediments of the practice are comparatively small. The flow of communications from patients and lower echelon staff toward the physician tends to be asymmetrical, with his own obligation to communicate and choice of communications being less inclusive than his expectations from others. In return, physicians ordinarily observe strictest confidence, to protect the 'privilege' of necessarily freer communication to him than is ordinarily allowed in social relationships.

In the Unit, as we have seen, doctors are enjoined to renounce the direct exercise of authority in the form of giving orders; they are expected to acknowledge the presence of indispensable skills elsewhere in the population and to function as coordinators rather than as dispensers of these skills; and they are expected to work publicly rather than privately in handling patients' communications.

Physicians who apply for positions in the Unit are, of course, a self-selected population of those who think, from whatever knowledge they have of the Unit's methods, that they would like to function in this context. So to some extent new doctors are individuals who at least feel themselves to be personally compatible with the Unit's modes of operation, and who are also positively motivated to try to function within this framework.

Before the new doctor enters the Unit to begin the working out of his own individual pattern of role performance a certain amount of anticipatory socialization occurs. Within the Unit, if the doctor is to take over the group of another doctor who is departing, some of the patients who expect to undergo the change may look forward positively towards it, expressing their dissatisfaction with their present therapist and optimistically idealizing the future one. Others, at the opposite extreme, may resent the new therapist's arrival, feeling acutely the loss of their present doctor. In some cases patients feel that the new arrival has pushed out his predecessor. Others range in between with various combinations of ambivalence toward the change.

The staff, too, look forward to the arrival of a new doctor with a good deal of feeling that plays a part in shaping his reception. For the social therapists, a bachelor doctor may be anticipated with positive feeling for personal reasons. Their interest may serve to make them receptive to the new doctor's gestures of friendship when the latter is seeking comfort and understanding in his attempt to deal with the dilemmas of his role in the Unit. The social therapists, chosen for their attractiveness, are particularly suitable in this situation, even though senior female staff may have more in common with the new bachelor doctor intellectually. New doctors often turn to one or the other or both of these cross-sexual informal staff relationships in working through their problems of adjustment to the Unit community.

The stage of anticipatory socialization for the doctor is rife with fantasy—both for the doctor (because of the excitement and uncertain quality of experience in an innovating centre like the Unit) and for those within the Unit (because of the importance of the doctor in the system). There is a diversity of relationships pending for each doctor within the Unit, and these vary with the composition of the Unit and the state of organization at the time of his entry.

When the doctor actually enters the Unit, he experiences a very great discontinuity from the point of view of all his earlier conditioning as a physician and psychiatrist. He gives up the use of a uniform, is not addressed by a title nor does he thus address others—Christian names being used almost exclusively; and he is asked rather direct and personal questions by patients and must perform publicly in handling the new situation. Whatever mode of handling the situation he chooses —e.g., interpretation of the questioner's motivations—will be publicly observed, for 'treatment' here occurs in larger groups, not in private. His style must be developed under the scrutiny of all the patients as well as his colleagues.

Paradoxically, it actually helps a new doctor to adjust to the Unit community if he is manifestly in a bit of trouble in the early stages. The slogan 'we are all patients here together' becomes virtually true, and by exemplifying it unashamedly early, not too severely, and not in a prolonged way, the new doctor actually demonstrates his adherence to the Unit's ideological stand.

An aspect of doctors' adjustment to the Unit that is very different from that in other hospitals is the degree to which social adjustment to the institution as a community is important in the actual performance of the doctor's professional role. In any hospital, doctors must get along personally to some extent with others in the system if they are to function well. But usually this may be kept to a minimal and routinized form, professional skills being clearly differentiated from the interpersonal relationship aspects of role performance. In the Unit, a doctor who does not make himself part of the Unit community, become socialized to its norms and way of life, and adopt a leadership position within it, cannot perform in his professional role.

Clearly, the new doctor has not only to learn aspects of the new system, but to *unlearn* his earlier ways of handling situations in his professional role. He must modify his ethical position on confidentiality of information communicated in psychiatric treatment; he must give up much of the detailed control of events in the treatment situation while retaining full formal responsibility; he must give up many of the symbols and prerogatives of status that protected him by creating social distance as well as gratifying him personally. In the stresses of the early attempts to reconcile the divergent prescriptions for his role and to assimilate the discontinuities, he may regress either professionally (by using modes of functioning appropriate to earlier contexts but not to this—e.g., becoming autocratic in his manner) or personally (e.g., by becoming upset or withdrawn).

On the other hand, the Unit provides many sources of support for the new doctor. The fact that he can, temporarily and mildly, 'become a patient' in the situation, may help, provided he does not take this idea *too* seriously or hold it for too long. The lowered and limited expectations for novices in the doctors' roles is also helpful. While a new doctor is confused and dependent on those who have learned to make their way in the system he is not expected to perform as an expert.

A problem for the new doctor from early on in his absorption into the Unit is that of assimilating ideal-real discrepancies that he observes. An awareness of these discrepancies may assist him in formulating his own pattern for resolving his role dilemmas, but initially it may be disturbing to him. While every organization has 'ideal-real' discrepancies, an innovating one that is experimentally applying its ideal principles, and one that has a formal substructure so different from its advocated structure is likely to be rather extreme in this respect. When a novice enters the Unit he can learn relatively easily what the ideal system is because the principles of 'democratization', 'permissiveness', 'communalism', and 'reality confrontation' are encapsulated in slogans that are easily communicable in package form. On the other hand, mastery of the informal system, according to which the qualifications are provided for the ideal precepts, and acceptable and tested solutions to the typical dilemmas are worked out, takes more time.

Between their early stage of comparatively passive observation, usually accompanied by a certain amount of confusion, distress, and anxiety, and their stage of stabilized role performance, doctors usually go through a transitional stage in which they try out patterns of participation initially as participant observers in others' groups, then as fledgling group leaders themselves. In this, the role models for the new doctors are not only the older doctors, but others of the core staff who demonstrate in their handling of events the 'Unit way', and who informally may be able to 'fill in' the new doctor with the informal lore and background of 'inside information' on the histories, personalities, and characteristic ways of handling situations of the key figures in the Unit.

Once a doctor has stabilized his pattern of role performance, he becomes part of the system, and his way of managing the tasks presented to him in the Unit becomes part of what everyone else must reckon with. A psychologist who visited the Unit for an extended period of time described the variations in doctors' patterns of role performance in the following terms:

> Each of the doctors has a different idea of the Unit, what it is about, where it is going, and so on. Dr C makes the point that the main thing about the Unit is that it permits a doctor to use what ordinarily goes to waste in a psychiatric hospital—i.e., a knowledge of the patients' behaviour in every aspect of their hospital life. . . . A knowledge of this gives the therapist data to understand the patient as a whole—showing up areas of consistency and inconsistency and difficulty in his behaviour. Furthermore, he feels that the group helps in producing information and in supporting the patient in getting him to cope with confrontations. The doctor, in his mind, operates as the key figure in all this, evaluating the information as it comes in. . . .

Dr B stresses more his response to group directives. . . . His main point is that the behaviour of these patients, like that of all patients, is disturbing, upsetting, and arouses terrible anxieties and guilt feelings in the staff. . . . In most hospitals they control this in various ways, like the formalism of staff organization. The Unit has begun to give patients freedom, but hasn't yet gone as far as it might because of the fears of those in authority. He feels that when patients are given freedom—even to acting out in extreme forms, something happens to them in groups that is therapeutic . . . but he is rather mystical about what this is.

Dr A has a similarly mystical feeling about the community as a whole, but as far as his handling of individual patients, he is more cautious than Dr B, preferring to see them individually rather than in groups where there are serious problems.

Dr B tends to underestimate the difficulties raised by using permissive-democratic methods, while Dr A overestimates them. Dr B says they're not real issues, and that patients' groups could cope. He tends to put their disagreements in terms of Dr A's personality, and he plays the demagogue with patients and some junior staff. Actually Dr A, being senior, has more responsibility and has to be more careful than Dr B.

Each of the doctors has a lot of leeway to work as he sees fit here. This is fine in some ways, but it has some disadvantages. For one thing it's important for a man to be a 'good community person' whether or not he's a good psychiatrist. It's difficult to know if a person is a good psychiatrist or not—because this kind of treatment isn't like the physical treatments or even psychoanalysis. They have more definite ideas about what constitutes treatment, and specific rationales. Things here have many conceptions and rationales. Ideas are drawn from psychosomatic medicine, psychoanalysis, sociology and so on. What each doctor does in his groups is up to him. Each must also adjust himself to the larger Unit situation without too much pain or trouble. Some do this by simply keeping their mouths shut except in their own groups. Others set up small empires of their own in rivalry with the main part of the Unit. Some, who are more vulnerable, suffer or leave.

There are also rewards in the interpersonal relations approach—coming to work in the morning, being part of groups—happy to see the people and so on. And the system of counterlocking groups, public performance, and so on does make for some checks on a doctor's performance built into the system. But, they don't get the specific rewards of being a good doctor—doing a competent professional job. . . . Competence in any good hospital is shown through studying dynamics, presenting analyses in case conferences, producing results. At the Unit, this tends to be very minor really—and they tend to stress the group's power so much that even if a doctor does do well it's difficult to trace his efforts. Interpersonal relations are stressed far more.

A nurse described the differences in doctors' policies in the following terms:

Each doctor has a different idea. B just about lets a patient die before he'll let him stay in bed. E is bit more stern about it too. A and F will pop them into bed more easily. If you work in the ward and a patient wants to stay in bed, you'd be more likely to go along with them and order breakfast if it were A's patient than if it were B's, because you'd know that B would more than likely be around to get them up or would react against their getting special treatment. The patients compare notes on this.

The ambiguities of role prescriptions can, in some cases, lead to undesirable results, as we have indicated above in our table of possible types. An example of a doctor who was comparatively well trained technically, but who found the amorphousness of Unit methods personally distressing (type C in *Figure* 9) follows:

(Nurse speaking): Dr F was a good example of a doctor who could not adjust because he couldn't share his problems. As things got more difficult for him, he'd get more anxious and arrange more private interviews with his patients so that he could feel that he had the situation under control. He wrote up the most thorough and detailed notes of any of the doctors, but finally he couldn't stand it any more and left to work on the other side of the hospital where he could confine his work to the controlled doctor-patient situation.

In this case there is no indication that his therapeutic results were not of a high calibre by any standard, and Dr F was personally popular among both patients and staff. His own anxieties at the diffusion of authority and the lack of concise methodology were, however, too much for him to bear.

Our type B is illustrated only by isolated episodes. None of the doctors observed in the period under study typified the self-satisfied malpractitioner in any persisting way, though illustrations of this type of behaviour were occasionally observed.

The following comments made by doctors about the behaviour of their colleagues illustrate this.

'Dr A has a counter-transference problem with (pretty, young, female) patient X. Spending so much time with her in private interviews is not going to help her relationships in the Unit as a whole.

'Dr C is just rationalizing his own feelings of guilt and inadequacy when he says that it was good for the patient's treatment when he (Dr C) missed an appointment on the ground that the patient has to learn to take these frustrations so common in life outside.'

Only one doctor during the period under study exemplified the all-round negative (type D) reactions. He was a visitor, personally disliked by many of the staff, lacking in leadership qualities, and inept in psychotherapeutic modes of participation. He was never given autonomous control of a group, since the permanent staff did not feel confidence in him; he did not develop any good informal relationship with other staff members that would have acted to guide and stabilize him and to give him a nucleus of support in group discussions. He was considered too persistently 'odd', and an 'outsider' even by patients to be effective on technical grounds. As the staff came to express it: 'He never found a role for himself in the Unit.' He left prematurely and unhappily after some weeks of marginal participation.

If any single set of dilemmas can be designated as focal in stimulating the emergent patterns of performance in doctors' roles, it is probably the set arising from the area of authority-responsibility. In the doctor's role more than in any of the others, there is a marked discrepancy between the formal basis for authority and expectations with regard to responsibility on the one hand and the Unit's ideological tenets on the other. This discrepancy makes itself felt and must be dealt with in all the doctor's activities. His pattern of role performance hinges to a very great extent on how he resolves the dilemmas implied in this discrepancy.

STAFF NURSE

Another set of adjustment problems is exemplified in the staff nurse role. Like the social therapists, staff nurses are expected to be in regular close contact with patients. Yet, unlike the therapists, they are permanent, medically trained personnel. Their training, however, is less applicable to the Unit situation than to conventionally organized hospital wards. In the Unit they handle medicines and equipment and administer the nursing station. Their ward-interaction functions are largely taken over by the social therapists. The social therapists, however, are not (by informal arrangement within the Unit) in the usual nursing hierarchy subordinate to staff nurses. This creates a situation in which the staff nurse is responsible for some of the social therapists' functions, but has no authority over the person performing these functions. While the staff nurse is urged to participate in Unit groups on the same basis as everyone else, the weight of clerical and administrative work, and the necessity for maintaining a perpetual vigil in the nursing station, tend to contravene this participation.

A further element discouraging the participation of the staff nurses in therapeutic groups is that these nurses are considered too well trained and experienced to get the kind of didactic attention the new therapists get; yet they are less trained and experienced than members of the core staff. This yields the situation where they are felt by core staff to be too well trained to get special attention, but felt by themselves to be not well enough trained to participate authoritatively in group psychotherapy. Actually, the point is that their training is in a different field—that of physical medicine—which is a necessary but relatively peripheral service to the Unit treatments. From the rehabilitation point of view, staff nurses, unlike social therapists (whose ordinariness and femininity are stressed), are not part of people's regular social networks.[7]

In a report on the role of the staff nurse Hector Smith worked out the following analysis in collaboration with members of the research team:[8]

There are areas of potential conflict to which each staff nurse must adapt:

(a) Any staff nurse coming into the Unit must learn to work within a type of environment that is different from that for which he is trained. Discipline, orderliness, routine, set channels of procedures for communication are subordinated to the attempts to create a more receptive, patient-oriented milieu. This difference requires radical readjustment of expectations, habits, and values for the staff nurse.

(*b*) The Unit's emphasis on equalitarian participation in group discussions for most forms of decision-making necessitates the staff nurse giving up elements of authority that have helped him to cope with difficult interpersonal relations with patients. He must learn other methods of coping.

(*c*) The Unit's treatment ideology recognizes that many of its procedures as well as the nature of the work itself will at times have disturbing effects on staff members. The recommended way of dealing with this is to discuss one's *personal* problems as well as technical professional problems in staff groups. This procedure requires adjustment of personal norms.

(*d*) The Unit's methods aim to develop in patients a sense of responsibility by giving them decision-making powers over many elements of treatment and administration in the Unit. Every staff nurse must learn to reconcile his wish to go along with this general treatment policy with the fact that he is responsible for certain very rigidly prescribed ways of handling things like drugs and medical equipment—some of which are essentially not open to discussion.

(*e*) Though the Unit has set up an extraordinarily full programme of group participation, meetings, etc., and these allow opportunities for dealing with many of the difficult problems already mentioned, there are loopholes, odd corners and time periods when the functioning of group events is interrupted—e.g., by holidays, weekends, certain hours between early evening activity and full night-staff control, —when the staff nurse is the only staff member available, being tied as he is to the nursing station. In such situations he may:

(*i*) Be scapegoated for absent staff.
(*ii*) Be expected to substitute for them, e.g., by acting as doctor.
(*iii*) Be confronted with an interpersonal crisis with neither the group support nor the conventional authority.

(*f*) While he is more experienced than the social therapists, he has no direct authority over them in their performance of many ward activities that are customarily in the staff nurse's province—unless they themselves turn to him for assistance. This latter eventuality may have its difficulties too, since the social therapists may be anxious, dependent, or displacing their feelings from other staff members in ways similar to those of patients.

(*g*) Every staff nurse in an innovating centre like the Unit must learn to reconcile his needs to remain part of his own professional group (who may tend to see his current practices as unorthodox, queer, not up to standard) and his need to be accepted in the innovating group who require adjustment to their norms.

Various adjustments to these potential conflict areas in the Unit situation are possible. The following reactions have been actually observed:

(1) Self-depreciation, uncertainty and insecurity. Because the medical aspect of Unit treatment has assumed a relatively minor place in the treatment programme, the staff nurse may feel *personally* of little importance to the work of the Unit. This will be particularly likely to the extent that he is not temperamentally inclined to the new methods, or lacks skills at them which he would consider appropriate to the permanent staff status in the organization. He may have been very skilled at the modes of treatment in physically oriented psychiatry, but be inarticulate in the kinds of verbalizing skills required in psychotherapy.

(2) Inappropriate over-resentment at other staff members—e.g., the social therapists, who he may feel have taken away the 'cream', or most rewarding aspects of his role, leaving him mainly grinding routine or awkward situations. Doctors, for example, may turn to the therapists rather than to the staff nurses for reports on the patient's ward life. He may react negatively to the doctors themselves, whom he sees as the instigators of the difficulty and as persons who, while retaining power and mobility themselves, insist that he be 'democratic', though tied to the nursing station and faced with difficult situations.

(3) Excessive passivity—feeling that the best way to safeguard one's position in the conflict situations is to do nothing. In fact, withholding of information or action may be one of the more effective ways of expressing the kinds of resentment mentioned above. The *routine* aspects of the role may be elevated to more than necessary importance, providing a kind of legitimate shelter.

(4) Recourse to patient groups. A staff nurse may identify himself with the patients and, in seeking their goodwill, allow himself to be

manipulated into positions that are perhaps satisfying to himself and to the patients in the short run, but incorrect therapeutically. He might find himself eventually in a position from which it is difficult to extricate himself. It is so easy to give a patient what he asks for. One feels needed, and is flattered by the patient's grateful thanks and assertion that you are the only staff member who really understands him. One may thus come to really feel part of the Unit and a useful member. When and if he perceives that the patient has been using him, he may be struck all the harder by the feeling of his inability to deal with patients and Unit situations. His reactions may take the form of despondency, or anger with the staff for not making him aware of the pitfalls that lay in the way.

(5) Recourse to external colleague groups. If a staff nurse feels left out, misunderstood, inadequate, or otherwise under stress, he may take the defensive course of beginning to associate with his colleagues external to the Unit to a degree that harms his Unit participation. He may genuinely resonate to their sentiments that the innovating Unit is on the wrong track, and seek by inappropriately identifying himself with them to bolster his self-respect. This could be maladaptive from the Unit's viewpoint, both through increasing external difficulties and through taking the staff nurse off his post for extended periods of time while he visits colleagues in other parts of the hospital on quasi-legitimate errands.

(6) Displacements. The staff nurse may displace expressions of affect in such a way as to be harmful. For example, if he has had to handle a series of difficult patients, and had little success in diverting their aggression into discussion group channels, he may explode at the next patient who comes to the nursing station, stating that he will *not* be used as an object of the patient's aggression. It might happen that this particular patient is very frightened of the idea of his being aggressive, and the error in timing may have harmful effects.

Such problems of recognizing and handling one's own feelings are routine among psychotherapists—but staff nurses are in a sort of in-between position where they often do not have the degree of training (including psychoanalysis) that more senior medical staff may have, *nor* are they sufficiently untrained to warrant the special supportive measures taken for the social therapists. Staff meetings are designed to handle such problems of the permanent trained staff, but they may not adequately do so, particularly in periods of heavy staff agenda, which is precisely when the staff nurse, too, is likely to be in trouble. Also, pride may keep a staff nurse from freely communicating his difficulties to the staff at large.

The staff nurses, thus, show many problems similar to those illustrated in the dilemmas and emergent patterns in doctors' roles. They also have certain distinctive features that result partly from the differences in dilemmas due to their different status, and partly from the differences in patterns of resolution open to them in this status. While the doctors, like the staff nurses, have been medically trained and must assimilate the radical discontinuities in cultural conditioning implied in entering the Unit, they have more control over the actual form their new environment will take. Unlike the doctors, the staff nurses cannot easily dispose of problems through authoritative action, nor can they regulate their presence or absence in the Unit to quite the same extent as doctors. They must thus find their most viable modes of resolution within the situation. Those observed included the adoption of a rather passive mode of behaviour, meticulous attention to administrative details like record keeping, and shifting primary affectual involvement outside the Unit itself.

SOCIAL THERAPISTS

The role of social therapist reflects, in its characteristic dilemmas and patterns of resolution, the problems raised by the ambiguities between treatment and rehabilitation aims.

The social therapists are chosen for their lack of formal training and for their youth. The lack of training is thought to be valuable in that it assures the staff that they will not have any preconceived ideas about treatment that derive from the traditional system and are therefore likely to be antithetical to those of the Unit. Their youth is thought valuable in making them more flexible and adaptive in the new situation and in giving the Unit a constantly refreshed stream of vigorous and optimistic participants. Other characteristics of the social therapists and the staff's rationales have already been mentioned.

From the social therapist's earliest exposure to the Unit, the ambiguities as to treatment and rehabilitation aims make themselves felt most acutely in her attempts to develop a suitable pattern of role performance. The ambiguity is expressed in the instructions given to the therapists on arrival—a paper containing both practical instructions and general, theoretical orientations to guide action:

The role of each individual therapist depends largely on the personality of the therapist concerned. The therapist should, however, always try to keep in mind that her contact with the patients has a therapeutic purpose and is part of treatment, even when the contact appears to be largely a social one.[9]

As one therapist put it, 'Dr B tells us to be ourselves; Dr A tells us to be therapeutic. Sometimes these two things don't go together.'

In a study of the social therapist's role, Marcella Davis[10] distinguished two main types of early anxiety corresponding to the two elements in the basic role ambiguity: about herself in the role and about the treatment methods.

1. The early anxieties about self-in-role included the following:

What am I expected to do? How should I start to talk? What should my attitude be? Will I ever be able to meet patients on an equal level? Will I ever be able to work with patients who are disturbed? What do I do if I am physically attacked by a patient?

Will I be able to do what is expected? Would I ever be able to talk with the patient as a social therapist (therapeutically)? How should I begin to relate to the doctors? How do you tell what your place is here?

Do I have the qualifications for the role? Am I too young; is this job only for older people? Will I ever be able to take all that talking? I feel too insecure ever to say how insecure I really am. There seems to be something in me that makes it difficult to contact patients.

2. The early anxieties about Unit therapeutic methods included the following:

Do the doctors know the answers to the patients' problems? I was shocked when the doctor said, 'I don't know what to do for this patient.'

Is it ethical to tell a patient in front of everyone that he is a homosexual?

Is it true that everyone has the same kind of psychiatric problems? I was worried about being told that we are all sick together.

Can it be true that it helps things to allow so much tension to develop? I feel upset when there is so much emotional tension in the groups.

Can it be true that the best thing is to let everyone say just what they feel? This seems too impulsive. People aren't aware of what they're doing and it goes on in the name of therapy.

Mrs Davis noted that social therapists went through three stages in resolving their anxieties in these matters and adjusting to their position in the Unit:

1. In the first stage, the therapist attempts to see herself in her role as a natural, normal person reacting spontaneously to people and situations. This line of thinking is encouraged by that element of the Unit senior staff's attitudes that stress the rehabilitative rationale that therapists are particularly valuable by simply being themselves—nice, ordinary persons who accept the patients despite their problems.

The following kinds of things were said by therapists to describe their images of themselves in the earliest stages of adapting to the therapist's role:

'I saw myself as (trying to be) natural with the patients.'
'(My job was) to cheer the place up.'
'(Our job is) to be normal people circulating among sick people.'
'To be myself.'

2. At some point in her exposure to the role, usually after about a month, there is a modification of this image. The therapist becomes more concerned with that aspect of her role that makes her an intermediary between the patients and the larger system, particularly the staff:

'To be on the ward as an object for the patients to tell problems to and to communicate relevant things to the staff.'

'To help patients to have enough confidence in other patients and staff for them to come into treatment and participate in different activities.'

'Ideally we are supposed to be the communicants between the doctor and the patients.'

3. In the third stage the therapists' image of their role, in ideal form, is a more sophisticated one, involving the desirability of establishing a specific kind of warm, interpersonal relationship with the patients:

'To be a person, to be able to be a woman, to be able to give and come near to the patients, and to do this without being aware (self-conscious) of what you are doing.'

'To understand and relate to patients in a warm way.'

Mrs Davis notes that superficial resemblances between first and third stages can be misleading. The third stage involves, indeed, the ideal of a warm and natural kind of relationship. However, it is within the framework of an awareness of the potentialities, limits, and pitfalls of the social therapist's role. In our terms, the social therapists in this stage work out ways of directly implementing the rehabilitative aims of helping patients to function in ordinary relationship ('be yourself') while also orienting their activities to assist with the treatment aims ('be therapeutic') that the larger Unit organization entertains.

The process of absorption of the social therapist through the phases described tends to be a potentially difficult one, and a great deal of attention is given in staff meetings and tutorials to the question of how they may be assisted in the transitions, so that the linked goals of their personal well-being and their adequate role performance may be jointly promoted.

Elsie Nokes, in another study of the therapists' role,[11] found that role conflicts tended to arise throughout the therapist's career in four different aspects of the role:

1. In relationships with the patients (ordinary).
2. In patient relationships with strong transference elements.
3. In relationships with strong counter-transference elements.
4. In group participation, as against individual relationships.

Mrs Nokes, like Mrs Davis, noted that the social therapist is soon disabused of her initial impression that naturalness and spontaneity are enough. While her own contacts with patients are more within the framework of 'ordinary' types of activities than those of other staff members, she must beware of some kinds of 'special' relationships and entanglements that may arise. The group allegiance problem involves the therapist's clarification in her own and others' minds that she is expected to 'feed back' information to the doctors as part of her role obligations and that this is not to be seen as betrayal of an intimacy (e.g., being an 'informer' or a 'stool pigeon').

In keeping with the injunction to be 'natural', the therapist might expect to relate to people in a way that is relaxed and willing to give and receive information of a personal nature; on the other hand, as a therapist, she is expected to be circumspect (i.e., cautious in giving personal details, joking too much, giving personal advice), to select information of therapeutic significance and to relay it, and to beware of possible sexual involvements.

The problem of interpersonal distance is a constant one for therapists —whether or not to accept gifts, dates, or pleas for special help. In the layman's terms of reference, ordinary kindness or protectiveness may be considered anti-therapeutic in the Unit because it keeps patients from facing 'reality' and recognizing their psychopathology.

While the staff considers one of the values of the social therapist to be her feminine attractiveness, they also suggest that she look at strongly positive or negative feelings towards herself on the part of patients in terms of transference components rather than as the 'real coin' of a love relationship. If she allows herself to encourage 'special relationships', or to respond too personally, she learns that she can get into a great deal of trouble. Some therapists find it onerous to be constantly a 'good object' —muting reactions of anger or depression and of love in the forms it might take in ordinary relationships.

In their studies, Mrs Nokes and Mrs Davis distinguish three elements in the situation that contribute to an adaptive resolution of the anxieties and dilemmas of the therapist's role:

1. *The uniform.* In keeping with the general principles of informality and status blurring of Unit ideology, the doctors and other core staff wear no uniform. The social therapists, however, wear a simple overall smock. This represents a compromise that has adaptive value for them. With regard to the use of this uniform, Mrs Davis has noted several kinds of characteristic statements made by therapists about how the uniform assists in adjustment:

It is practical ('keeps clothing clean').
It defines ('helps you to play the role of social therapist').
It depersonalizes ('patients relate to a uniform and what it stands for rather than the person').
It levels ('keeps us all looking alike and prevents competition in clothing').
It identifies ('from the patients' point of view, it is the only distinction we have from the female patients').

It clarifies ('makes it clear to you and the patient that you are the social therapist and he is the patient. It separates you from the patients').

It desexualizes ('if we were in the role of a woman, staff anxiety would be high.)'

It protects ('helps the therapist to retreat behind').

2. *'Official' groups.* The formal groups in which therapists can deal with their anxieties in adjusting to their roles include staff meetings, therapists' tutorials, and a special therapists' tutorial with one of the doctors who has made it available for supportive group therapy. Each of these groups has teaching functions as well as therapeutic functions in assisting the therapists' adjustment to the Unit. They also differ among themselves in the type of relationship offered. Tutorials run by junior staff, for example, tend to have more easy interchange of information in them than those run by senior staff. The tutorial run by the director is never fully freed of the underlying awareness that he has more power over the social therapists' occupational careers than do other staff members. The tutorial with Sister tends to be seen as an opportunity for a relationship with a warm mother figure and is specially helpful to those who are responsive to this.

3. *Informal relationships.* The informal contacts include spontaneous group discussions among the therapists themselves, individual contacts with permanent staff members, relationships with patients, and activities outside the Unit. The degree to which the therapists as a group are mutually supportive varies. There are always some special friendships in the group. Sometimes there are conspicuous enmities and rivalries. The overall *esprit de corps* varies greatly. The relationships among the therapists vary with their own internal composition, but also with the kinds of relationships other staff members make with them. Different kinds of relationships have different implications for the therapists as a group. A therapist's friendship with a senior nurse or a secretary or an instructor might not entail special ramifications among the therapists' group. However, when a bachelor doctor shows a special interest in one or another of the girls, rivalries are apt to develop. Relationships with the patients are often supportive for therapists, even within the bounds allowed in avoiding transference relationships and other emotional

entanglements. The amount of support the social therapist derives from contacts outside the Unit varies greatly.

With regard to their interstitial position between staff and patients, one pitfall occurs if a therapist becomes attached to a patient and fears the consequences of bringing his problem up in a group discussion. Each individual therapist works out her own way of handling such situations to save her from difficulties in her various relationships. She may keep quiet about him even if she knows it is inappropriate to do so, according to Unit ideology. She may, in such a case, be less afraid of being hurt herself by members of the permanent staff, than that the patient with whom she is involved would be hurt. If either the therapist or the patient sees the permanent staff as destructive, she may protect the patient or protect herself from his anger by not relaying information on him to the staff. She knows that this is wrong according to Unit ideology, but she has various ways of rationalizing it: (*i*) she may create a counter-ideology of her own, where she believes that a case like this should not be handled that way, or (*ii*) she may introduce a qualification to the dominant ideology. For example, the dominant ideology is all right in general but this particular patient is not ready yet; there is a timing problem rather than a complete rejection of the ideology. Or another device is to bring up a 'smokescreen problem'— bringing up someone or something else to protect the real object of concern.

'Finding one's own role in the Unit', then, tends to mean for social therapists finding a way to reconcile the twin directives of 'Be natural', and 'Be therapeutic'; and to balance the demands made by the staff with those made by the patients. As one therapist put it, 'the role of social therapist is to please everyone from the cook to the medical superintendent'. In learning to do this she is helped by being given a special status that is granted a good deal of recognition by both staff and patients as being important in the whole enterprise (and symbolized in the therapist's uniform); and she is provided with groups of various kinds to learn what is going on and to 'ventilate' her feelings and difficulties. On the other hand, the special recognition may prove a problem in that being idealized sets standards and prohibitions that are sometimes onerous; the group sessions may provide problems about how to handle information in complex interpersonal fields where loyalties to patients as persons according to the norms of 'ordinariness' may conflict with loyalties to staff according to the norms of the therapeutic ideology.

Each therapist works out her own way of handling all these problems in such a way as to minimize conflict and discomfort. In general, though groups of therapists vary widely in this regard, they tend to be comparatively passive and non-communicative verbally in groups where staff and patients are involved together—despite all efforts to make them talk more. This can be understood in the light of the field of forces in which they are involved, and their own characteristics as part of no authoritative professional group, and having no external stabilizing relationships. If a therapist raises a problem, it may be taken to be a reflection of her own personal problems, and she has few ways of gauging this during her stay in the Unit because therapists are usually heavily involved in the Unit's life. The forces making for equilibrium in the Unit often seem so delicately balanced, that many social therapists seem to feel it best not to interfere—especially given their lack of training and their transiency.

SUMMARY

In general, then, it may be said that the system of roles that is at the core of the Unit's treatment instrument (i.e., its social structure), is an emergent system, not entirely like the 'as if' system of the Unit's ideology, nor like the conventional system prescribed by the National Health Acts. It is not an equalitarian group living together and sharing the work task, the power and responsibility and the perquisites of the organization, with each person contributing in the way best suited to him as an individual; nor is it the formal specialized segmented and hierarchical organization prescribed in the statutes. It is, rather, a social system made up of relatively tightly-knit and interconnected subgroupings, each of which may contain individuals who, though of different professions, may perform one another's functions to some extent interchangeably (as with the 'core' staff), or who have similar kinds of functions from the treatment/rehabilitation point of view (ancillary-permanent staff).

Each individual who comes to the Unit enters in one of the formal roles, and must work out within the limits available to him in the formal system some 'blend' of behaviour consistent in some ways with the ideological principles of the Unit, and in some ways with the prescriptions of the larger hospital system.

Usually this process of socialization of new staff members to the Unit is preceded by an anticipatory stage in which both the novice and those who are to receive him into the Unit develop certain expectations that will contribute to the factors affecting the pattern with which he eventually emerges. Because the Unit is so different both from the kinds of professional settings from which the trained staff come, and from the kinds of 'ordinary life' settings from which the untrained staff come, there is usually a period of 'culture shock' in which the discontinuities of entry into the Unit must be absorbed by the individual.

Once in, the novice experiences certain additional stresses built into the Unit system, but also enjoys certain sources of support and reward. In working out patterns that are on the one hand personally rewarding and on the other hand acceptable to others in the Unit, members of different roles have somewhat different, though overlapping, problems, and may develop patterns of role performance that have different therapeutic implications.

The primary problem facing doctors, for example, is that of reconciling the formal medical system of authority with that advocated by the Unit. This is difficult not only because of their long training and conditioning in the authoritative system, but because of the fact that they retain formal responsibility for what goes on in the Unit. Furthermore, in many situations it seems to them more therapeutic to be authoritative. If larger therapeutic goals rather than Unit ideology are to remain paramount, 'non-U' behaviour is often called for. Different doctors work out different ways of meeting these problems, and some of them have been described above.

For staff nurses, illustrating the ancillary permanent staff group, the problem is somewhat different. They have many features in common with the doctors in that they are formally trained in the medical way, and retain certain formal responsibilities that cannot, essentially, be passed around democratically. On the other hand, they do not have the power of the doctors to control the flow of events—with the negative implication that they must face the dilemmas implied in the authority-responsibility conflict at a more immediate interactional level. Since they retain only partial responsibility—i.e., for medicines, etc.—and not for the administration of the treatments as a whole, the staff nurses can work out protective adjustments in enclaves within the system rather than, like the doctors, affecting the entire system by the particular resolutions they choose. Some of these adjustments have been described.

The social therapists provide illustrations of the problem of potential conflict between treatment and rehabilitation aims *par excellence*. As ordinary nice girls with whom patients may form warm trusting relationships they seem to implement rehabilitation aims—following through the ideal of revising the traditional environment in the hospital. According to this they are to be 'natural', and to relate to patients as they would to people of these types in the outside world, only perhaps with more kindness and sympathetic tolerance than is the general norm. On the other hand, to the extent that they are seen as agents of the treatment régime—drawing communications that are of a transference nature, they run into complexities in their relationships with which they are not equipped technically to deal. By *not* responding directly to patients' gestures of hate, fear, love, and so on, but merely drawing these communications into group contexts where they can be dealt with, they are implementing treatment, but contravening their 'natural' modes of relating. Being natural implies responding spontaneously in a variety of ways from extreme negative rejection or retaliation (which goes against permissiveness) through extreme positive involvement (which goes against communalism). In such cases, the emotional involvements are to be seen as 'transference', a concept that is barely graspable intellectually during the short period of the therapists' residence in the Unit, and often very difficult to translate into a course of action that will satisfy the various forces in their interpersonal fields. How to deal with the fact of loving a patient, feeling a doctor is not doing his best to help him, being obliged to bring up what the patient says in public group discussions, and to relate to all patients without special favouritism—these and comparable problems are the stuff of social therapists' role dilemmas. We have mentioned some of the ways in which they tend to cope with them, and the patterns of role performance that emerge in the Unit.

It must be noted here that the patterns of role performance described as relatively stabilized patterns forming an overall social structure, are patterns that are discernible in the flux of Unit life. They do not exist simultaneously neatly arranged with reference to one another in any static crystallized sense. They are, rather, in constant flux, forming ever-changing kaleidoscopic arrangements in response to a number of recurrent forces in the situation. Some of these will be discussed in the next chapter.

NOTES AND REFERENCES

1. Jones, Maxwell, and Rapoport, Robert N.: 'Administrative and social psychiatry.' *Lancet*, **2**: 386–8, 1955.
2. Merton, Robert: 'The role set: problems in sociological theory.' *Brit. J. Sociol.*, **8**: 106–20, 1957.
3. Jones, Maxwell: 'The role of the social therapist' (mimeo).
4. Skellern, Eileen: 'A therapeutic community.' *Nurs. Times.*, April–June, 1955, p. 9.
5. Parker, Seymour: 'The doctor and patient roles in a therapeutic community.' *Psychiat. Quart. Supplements*, **31**: 112–28, 1957.
6. Jones, Maxwell, and Rapoport, Robert N.: 'The absorption of new doctors into a therapeutic community' in Greenblatt, M.; Levinson, D. J.; and Williams, R. N.: *The Patient and the Mental Hospital*. Glencoe, Ill., The Free Press, 1957.
7. To some extent this first, though not the second, source of difficulty applies to instructors and other permanent ancillary staff members.
8. Smith, Hector: 'Some problems in changing psychiatric nursing roles.' Unpublished ms.
9. Jones, Maxwell: 'The role of the social therapist' (mimeo).
10. Davis, Marcella: unpublished paper on the role of the social therapist.
11. Nokes, Elsie: unpublished paper on the role of the social therapist.

CHAPTER 6

Selected Social Processes

The foregoing description of the Unit's social structure gives only part of the material necessary for understanding the relevance of social factors for treatment in the Unit. To use a well-worn metaphor, we have presented a description of the skeleton and anatomy of the creature, but we still lack important information on its physiological processes if we are to understand how it actually works.

In the Unit, as in any social system, there are a number of key processes, deriving from the structure and composition of the organization that give it its unique quality. In this chapter we shall consider four processes which, while observed in the unique context of the Unit, are analysed in terms of their generic relevance to therapeutic community functioning. One of the processes, that of *oscillation* in the state of social organization,[1] we shall treat as a global process affecting Unit functioning pervasively. The other three processes—the staff's variation in usage of the crucial designation 'constructive' vs. 'destructive' for the behaviour of Unit participants, the formation of cliques with substructures within the Unit, and the tendency of individuals to 'pair-off' with other individuals—are all analysed in the context of the overall oscillatory process. The process of oscillation is not one that is deliberately induced by the staff of the Unit, indeed, it is one that functioned out of explicit awareness of the Unit's participants prior to the research. It is abstracted through observations of repetitive regularities in the *variable* handling of specific events. Hypothetically, this process is one of social control, according to which members of the social system behave differently at different times, unselfconsciously, to act for the preservation of the social system. In a system like that of the Unit, where disruptive forces, are actively at work and the overall state of organization is highly labile, one finds a great range of variation in behaviour necessary to equilibrate the overall system. The variations are manifested in the way the staff behave to the patients, the way the patients react to the staff's behaviour, the extent to which the ideological themes are put into practice, and, ultimately, the patients' fate in treatment and rehabilitation.

At different phases of the oscillatory process, any given event may be perceived differently and different courses of action may be prescribed. To embrace this heterogeneity within a single conceptual framework, the staff distinguish abstractly between 'constructive' and 'destructive' participation—the former putatively having therapeutic implications, the latter the reverse. While the use of these terms may help to decide or explain choices made among alternative courses of action, they seem to be used in a variable way, but with sufficient regularity of variation to be termed a social process. We shall analyse the processes of clique formation and 'pairing off', two types of occurrence that have been observed to have different implications at different points in the oscillatory process. In doing so we shall again indicate some of the complexities and pitfalls in the usage of the terms 'constructive' and 'destructive'. Our focus throughout will remain the larger implications for patients' treatment and rehabilitation.

OSCILLATIONS IN THE STATE OF SOCIAL ORGANIZATION

The concept of social organization has to do with the inter-relatedness of persons representing parts of a social system at a given time. A state of perfect organization, only hypothetical in any social system, would exist when every participant performed his social role in such a way as consistently to fulfil the expectations of all the others. In this equilibrium state, the system would function harmoniously and would efficiently attain the goals and values according to which it was organized. Complete disorganization, on the other hand, would mean the termination of the social system through the death of its members, their absorption into other social systems, the cessation of their motivation, or other defections of behaviour crucial to the survival of the system.

Both poles of the continuum may be conceived of as extremes between which actual social systems function. Particular social systems vary in the degree to which they maintain a stable equilibrium between these poles or fluctuate in their state of organization. An organization like the Unit, with its many socially disruptive patients, its permissive ideology, and its interlocking social groups, seems to foster an unusual magnitude and variety of fluctuations in the overall state of social organization.

The Unit's 'emotional climate' varies very greatly from time to time. At the community meeting one morning, a query about a relatively routine and apparently innocuous topic such as why a patient did not go to his workshop might be taken as an attack and be dealt with not only by the patient but also by the group defensively, by counter-attack, withdrawal, or an emotional display. On another morning, what would appear to be a far more disturbing topic—e.g., murder or incest—might be discussed calmly and rationally by all who had something to contribute to the understanding of the problem. The impression that the differences cannot be explained in terms of the disturbance-value of the content is further sustained on observing that similar problems—e.g., the use of a ward kitchen—are differently handled on different occasions. Furthermore, it is noted that there are wide variations in attendance at groups, in quantity and quality of participation in activities, and so on. Even more striking is the observation that there is a wide range of variation in the degree to which the staff put Unit ideology into practice. On some occasions a given situation is handled, by any criteria, more democratically, permissively, communally, and realistically than a similar situation on other occasions.

Just as it proves fruitless to attempt to find a comprehensive explanation for these variations in terms of any single factor (such as content of the discussion or activity), so it is fruitless to demonstrate their association with an all-embracing process. Individuals or small groups within the Unit relate to one another in many ways. Different kinds of real and imaginary alignment cut across the social structure, and these relationships change somewhat, independently of the other processes in the organization. However, it may be useful for us to think of a type of process called *oscillation*. By this we mean the process of fluctuation in the state of social organization between the two poles of perfect equilibrium and disintegration. This process may occur in a social subsystem of any magnitude, from the smallest (relationship between two individuals) to the largest (the total Unit social organization).[2] We shall focus here on the cyclical processes which involve the Unit as a whole. The details and arrangements of phenomena in the process are hypothetical, but have partial empirical support.

Oscillations may be conceived as varying around the basic pattern represented in *Figure* 10.

FIGURE 10 *OSCILLATORY PATTERN*

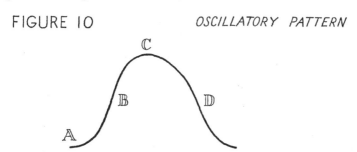

Phase A. This is the point of relatively greatest equilibrium and integration. The members of the organization are performing their social roles most in accord with the expectations of others. Intra-personal tensions and environmental stimulations of interpersonal tensions are at a minimum. Behaviour tends to be consistent with ideals. It does not arouse anxiety for staff to be permissive, since the amount of socially deviant behaviour occurring is small and is easily handled within the treatment framework. Group decisions are likely to be taken in the best interests of the social system as a whole, so that staff need not be apprehensive about having diffused responsibility for Unit affairs through its entire population. Consensus is relatively easy to reach, and the social climate is a relaxed one that fosters trust.

In this phase the interests of treatment and those of rehabilitation seem to come closest together. Since all the patterns of behaviour described for this phase in the Unit are taken to be indicative of a good general capacity for social adjustment, those patients who have consistently shown socially integrative behaviour are encouraged to resume ordinary social roles outside the Unit.

Phase B. As 'constructive' patients are discharged and replaced by new patients who bring with them predispositions to disrupt their interpersonal contacts, the potential for disorganization mounts. Patients are permitted to act out, in keeping with Unit ideals, and interpersonal tensions begin to mount. The new patients are not the only ones who contribute to these tensions. Sometimes older patients who have come through Phase A have interpreted the relative inactivity of the staff as neglect or rejection, and engage in deviant behaviour in an effort to gain attention. Interpersonal tensions generated around any particular focus, e.g., a ward, tend to ramify into the workshops, socials, and other groups. The interlocking group structure which implemented therapeutic communications now operates to diffuse tension. As personal anxieties intensify, defensiveness, aggression, and withdrawal mount, trust and constructive communication decline, and the fulfilment of social role expectations is impaired. Attendance at groups falls off, participation becomes defective, communications through the regular channels are inhibited through fear and distrust. This last blockage cuts down the flow of spontaneous information on which the staff depend for their own feeling of security about the diffusion of responsibility among the Unit community. Indeed, the problems increasingly exceed patients' ability to deal with them, and their competence becomes decreasingly matched to the responsibility informally delegated to them.

New patients are not as effectively absorbed or welcomed by the old ones, who have become sceptical of the value of Unit treatment and concerned with their own personal problems. Patients who tend to withdraw under stress isolate themselves, sometimes leaving the Unit altogether by taking their own discharges. Even some of the patients whose problems do not centre on authority relations are likely to resent the staff's failure to intervene decisively to solve interpersonal problems. Those patients who had been staunch upholders of Unit ideology become substitute targets for the aggressiveness of others who are hostile towards the staff. The patients who symbolize staff members among fellow-patients are more vulnerable hate-objects onto whom aggression against the staff can be displaced. Prestige among the patients is gained increasingly through demonstrating 'anti-Unit' values—defiance, symptomatic acting out (drinking, taking drugs, fighting, etc.). Patients who communicate openly or take staff-like attitudes in meetings are negatively sanctioned. Staff members are seen as 'snoopers', 'Gestapo', 'incompetent', 'exploiting', 'hypocritical', or 'callous'.

In this phase patients tend increasingly to see adjustment to society as undesirable and those promoting it as loathsome. According to the new values asserting themselves in the crisis, individuals see social adjustment as antithetical to personal happiness. They discredit staff assertions that personal rewards may more dependably flow from minimal social conformity and that this does not necessarily imply the compromise of individual integrity. Some feel that the Unit, which they trusted, is failing them. Patients tend, now, to see the aims of treatment and rehabilitation as either incompatible with one another or unacceptable.

Phase C. The crescendo of tension has mounted to such a pitch that a turning-point must be reached if the health of individuals is to be safeguarded and the perpetuation of the institution assured. Some characteristic turning-points are:

Complaints from outside may threaten the existence of the Unit—from local citizens about housebreaking, from the local police about public indecencies, from the larger hospital system about disturbance to other patients or damage to hospital property.

Internally, the threat of disintegration, personal and social, may reach alarming proportions. A patient may attempt suicide, another may show intensified psychotic symptoms, meetings become so poorly attended and so unproductive as to cause staff alarm, disturbances in the wards at night place severe strain on the night staff.

At this stage there is a breakdown of effectiveness of Unit themes and a necessity to take steps to re-establish an equilibrium. The system tends now more easily to expel extreme deviants in order to bring the situation under control. Staff may 'certify' a patient, sending him to a mental hospital for his own protection (if he is suicidal) or to safeguard others (if his behaviour threatens to become uncontrollable). The director may insist on the discharge of patients whose behaviour is disturbing the external authorities or the local community. The 'pruning' process becomes more than usually active. Staff take steps to discharge 'dead wood', 'untreatables', and others defined as 'too ill' to be helped by Unit methods, too unmotivated to receive treatment really to participate, or too disruptive during a phase of disequilibrium to be tolerated in the interests of the community as a whole or of other patients who might benefit if relieved of pathogenic influences.

At other periods the staff would seek positive sanctions from the entire Unit before performing such authoritative acts. At points of external threat or internal disintegration, it becomes increasingly difficult to count on patients' willingness or stability to assume responsibility for the action deemed appropriate by those with formal responsibility; and it becomes increasingly difficult and time-consuming to reach consensus in discussions. When the staff perceive threats as sufficiently severe to warrant action regardless of internal sanctions, they act authoritatively. In this sense they evoke their 'latent' or 'submerged' authority, formally vested in them by the hospital system but more or less obscured in the ordinary functioning of the Unit according to its ideals of equalitarian democracy.

The trend may also be reversed without authoritative action by the staff if there is an unusual display of leadership by patients who succeed in mustering courage and support even in the face of severe opposition; through timely and astute interpretations by staff members or by constructive patients; or by more active efforts of staff members to absorb anti-social patients into the Unit life through non-authoritative, informal contacts.[3]

It is during this phase that the staff differentiate most between treatment and rehabilitation. Patients who are 'too sick' for the Unit are either discharged or sent to mental hospitals for other forms of treatment. Even some of those kept within the Unit are seen as needing more expert attention. The view that fitting in to the Unit régime is rehabilitative is less relevant, because the régime is clearly disordered and in need of social reorganization. Metaphorically, the 'treatment instrument' needs repairing. In the interim, individual patients require attention *as individuals* towards restoring their personal capacities for social participation.

Phase D, the reorganizing phase, gains momentum as reparative forces come into play. The discharge of disruptive patients in itself alleviates some interpersonal tension. Some of the remaining patients who identify with those sent to mental hospitals become less resistant to treatment if they see this fate impending for themselves. Others, feeling guilty that they have failed in their responsibility as informal therapists, or because they have contributed to the precipitation of disturbances so vividly experienced, feel a strong wish to 'repair' the damage.

The staff, too, sometimes feel guilt at their own departure from their ideological tenets, though they may have acted in accordance with another set of principles—e.g., those of medical ethics. Having acted autocratically and lowered their standards for communality and communications to deal with what they perceived as 'reality' problems for the social system as a whole, they now intensify their efforts to re-establish a social situation that will once again allow a greater degree of permissiveness, democracy, and communality. Ideally this is both assisted by and fosters 'reality testing' for individual patients who survive the upheaval. Staff are more active and didactic in group discussions. By removing the most severe social irritants and then reasserting the outlines of the social structure, they provide conditions for the reduction of tensions. 'Pro-Unit' leaders among the patients now feel secure to speak up. Consensus becomes easier to reach, Patients' atti-

FIGURE II   SOCIAL FUNCTIONING AND THE OSCILLATORY PROCESS

	Phase A	Phase B	Phase C	Phase D
Interpersonal Relations				
Role Performance	Conforming	Deviancy mounts	Deviancy peak	Strain to conformity
Social Organization	Integrated	Disorganiza-tion mounts	Disorganiz-ation peak	Reorganiza-tion
Mood	Relaxed	Tension mounts	Tension peak	Tension abatement
'Ideal-real' Relations				
'Permissiveness'	Free	Limits strained	Limits set, deviancy repressed	Restoring freedom
'Democracy'	Universal participation	Staff anxiety mounts	Emergence of staff 'latent authority'	Staff leadership
'Communalism'	Community	Cliques form	Fragmenta-tion	Surging together
'Reality-Confrontation'	Consensus	Disagreement mounts	Dissensus	Eagerness for agreement
Goal Attainment				
Treatment and Rehabilitation	Effective merging of treatment and rehab. goals and methods	Treatment and rehab. begin to deteriorate as goals*	Treatment and rehab. begin to split as means†	Re-synthesis of the two goals with the Unit as means

* E.g., patients feel that adjustment to the Unit or to society is difficult or not related to one another or undesirable.

† E.g., staff feel that some patients need treatment in a more sheltered environment than the Unit, and refer them to mental hospitals. Patients feel that the Unit is making them worse and leave.

tudes toward one another are more positive. Participation in the Unit's round of activities improves and becomes more constructive. The staff work to restore a social system in which rehabilitative as well as treatment aims will simultaneously be fostered by participation in the Unit. Phase A is once more regained.

The general picture is summarized in *Figure 11*.

EMPIRICAL SUPPORT FOR THE OSCILLATIONS HYPOTHESIS

The tendency towards recurrent oscillations in the overall state of social organization of the Unit has partial support from empirical studies done in the Unit. In his study of a ward, reported in the last chapter, Parker found sociometric support for the hypothesis that the discharge rate increased, particularly discharges among newcomers to the Unit, during the periods of mounting disorganization. We may thus regard a high discharge rate, particularly of 'prematurely' discharged[4] patients, as ordinarily indicating a condition of social disorganization.

We plot the incidence of 'premature discharges' by counting the percentage of discharges in each period that represents patients who stayed twenty-five days or less. This is done in *Figure 12*.

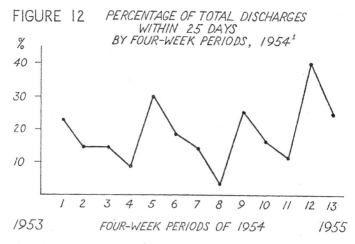

FIGURE 12 *PERCENTAGE OF TOTAL DISCHARGES WITHIN 25 DAYS BY FOUR-WEEK PERIODS, 1954[1]*

[1] From a study made by Peter Nokes of discharges in 1954. This curve tends to be positively associated with the curve indicating total discharges, and negatively with the mean length of stay curve. Premature discharges thus occur more frequently at points of high general discharge and thus tend to bring down the mean length of stay figure.

The high points of premature discharge occur at periods 5, 9 and 12.[5] Nokes, in his study of discharges over an entire year, found that one kind of disorganizing force affecting discharge rate is the arrival and departure of doctors.

Towards the end of period 3, two doctors left the Unit. There was a gap following their departure before the two new doctors arrived. Observations in the Unit and an analysis of each doctor's early discharge rates indicate that the peaks at period 5 and 9 are associated with the turnover of doctors—more specifically, the arrival of new doctors. The following seem to be some of the factors involved in the process:

Just before leaving, especially if no replacements are in sight, doctors tend to terminate the treatment of many of their patients in order to avoid the problems associated with change of doctor. This would account for the levelling off of the declining discharge rates in periods 2 and 3. Following the departure of a doctor, if he is not immediately replaced (and the two who left were not), there is a brief lull in discharges because the Unit's patient load is smaller to correspond with the smaller staff. Some of the departed doctor's patients who remain and are assigned to one of the Unit's other doctors are dissatisfied with the situation in their new group and leave—but others have their stays lengthened by 'beginning all over again'. When the new doctor arrives circumstances promote a rise in discharge rate. This is the period in which new doctors are learning about the methods of Unit treatment and patients who are newly arrived tend to feel that they have not got the best possible therapists. One new doctor arrived in period 3, and another in period 8. In period 12 we find that seven of the eight premature discharges are of patients assigned to the two new doctors, while the two more experienced doctors have only one such discharge. The discharge phenomena of periods 9 and 12 seem to exemplify a condition where overall disorganization flows from relatively localized discontinuities in particular doctor's groups.

Any institution functions with a certain amount of staff turnover as part of the normal processes of institutional life. The data here indicate that the coming and going of doctors has an especially important effect on the problem of holding new patients in the Unit.

In the year described, many of the peaks in the premature discharge rate seem associated with the turnover of key staff, although this indicator of social disorganization may be associated with a variety of factors.

Seasonal Factors

From general observations it would seem probable that seasonal variations are also at work producing variation in the discharges pattern. There seem to be tendencies towards increases in discharges in midwinter, early summer, and autumn. At these periods factors at work tend to stimulate patients to leave regardless of staff turnover. In autumn, for example, the harvesting season calls for temporary labour in the rural areas, with 'quick' money and no lasting obligations; the winter seems to affect the morale of some patients adversely, and hence their motivation to undertake therapy;[6] the summer seems to give some patients an urge for the 'great outdoors'. A more purely internal factor connected with seasonal differences is the fact that staff take their vacations more frequently in the summer. This accounts for a tendency for peaks at that point. In the winter, in addition to the weather, observations indicate that the Christmas holidays play an important part in the therapeutic careers of patients. It is at this time that patients feel especially left out and homeless, if they do not have homes to go to. To the extent that staff take holidays during this period, rather than creating a homelike Christmas atmosphere (a situation that varies from year to year), patients are likely to feel the impact of the season even more, and discharge rates are likely to rise. All these have been recorded as verbalized tendencies in the different seasons, but we have no data to indicate how powerful are the seasonal influences in and of themselves. In general these factors illustrate the influence of pervasive external factors on the internal organization of the Unit.

Patient Composition as a Factor

Patient composition seems to be another factor that affects the oscillatory process. Patients of some personality types become more disturbed under certain circumstances than others. When new patients of exceptionally disruptive or psychotic personality enter the social situation, certain others whose defences are hard-pressed may respond to their presence by becoming more disturbed. It seems that the Unit can accommodate only a certain proportion of each type of patient—e.g., manics, or homosexuals, or alcoholics, or aggressive psychopaths. When this balance is tipped by the addition of new patients, tension may mount precipitously from the anxiety of others. While this general 'balanced aquarium' concept is implicitly recognized by the staff at such points by 'pruning' patients in periods of disorganization, or in admitting new patients,[7] there is no explicit set of ideas and policies to regulate the patient composition. Intuitive actions are taken at points of stress or trouble to restore an equilibrium.

Social factors external to the Unit may also contribute to this picture. On the staff level, the kinds of external pressures described below by Parker influence internal Unit policy. On the patient level, aside from the seasonal occupational factors mentioned, it is important to note that family influences are operative in a variety of ways. Some data on this will be introduced in later chapters.

During another year (1956) reports from the nursing records were coded to count the sheer number of patients' complaints of various kinds, and these were classified and tabulated against crude discharge figures. We classified them into three categories:

(1) *physical complaints* (i.e., headaches, pains, medications administered for physical complaints, and so on).
(2) *psychological complaints* (restlessness, depression, hysterical outbursts, strange behaviour—for which no medication was prescribed).
(3) *social disturbances* (e.g., altercations, drunkenness, abusiveness etc.).

The greatest number of entries was in the first category, and the others followed in the order listed. Physical and psychological complaints seemed to be closely interrelated in their fluctuation, while social complaints were less associated with either of the other two. When plotted against crude discharge rates, it seems that in both years there was a tendency towards an obverse relationship between total complaints and total discharges at any particular period, with the latter lagging behind the former. This is indicated in *Figure 13*.

Hypothetically we have here a process in which disturbances mount to their peaks and discharges follow after a small intervening period of time. One gets the picture of a build-up of tensions manifested by and contributed to by these recorded incidents of disturbance, followed by a discharge of patients. This supports our observations on the tendency of disturbance to be associated with discharge in the oscillatory process.

It appears, then, that build-ups of collective disturbance occur periodically for a variety of reasons, and are followed by increased discharges. A high general discharge rate seems accompanied by a high discharge rate for short-term patients. The latter show (cf. below) the least improvement, so, high discharge can be said to be ordinarily related to therapeutic loss from the point of view of the Unit's aims. Aside from the factor of turnover of medical staff, there seem to be other determinants of tension build-ups. There is a seasonal factor. Early summer, early autumn, and mid-winter seem to be peak periods of discharge for a complex of reasons. Patient composition of the Unit at any given time and the influence of external relations of Unit members are other factors.

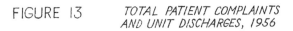

FIGURE 13   *TOTAL PATIENT COMPLAINTS AND UNIT DISCHARGES, 1956*

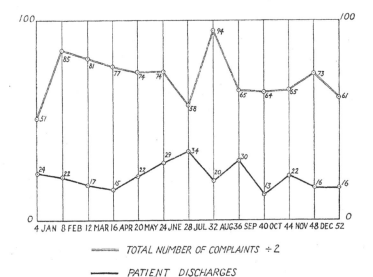

Thus, we have seen that Unit policy varies with circumstances, though its ideal goals and methods remain relatively constant. One way in which we can see these changes in policy is through the manner in which the terms 'constructive' and 'destructive' are applied to different kinds of behaviour at different points in the oscillatory process.

'CONSTRUCTIVE' AND 'DESTRUCTIVE' PARTICIPATION

It is clear that milieu therapy, as it is actually practised in the Unit, is a far more complex matter than simply establishing a social organization in which the staff and patients can practise permissiveness, democracy, communalism, and reality confrontation. Because of the composition, structure, and external relations of the Unit, numerous factors are constantly at play that bring about a social process of oscillations in the state of organization. At the disorganized end, the process is reversed because of measures taken for system preservation; at the organized end, the situation tends to be unstable because of the composition, aims, and policies of the system—to discharge 'improved' (adjusted) patients and take in new, disruptive ones who are then allowed to 'show' their problems for treatment. The idealized therapeutic milieu conditions, then, are in a constant state of 'becoming'. Any particular action tends, in accordance with this, to be evaluated in terms of how it contributes to the goals of the system—therapy of individuals, rehabilitation of patients to ordinary patterns of social intercourse, and system maintenance. Actions that contribute to these goals are termed 'constructive'; actions that contravene them are termed 'destructive'.

As we have noted, the Unit staff tend to value the merging of treatment and rehabilitation goals, and consequently they feel it unnecessary to distinguish between constructive and destructive participation contributing to one of these to the exclusion of the other. Similarly, since Unit ideology aims at making the Unit social system a microcosm of the 'real world' and, thus, adjustment to the Unit correlative with adjustment to life outside, they do not distinguish between measures that are constructive with reference to Unit system preservation and those that are necessary for social existence in the outside world. The argument of this section is that three senses of the terms 'constructive' and 'destructive' are conceptually distinguishable, and in different stages of the oscillatory process they are used with different meanings by the staff without explicit awareness. We contend that the effective utilization of social processes for therapy would be enhanced by making the distinctions explicit.

Assuming the use of the terms 'constructive' and 'destructive' in the intended or exerted sense (rather than in the sense of effective or impinging influence), we can illustrate the three different senses in which the terms are used, and then indicate how they are applied differently in the oscillatory phases.

First, where the referent is the individual, a patient may be said to be acting in a constructive way if his motivation is judged to be consistent with his treatment requirements. The expression 'coming into treatment' implies this kind of involvement. An individual, sincerely wishing to act in such a way as to contribute to his own therapy, does what is considered necessary for this in the Unit—participates constructively, e.g., by communicating his own feelings about what is going on, listening to the interpretations of others about the same events, and so on. A part of treatment is contributing to the treatment of others, so the terms also have an individual therapy referent when they refer to the particular patient's intentions with reference to another patient. A patient is 'constructive' in the sense of aiming to contribute to his own treatment if he treats another patient in the prescribed therapeutic way. Levels of conscious awareness complicate this situation. A patient who '*thinks* that he is trying to help another', but is judged by the staff to 'be *really* demonstrating his sadistic impulses' might be said to be consciously behaving in a constructive way, but demonstrating unconscious destructive motives. The terms are, of course, manipulated and abused by patients, who consciously 'beat up' other patients while stating to staff members who observe the aggressive behaviour that they were 'only trying to *help*' the other. The situation is even further complicated by the Unit's prevailing idea that 'You've got to get worse to get better', which implies that the feeling of discomfort is not a satisfactory criterion for establishing whether an action is constructive or destructive. Constructive actions can cause pain, and it may be destructive in terms of an individual's therapy to gratify him—e.g., by taking him out drinking if he is an alcoholic, or having a sexual affair with a patient whose problems involve promiscuity.

The second sense in which the terms constructive and destructive are used has reference to rehabilitation—fitting into socially acceptable forms of behaviour. Thus, a patient may be said to be constructive if he is punctual at group meetings, produces well in his workshop rather than wasting time and materials, gets on well with his peers and foreman rather than having discordant relationships with them.

The rehabilitation sense of the terms is usually related to the third referent: the relevance of the behaviour for the maintenance of the Unit as a social system. Consider the case of the individual who smashes up the flower-pots of the hospital Matron. This smashing-up may be considered 'constructive' from the treatment point of view in that it expresses symbolically some problems of the patient which he then discusses in therapeutic groups, gaining insight and subsequently improving his personal capacities for certain kinds of relationships. If the individual were to pay for the damage, his activities might not even be considered too destructive from a rehabilitation point of view. If, on the other hand, this incident came on top of several similar ones and the patient knew that the Matron was feeling annoyance at the Unit and its methods such that she might take some action to interfere with the Unit's functioning, the patient's act has clear destructive components with reference to the Unit's functioning as a system. Consider, again, the case of the patient who proposes a system for handling ward laundry that is technically much superior to the prevailing one—with the motive of destroying the staff's prestige through exposing them as incompetent. His aim with reference to the staff (and thus therapeutically for himself) is destructive; with reference to the functioning of the social system, constructive.

Obviously, many, if not most, actions are mixed, particularly since most patients are individuals with problems of ambivalence. Yet the establishing of judgements as to the relative constructiveness or destructiveness of each activity and transaction is useful for therapy and system maintenance.

There seem to be two distinct kinds of problems associated with establishing these judgements: (a) a perceptual problem, and (b) a conceptual problem.

The first is the kind of problem that is indicated when an individual feels confident that he could evaluate an act as constructive or destructive if he were sure that his perception of the act were correct. The system of interlocking group membership, continuous group meetings, and 'healthy' staff participation all contribute, in the staff's minds, to the accuracy of perceptions. 'Official' groups are considered more satisfactory than self-selected cliques, larger groups more satisfactory than smaller ones in sorting out the 'facts' of what is going on. Though the Unit has an expression in support of the democratization theme that 'the staff are sometimes sicker than the patients', this situation, if it ever does occur, is expected to occur less frequently, less intensely, less sustainedly, than the prevailing situation where the staff can serve as stabilizers for perceptual distortions that might be current among patients. The nagging awareness that on some occasions no one and no group in the Unit can be relied on to appraise the 'reality' situation accurately is occasionally expressed in the view that a detached expert should be brought in at times of such crisis and discord to analyse the situation. This, however, is not done systematically, though visiting professionals are sometimes informally used for this purpose. The problem of understanding covert levels of meaning in Unit affairs is one that is mentioned against bringing in analysts of the situation for brief periods.

The second kind of problem—that associated with conceptual ambiguities in the judgements as to constructive and destructive participation—may be illustrated in the problem of the administration of sedatives in the evening. If a night nurse gives drugs to a disruptive patient, the nurse may be behaving constructively with regard to the patient's therapy if the patient is so much in need of rest that he would otherwise suffer physically; the act may also contribute to others' therapy by enabling them to get rest; it may contribute to the nurse's comfort and morale, thus being constructive for the functioning of the staff. On the other hand, it may be destructive from the point of view of keeping the patient's tensions up so that the kind of involvement advocated in the Unit ideological tenet of reality confrontation will be fostered; it may be destructive to the individual concerned if he is an addict; it may be destructive for the other patients' therapy in that favouritism is shown; it may be destructive of staff organization in contravening the policy of the particular doctor concerned. Many points here are at issue—e.g., the advisability of rapid *v.* gradual withdrawal of drugs from an addict; the place of rest *v.* tension in psychotherapy, etc. In the absence of empirical validation for many of the alternative courses of action proposed and used within the Unit, a great deal of autonomy is allowed each doctor to follow variant patterns. It may happen in this situation, however, that a particular nurse finds herself considered constructive by one doctor and destructive by another, while pursuing the same policy with patients.

While it is not possible here to sort out every problem of theoretical importance, the interests of conceptual clarity may be promoted by indicating more precisely which of the rationales mentioned are invoked in judgements of constructive or destructive behaviour. Thus, if a nurse feels that the most constructive thing to do in a situation is to give drugs, it should be clear, if misunderstandings are to be avoided, which kind of constructiveness she has in mind—promoting her own capacity to function in her role, promoting the patient's capacity to participate in the community, promoting the other patients' capacity to cope with troublesome patients, or some other purpose.

Let us consider now how these terms tend to be used with different meanings in connexion with the oscillatory process. We have hypo-thesized that the oscillatory process may be viewed in terms of its therapeutic potentials as well as its sociological inevitability. In the phase of social reconstruction, several kinds of things characteristically occur that would support this view.

Patients sometimes partly identify with the 'casualties' of the process and feel that 'but for the grace of God' it might have been they who had gone to the mental hospital. This may lead to behaviour that is called constructive in treatment terms (e.g., 'coming into treatment' to avoid this eventuality) or destructive in treatment terms (e.g., giving up hope, breaking down, running away), or constructive in organiza-tional terms (e.g., increasing participation in groups and socials to help 'make the Unit work' better), or destructive in organizational terms (e.g., attacking the staff as hypocrites, who use the patients as guinea-pigs and treacherously send them off to mental hospitals when things get awkward). Patients who identify with the staff, feel guilty about not having helped the patient who was sent away, or about not having behaved consistently with Unit ideals, may similarly act in ways classi-fiable as relatively constructive or destructive.

In order to treat patients of the types described above most effectively it would seem necessary to sort out very carefully the ways in which each is being constructive. Aside from the consensual problem, which is both assisted and hampered by the Unit's structural property of catching the matter 'while it is hot' for interpretation, there is, once again, the conceptual problem. Take the case of a very disruptive patient who, after another patient with whom he identified was sent away to a mental hospital, took his own discharge. The motivation of this patient may have been destructive with reference to the Unit as a social system, in his fantasy striking a blow at the system and those in it by leaving prematurely. From the point of view of the actual func-tioning of the Unit, it may be 'constructive' for the patient not to be there, and the staff may rationalize the premature discharge as being a good thing not only for the harmonious functioning of the Unit, but for the patient himself who is 'too sick' to benefit from this form of treatment. If, on reflection, the patient reapplies for readmission to the Unit, he may be refused on the basis of this opinion, which may have been formulated in blanket terms of destructive participation, confusing the issues of the Unit's good with the patient's good.

Confusions of this type seem to be functional in some sense in the

Unit. This can be seen in collusions among the staff. When tensions mount within the Unit, patients are reacting in their various ways, flight, conformity, or on the other extreme with aggressive action against the system or some part of it; staff are also reacting, but in ways that are somewhat more muted behaviourally. They do not show as many or as severe psychiatric symptoms, but malaise and psychosomatic complaints may arise; they do not take their leave of the situation so easily, being bound by professional obligations, but fantasies of flight, of changing jobs, or of changing careers occur and pervade conversations. Perceptions of the situation may be clouded or distorted by personal tensions. Where the distortions gain sufficient group support to be carried into action, they may be called collusions. Two types of collusion have been observed in connexion with the process described: that of collusive anxiety and that of collusive denial. Their implications are discussed in connexion with *Figure 14*.

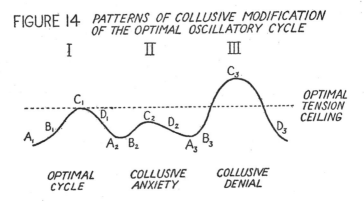

FIGURE 14 *PATTERNS OF COLLUSIVE MODIFICATION OF THE OPTIMAL OSCILLATORY CYCLE*

In the first cycle presented in *Figure 14*, the hypothetically optimal pattern is achieved. The staff allow deviation and disorganization to occur and tension to mount until the therapeutically 'optimal tension ceiling' is reached. While there may be losses through self-discharge and through pruning and unproductive emotional disturbances, these seem minimal and unavoidable; the net gain in the direction of didactically utilizing the tensions of the equilibrating phase (D1) seems maximized at this point.

In the second cycle, where collusive anxiety is graphically portrayed, authoritative action is taken prematurely by the staff because of an exaggerated perception of danger. The collusion might occur, for example, in the following way. A member of the permanent staff, perceiving possible danger because of a patient's destructive behaviour in the neighbouring community, might feel more alarmed than another, less permanently established, less formally responsible member of the staff. A third, however, might share the alarm through identification with the first; another might resonate to the sense of danger, possibly displaced from another source, e.g., a feeling of being out of touch with his groups (which would usually indicate the kind of inhibition of communications characteristic of Phase C), and so on. If an effective coalition is formed around this sense of alarm, premature action may be taken (C2) on the basis of the patient's 'destructiveness', e.g., by asking the patient to leave without strong patient support for the staff action before the optimal tension ceiling had been reached. This premature action might hamper the utilization of the tensions implicit in the oscillation. Aside from the unnecessary loss of the patient through staff action, there may be other effects. The maladaptive tensions of patients who remain, e.g., anger and disillusionment at what seems to be the unreasonable abandonment of valued ways of operating, would be higher than necessary. Their trust and confidence in the staff's sincerity might be undermined, and communications essential to therapeutic relationships inhibited. Moreover, there is the loss of the tension itself, which might have built up to a more powerful pitch to be harnessed productively in the ways outlined above.

In the third cycle, collusive denial is pictured. This might, for example, occur if a particularly influential member of the core staff group, for conscious or unconscious reasons, idealizes the state of affairs. He might, for example, assert that everything was quite all right, that the patients were handling things adequately in a 'constructive', communal manner, and that there was nothing to worry about, while in fact the optimal tension ceiling had been exceeded. The idealization might become collusive if staff consensus is reached for inaction—one person giving silent pseudo-assent through a personal fear of contradicting the idealizer; another remaining silent because of a feeling of newness in the situation; another because of the feeling that his loyalty to the ideals was in question; another because of deference to the social status superiority of the idealizer. If, in such a situation, real dangers were present in the Unit, grave difficulties might go unattended until something of a very serious nature occurred—e.g., a suicide, a psychotic breakdown, or an episode involving extensive destruction to property or disturbance to the neighbouring community. Unnecessary losses in patients, confidence, energy-utilization, and so on, would be experienced here as with collusive anxiety.

In the sections that follow, we shall deal with phenomena amongst patients in terms of 'clique formation' and 'pairing-off'. These groupings, too, have characteristics akin to those we have termed 'collusive' for staff, but in describing them we shall use the Unit's terms of 'constructive' and 'destructive' participation, interpolating our own analysis of the different senses in which these terms are used.

CLIQUE FORMATION

As we have noted, the type of clique formation and attitudes of the staff towards it vary with the oscillatory process.

Within any kind of social system, informal groups tend to form that are not identical with the officially prescribed groupings. Obviously the degree to which these informal associations deviate from, or even work at cross-purposes with, the formally prescribed activities and relationships, depends on numerous factors. One factor is the degree of crystallization or institutionalization of the established formal system. This alone does not, however, wholly determine the pattern of clique formation. Some systems that are in the process of being formed may curb spontaneous patterns of participation less than those in which the institutionalization has been long established and many of the interaction patterns formally prescribed. On the other hand some long-established and highly structured systems are secure enough to allow great scope for informal group formation. Institutions that operate according to a coercive mode—e.g., prisons—are more determinant of their participants' behaviour patterns than those that are permissive—e.g., a summer holiday camp. Participation in institutions that are selected by the constituents probably entails less hostility than in those that are imposed on the individuals concerned.

In the case of the Unit we have a special situation in which the staff recognize and are actively interested in informal group formation rather than simply harbouring it as a necessary social phenomenon accompanying any form of organization. The Unit's ideology stresses the importance of spontaneous group formation as a legitimate adjunct to treatment.

Cliques and informal groups within the Unit form on a spontaneous basis both among the staff members and among patients. Stable informal groupings between staff and patients are rarer and tend to be discouraged, except within the context of the regular round of Unit life—e.g., social therapists chatting with patients in the wards between tea time and supper time (but not after lights out); doctors chatting with patients in the workshops or socials (but not in patients' London flats or in pubs).

In this section we will consider only the formation of informal groupings among patients. One characteristic of Unit patient groupings is their continually shifting character. The emotional pitch at which Unit life is lived, the transiency of its population, and the tendency of many of its members to be rather unstable in their affectional bonds, makes for a kaleidoscopic quality of group formations.

Seymour Parker, in his studies of group formation within a male ward,[8] found this relatively shifting pattern reflected in sociograms. He found that the patterning is not random in nature, but fluctuates according to discernible factors in the continuing life of the overall Unit. During a three-month period, Parker noted changes in the composition, communication patterns within and between groups, leadership patterns, orientation to staff, and role performance. These all seemed to be interrelated, and to occur as a patterned response to disruptive forces external to the Unit impinging on the Unit's senior staff members.

Early in the period under study, the ward of about twenty-five patients was divided into three definable sub-groups. Five individuals were distinguishable sociometrically as leaders within the ward.[9] The groups tended to convene in the ward during the hours in which 'official' groups were not scheduled, and to interact in their own ways. Of the twenty-five ward members, sixteen affiliated themselves with one or another of these groups.

One of the groups was known among the patients as the 'intellectuals' and contained two of the leaders. These leaders were skilled in giving their 'expert' opinions and advice on psychiatric matters. The level of education of members of this group was comparatively high and a considerable knowledge of and interest in psychodynamics was shown in their discussions. Their group tended to resemble Unit 'doctors' groups'.

A second group gathered round another of the leaders who was regarded as a 'regular fellow'. Here salty tales were popular and light conversation was the rule.

A third group that met three times weekly was known among the patients as the 'cockney psychiatrists'. Its members consisted mainly of patients from the lower socio-economic level of society with relatively little education. This group tended to give supportive attention to individuals who had been 'pinpointed' in the regular Unit groups and gave them supportive assistance along common-sense lines. This group did not have any recognized leader.

The two other leaders who were recognized sociometrically within the ward were not associated with definite stabilized sub-groupings. One of them was called by patients 'the preacher' (and by the staff, the 'ward's superego'), and he would give moralistic sermons to those who broke the rules. The other highly-chosen individual sociometrically was an older patient who took it on himself to organize activities and to help with arrangements to fulfil such responsibilities as preparation of refreshments for evening socials.

In this early phase of the study, the leaders were considered 'constructive' in every sense. They were, on the whole, friendly among themselves, positively oriented towards the staff, active in communicating informal ward affairs to everyone in the community meetings, and effective in attempting to integrate new patients into the ward routine. The leaders were important in maintaining patient confidence in the staff and in linking the staff with the flow of patient life.

Parker illustrates the functioning of these relationships at this time by describing the following incident:

'One of the newly arrived homosexual patients suddenly announced to a few of his wardmates that he could not tolerate the Unit any longer and planned to leave immediately. He refused to divulge his reasons or to discuss his feelings with other patients or members of the staff. A day previous to his departure, one of the ward leaders approached this patient and told him that his decision to leave would upset and discourage others in the ward, as he was so generally liked. After discussing the possible effects of his departure, he confided to the leader that he had fallen in love with another male patient and was reluctant to speak about it for fear of being rejected by the object of his affection and by the entire community. His fear had mounted to such heights that he could not even tolerate the thought of discussing his problem at the community meeting or with the patient he was fond of. The leader promised that he would not make the situation public without his consent. However, he asked the homosexual patient whether he objected to his discussing the matter with the other involved and then, if he agreed, to bring the matter before the group. After successfully completing his mission as an intermediary, the leader spoke about the affair at the community meeting the following day. Here it was handled sympathetically and served to encourage other patients who had experienced (or were experiencing) similar problems to speak up and help convince the disturbed patient to stay. The reaction of the group enabled him to talk about his feelings and remain in the Unit. It also facilitated the handling of ward problems created by homosexual attachments, as well as giving the staff an opportunity to learn about some of the reasons for tension in the ward.'

During this period the regular Unit groups were functioning well, inter-group conflicts and negative transference were being handled therapeutically, and premature discharges were at a minimum. The overall emotional toning of the Unit was positive and it was generally felt that the treatment was productive, and that fitting in well to the Unit life presaged social adjustment after discharge.

At the same time, however, pressures external to the Unit were being exerted on the senior staff members to exercise more control over the activities of patients and to organize staff activities in a more regular and disciplined way. On one occasion, when Unit patients acted out in such a way as to disturb external authorities (though still within the limits of the Unit's permissive policies), effective pressures were put on the Unit staff to discharge the patients from the hospital. During this same period, three of the important ward leaders requested and were granted discharges on the basis of their length of stay in the hospital and apparent improvement. Thus stimuli were introduced into the functioning of the Unit of a kind that aroused a great deal of antistaff sentiment, while the individuals among the patients who might have served to ameliorate and re-direct these feelings were absent, leaving a dearth of 'constructive' leadership.

There ensued within the ward a period of dissension, rivalry for leadership, guarded communication, and general tension. To add even further to this list of disorganizing factors, Parker reports that among the new admissions were two extraordinarily hostile and aggressive patients. One of them had a history of physical violence, a reputation for toughness (which he quickly affirmed by threats and actual fights). While the leaders who remained within the ward retained some influence in two of the sub-groups, participation in the groups dwindled and there were marked signs of hostility between the groups. There was less visiting between the sections of the ward, and intimate, spontaneous communications tended to be confined to smaller groups or pairs. Communication to the staff in the way that had been seen even by patients as commendable in the prior stage was seen as 'squealing'. Helping an uncommunicative patient to discuss his problems in groups was now seen as 'needling'. Quarrels within the ward increased and informal activity to curtail acting out and to encourage participation in the socials decreased. In other words, activities that were defined as 'constructive' by the staff in terms of therapeutic ideology tended to be seen by many patients as 'destructive' in terms of their own norms and comfort.

The staff noted in their reports during this period that the patients were being more careless about keeping the ward tidy and less interested in taking an active part in such patient-run activities as the distress fund and the informal participation in absorbing new patients. There was a general increase in anti-staff and anti-treatment sentiments. Where the Unit was seen before as a courageous innovating treatment centre, it was now seen as a place that was making 'guinea pigs' of patients. Where staff non-participation was formerly praised by patients as being 'permissive' and 'democratic', it was now condemned as showing poor leadership and a lack of confidence in treatment methods.

During this period the percentage of reciprocated choices among patients in sociometric tests dropped sharply; there were still recognizable leaders among the patients, but the new leaders were characterized by the staff as 'destructive'. They were described as belligerent and anti-staff, and Parker noted their lack of communication among themselves. Premature discharges rose in number, partly in response to the level of tension in the Unit, and partly because of the defection of patients in their roles as reception committee members responsible for fostering a positive orientation to the Unit. Patients gained less prestige among their fellows for participating in the staff-prescribed way and there was a reduction of communication as well as of consensus on how various ward programmes should be handled. The number of violations of Unit regulations (e.g., being in the ward in pyjamas by nine o'clock as reported in the nurses' records) almost doubled; the social therapists became increasingly distressed about their difficulties in performing in their role.

Gradually the staff worked through many of these difficulties by acting more authoritatively, to restore equilibrium, by 'pruning' the most disruptive elements, and by mustering their skills and resources for forming relationships with patients and resolving intergroup tensions in ways that were both 'constructive' for the ward as a whole and therapeutic for individuals. By taking these steps, they not only sought to eliminate troublesome 'pathogenic' patients by discharging them, but sought to establish a more favourable patient image of the staff by being better exemplars and communicants themselves. In fact, Parker reports that *permanent* structural changes emerged as a result of the staff's efforts to adjust to the crisis situation.[10] For example, one doctor began as a regular part of his practice to attend afternoon workshops and work alongside patients. We have an illustration here of a change in methods being fermented in the oscillatory process. According to this staff's efforts to make their own participation more 'constructive' led to the stabilization of new techniques.

The vicissitudes of clique formation are only partly encompassed in this analysis of a crisis, remarkable as it was for exposing many of the salient and recurrent elements in the Unit's functioning. A fuller typology of cliques would include cliques based on interests (e.g., the play-reading, footballing, or pub-crawling cliques) or on activity localized in some particular place in the Unit (e.g., the ward kitchen—which was also used as a focus for analysing spontaneous group formation and its consequences[11]), or on a style of life (e.g., 'nob' cliques *v.* 'slum' cliques). In every case, the nature of the clique's activities, its leadership and composition, and the overall Unit context of the clique all play a part in determining the way the clique fits into the Unit's overall functioning, which, in turn, affects the treatment of its individual members.

PAIRING OFF

'Pairing off' is a special case of clique formation, explicitly recognized in the Unit and worth separate attention. The term 'pairing off' is frequently heard in the Unit as referring to any two individuals, usually of opposite sex, taking a special interest in one another. In early phases of the development of the Unit, the staff attitude was unequivocally that 'pairing off' was therapeutically a bad thing—'destructive' in every sense. Every hospital and, indeed, every community is familiar with neurotic attachments that can draw together inadequate or paranoid couples—'against the world', or even, as in suicide pacts, precipitously 'out of the world'. There was also the fear of possible awkward consequences in a situation where male and female patients could develop sexual relationships. Other moral questions in this type of situation tended to involve individuals who were married (usually with difficulties in the relationship) developing illicit relationships in the Unit. Perhaps more germane was the feeling that pairing off usually meant withdrawal from involvement in the community, and hence from treatment. Communicating one's problems to a confidant who does not relay the information to groups is thought to sidetrack the individual from the larger pattern of potentially therapeutic relationships. In addition, this kind of involvement is considered detrimental to the functioning efficiency of the groups, which depend on everyone's participation.

Gradually the staff position on 'pairing off' has been somewhat modified, and it is no longer considered unequivocally bad. Some of the factors that contributed to this change of attitude were:

1. The growing sense of confidence that social pressures applied among the patients themselves provide strong deterrents to pairing off in adulterous relationships.

One woman, for example, who had paired off with a married man within the Unit, came under impassioned attack by another woman, and nothing could have been more effective than her tearful account of the emotional consequences of such an affair for the unlucky wife and family. Another patient put the situation more generally. He said that, on the whole, the patients leave couples alone if they feel the relationship is all right; but if the patients feel that the couple are up to no good—either for themselves or for others—they apply sanctions. From the staff point of view, this aspect of the change reflects the staff's conviction that patients have a store of social wisdom that can be effectively mobilized to achieve the same goals as the staff themselves hold for patients.

2. There seems to have been an impressive tendency for male patients to show a sense of chivalry about taking advantage of easy sexual relationships with some of the women patients. As one patient put it: 'Loveless fornication with highstrung women is, or should be, *out*'. While this is obviously not dependable as a form of control, the staff reason that in an open hospital with patients of this type, the use of diffuse social controls, rather than autocratic dictates, is the more effective course. Some patients showed promiscuous behaviour as a symptom or as a form of acting out. The staff view was that these symptoms, like alcoholism or other behavioural symptoms, were to be analysed and the patient presented with the social consequences rather than suppressed. Sexual behaviour presents special problems not only because of inhibitions on communicating about it (which were impressively lacking within Unit culture) but because a satisfying sexual life (unlike alcoholism, crime, or other symptoms) is one of the key goals of treatment. Distinguishing between abnormal, injurious, or self-defeating forms of sexual behaviour and more acceptable forms is one of the 'tricky' jobs in therapy. However, the staff argue that even with some 'accidents' there is no reason to believe that the hospital rate in such affairs exceeds that among the public at large, and the job of the hospital is not, primarily, to suppress such occurrences immediately, but to provide therapeutic and preventive influences.

3. There is a growing recognition of the beneficial effects of some pairing off. Pairing off can sometimes contribute to therapeutic progress by providing a testing ground for learning new relationships.

For example, an inadequate male patient who had never been able to have any sort of relationships with members of the opposite sex, developed new confidence and trust through pairing off with a woman who helped him to grow up emotionally. They apparently helped one another to develop a self-esteem and an incentive to recover. Same-sex pairs have also helped each other in some circumstances. Elderly pairs of men or women who tended on their own to feel left out; teenage boys who felt that most of the others couldn't understand them; mother-daughter or father-son types of relationship in which patients compensated for missing or painful elements in their own lives, have all been observed to have therapeutic outcomes.

An examination of many of the relatively stable pairs that emerged among patients recently treated in the Unit has led us to conclude that it may be an undesirable occurrence in the Unit's treatment framework, but that it tends to have favourable consequences for the individuals in the long run. There is some empirical documentation for this observation, reported in Chapter 7.

The ways in which pairing off is undesirable within the Unit are:

1. Turning attention and communication out of general community channels (and thus losing the effects of social pressures, the wealth of the group's ideas, the group audience for talking out problems, etc.).

2. Giving a patient reinforcement for taking a destructive position within the treatment community:

E.g., staying out drinking or love-making together after hours, missing meetings together, providing a sympathetic audience for hostile analyses of the staff or the treatment programme, etc.

3. Shielding a patient from the communications and social pressures of other patients:

E.g., one patient does the thinking and talking for another, never allowing the other to face the difficulties of any situation. In one case, for example, an aggressive patient, threatened another with physical violence if he 'picked on' his girl friend again in a group meeting. What this patient construed as 'picking on' his girl was seen by the staff as 'constructively bringing her up'—an indispensable part of her therapy.

4. Reinforcing neurotic tendencies:

E.g., alcoholics or drug addicts, who procure materials for one another; homosexuals; in some cases where complementary difficulties lead to mutal exploitation—e.g., where an unstable female patient paired off with a passive leucotomized male and used him as a sex-object, companion, and general lackey with no apparent enduring advantage to either of them; gratifying immediate impulses and diminishing the pair's responsiveness to group influences.

On the favourable side, we might list the following:

1. Pairing off may be seen as part of the course of unfolding of symptoms. In such situations, the 'acting out' aspects of the pairing can be interpreted to advantage and brought into treatment:

> E.g., one girl with a strong positive transference to her psychiatrist engaged in a series of transitory romances, which were interpreted as designed to rouse the psychiatrist's hostility. The aim of this was interpreted to be the desire to alleviate her guilt (which came from an earlier source) by having the psychiatrist punish her for her promiscuity. This girl seemed to change to a more socially acceptable pattern of cross-sexual relationships after this series of events.

2. The difficulties of each of the pair may be seen as complementary to those of the other in the direction of a *better* adaptation to society:

> E.g., a case where the male was a very effeminate psychopath who feared most women, and the woman was a very 'masculine' homosexual woman. They were attracted to one another and developed a relationship in the Unit in which they used one another's deficiencies to mutual advantage. They discussed their relationship at length in Unit groups, and eventually on discharge they were married. Between them they were apparently able to face society with a total inventory of characteristics approaching that of a normal couple, even if the total was arrived at by unusual apportionment.

3. The pairing off may be seen as marking the development of a significant two-person relationship when the lack of this had been a basic problem:

> E.g., a patient posed his problem in terms of his inability to pair off, saying that he had always been unable to form meaningful two-person relationships. When he finally did so in the Unit, it was felt that he was well on the road to improvement. (A psychiatrist commented with reference to two of his other male patients that if they could establish significant two-person relationships with *anyone* in the Unit, he would be very happy, because it would mark the beginning of a capacity to form some kind of satisfactory object relationship.)

Distinguishing between lastingly beneficial relationships and those based on 'transference' is, of course, a major problem. Frequently patients 'fall in love' with social therapists. Sometimes the social therapists 'fall in love' with patients. Most frequently intense transference phenomena focus on psychiatrists. Here, too, counter-transference is observable and is a frequently discussed pitfall in a treatment situation that explicitly stresses levelling of status hierarchies and blurring of formal differences in a communalistic ethos.

There is a feeling in the Unit that even within the staff pairing off is bad, because it diverts energy from the common goal of participating in the community. This is another element that is consistent with what has already been said above about the Unit. It relates, for one thing, to the quasi-religious spirit of the Unit's ideals, where at least some members of the staff feel that total energies should be turned inward to the task at hand, almost in the manner of celibate priests. The social therapists, who are perhaps more involved in the life of the Unit than anyone except the director, are often jokingly referred to with such terms as 'the vestal virgins'.

Special alliances within the staff set up a source of uneven distribution of affectual ties, creating bonds that could complicate efforts to use each uncommitted person for the goals of the Unit as a whole. There is a great effort to keep the locus of staff members' cathexies, and hence their creative therapeutic potentials, from becoming concentrated on a person rather than being diffused into the Unit as a whole. An example of the pitfalls in this might be if a social therapist or nurse is in love with a psychiatrist and, feeling rejected by him, acts punitively towards his female patients that she fantasies are receiving more affection from him than she is; or if she transfers her affection for the psychiatrist to one of his male patients, loses control of her feelings, and perhaps becomes involved with him outside the hospital in a way that is likely to detract from both the therapist's and the patient's ultimate adjustment and happiness.

In general, in pairing off and clique formation involve social groupings comparable to those prevalent in ordinary life (and therefore desirable in rehabilitation terms); but at the same time these phenomena may divert involvement in the larger community (and therefore contravene the ideal of communalism). Judgements made as to the 'constructive' or 'destructive' character of the pairing off process are linked to the oscillatory cycle as well as to the individual's psychodynamics.

Thus, if many couples are pairing off at a time when the staff are anxious about the state of overall functioning of the Unit, and it is not easy for 'constructively' minded patients in this position to 'use the community', their pairing off may be construed as the withdrawing, therapeutically 'destructive' type, and action taken to disrupt it. It seems that the conditions approximating phase A are the best ones for appraising the multiform dimensions of the phenomena, while the phenomena of fragmentation themselves occur most profusely in phase C.

SUMMARY

Though the Unit staff conceive of their treatment as a relatively constant influence administered impartially and with sustained fidelity to ideological principles, we have observed that the Unit actually functions in a somewhat different manner. Patients react in a variety of ways to the comparatively constant stimulus of the Unit's organisation of activities and system of roles, and these variegated reactions contribute to a mounting discord in the overall organization. The carefully constructed feed-back channels in the Unit's social structure contribute to this trend, ramifying whatever disturbances appear in the system so that they periodically reach the dimensions of collective disturbances.

When the collective disturbances within the Unit mount to a point beyond which the staff feel that the Unit's integrity as a social system will be threatened, action is taken to preserve the system. This action may or may not be consistent with the Unit ideology of treatment and rehabilitation, but at this point system preservation becomes the focal aim in the staff activity.

The tide of social disorganization may be stemmed by a variety of actions, including the reinstitution of authoritative leadership, the pruning of discordant and apparently unassimilable members, the skilful use of interpretations, or the intervention of some external agency such as the hospital authorities. The work of social reconstruction within the Unit ensues as staff and patients restore a collaborative basis for social action. It is only when a state of relative social organization is restored that the staff are able once again to behave consistently with their ideals of democracy, permissiveness, communalism, and reality-confrontation.

With regard to the implementation of the aims of treatment and rehabilitation, it seems that it makes most sense to talk about treatment and rehabilitation aims and methods coinciding at the state of best organization. Here the social system functions at its closest point of resemblance to ordinary social life. Adjustment to the Unit seems at this point not only comparable to adjustment in the outside world, but feasible in terms of the potentialities of individual patients. At this point they seem most in control of their instinctual life, and environmental provocation is minimal.

In the disorganizing phase the goals of treatment and rehabilitation seem to lose effectiveness in various ways. The disorganizing effects of the disturbances make life in the Unit decreasingly like life outside. Patients raise serious questions about the desirability of adjustment to the world outside and about the relevance of adjustment to such an abnormal mode of life for the resumption of an ordinary life outside. It is only at the stage of greatest disorganization, however, that the staff not only share the mounting scepticism about this point but also take the view that different means must be provided for different patients to realize the ultimate therapeutic goals; then and some patients are transferred to other hospitals or discharged at staff instigation.

At the extreme of greatest disorganization the aims of rehabilitation through socialization to the Unit do not make so much sense. Adjustment to the Unit is difficult, given the level of tension and the lack of supportiveness, and it seems of questionable relevance to adjustment outside. At this point neither adjustment outside nor treatment seems to be entailed in adjustment to the Unit. The individuals taken separately do not seem able, in many cases, to control their impulses, modify their behaviour, or bring themselves generally to participate in socially acceptable ways. The psychiatric personality model used by the staff tends increasingly to favour a static one, and more patients are seen as constitutionally incapable of receiving the treatment or in need of some kind of shelter or of biophysical intervention. At this point the staff act in such a way as to imply a policy of separating treatment from rehabilitation. Some patients are seen to need other treatment before they can be considered for rehabilitation.

The cycle of mounting disorganization and alternating social reconstruction is a hypothetical one only partly supported by empirical observations. To the extent that this cyclical process can be said actually to be operative within the Unit, it need not be entirely seen as undesirable despite being unsought. Forces of potential therapeutic value may be mobilized in this cycle and seem often to lead to results favourable to patients. Our aim has been to indicate the apparent presence of these cycles, their favourable and unfavourable outcomes, and to advocate not the elimination of cycles but their careful study, so that if they are to be used or cannot be avoided, they may be controlled to the extent of utilizing their therapeutic and minimizing their antitherapeutic potentials.

The oscillations of the general type noted seem part of the intrinsic social functioning of an organization with the Unit's constitution— transient disruptive patients, permissive staff attitudes, structural fostering of heightened communications and the goal of discharging patients who are most capable of acting as the staff allies in therapeutic practice. However, it has been noted that as well as the repetitive oscillatory pattern of functioning these collective disturbances may occasion structural changes of a more enduring kind. These structural changes became part of the general evolution of the Unit's social system as a treatment instrument.

Collective disturbances seem rather general in psychiatric hospitals,[12] and further study of their causes, concomitants, and effects may lead to development of attitudes toward them entirely different from those that have tended to prevail—namely that these are phenomena that are to be avoided and that have almost exclusively disastrous effects therapeutically. Further study is called for to enable us to specify in a more detailed way exactly what these effects are under what conditions so that the oscillatory tendencies may be fostered or curbed according to rational plans.

NOTES AND REFERENCES

1. Periodic episodes of 'collective upset' in mental hospitals have been noted by Stanton and Schwartz, Caudill, and others. For a good recent review of the way this phenomenon, somewhat akin to but differently conceptualized than our 'oscillations', see Caudill, William A.: *The Psychiatric Hospital as a Small Society.* Cambridge, Mass., Harvard Univ. Press, 1958, Ch. V. For an early statement of our own view, cf. Rapoport, Robert N.: ' Oscillations and sociotherapy'. *Hum. Relations,* 9: 357–74, 1956.

2. The oscillations observed were of varying scope. The smallest social system in which they were observed was in two-person relationships in which patterned expectations were operating. More often they were of larger scope. The ramifications of any given interpersonal disturbance are increased by the personal sensitivity of the Unit population, their 'inward-facing' and 'interlocking' group structure. This is illustrated substantively in an episode described in Rapoport,

Robert N., and Skellern, Eileen: 'Some therapeutic functions of administrative disturbance.' *Admin. Sci. Quart.*, **2**: 82–6, 1957.

3. Parker, Seymour: 'Changes in the administration of psychotherapy during a collective upset.' *Hum. Organiz.*, **16**: 32–7, 1958.

4. It is acknowledged that many patients who stay this short period of time benefit from Unit experience and therefore ought not to be called 'premature' without more detailed examination. However, there seems to be a clear tendency for patients in this category to be extremely heavily loaded with 'non-improved' ratings from the viewpoint of the staff members who have observed them. This will be documented in a later section. For our purposes, this group is taken to be comparatively unproductive therapeutically.

5. The peak at period 1 was a continuation of a downward trend from late in the previous year. One doctor left the Unit in December 1953.

6. For other data on the effects of season on the 'drive to live', and hypothetically the 'therapeutic drive', cf. statistics on suicide in Henry, Andrew F., and Short, James F., Jr.: *Suicide and Homicide*. Glencoe, Ill., The Free Press, 1954.

7. Parker, Seymour: 'Changes in the administration of psychotherapy . . .', *op. cit.*

8. Parker, Seymour: 'The natural history of a crisis.' *Psychiatry* (in press).

9. Parker, Seymour: 'Leadership patterns in a psychiatric ward' *Hum. Relations*, **11**: 287–302, 1958. Also cf. Polansky, Norman A., White, Robert B., and Miller, Stuart: 'Determinants of the Role Images of the Patient in a Psychiatric Hospital', in Greenblatt, M., *et al.*: *The Patient and the Mental Hospital*, Glencoe, Ill., The Free Press, 1957, pp. 380–401, for a discussion of processes related to those here described.

10. Parker, Seymour: 'Changes in the administration of psychotherapy . . .', *op. cit.*

11. Rapoport, Robert N., and Skellern, Eileen: 'Therapeutic functions of administrative disturbance', *op. cit.*

12. Caudill, William A.: *The Psychiatric Hospital* . . . , *op. cit.*, and Stanton, Alfred, and Schwartz, Morris: *The Mental Hospital*. New York, Basic Books, 1954.

CHAPTER 7

Patterns of Patient Reaction to the Unit

In preceding chapters we have been mainly concerned with describing the Unit from the point of view of understanding its functioning as a social system. In the present chapter we shall focus on patients. As we indicated early on in the book, patients come from a variety of backgrounds, with a variety of complaints and clinical characteristics, and aspire to a variety of ultimate personal and social goals. The Unit staff reduce these diversities to a comparatively simple paradigm of psychiatric illness, according to which most of their patients are seen as manifesting in various ways a single underlying form of anomaly in personality development. For the treatment of this they provide a single ideology and a single social structure within which variable handling occurs and variations of functioning can be observed.

In the present chapter we shall critically examine the implicit assumption on which the Unit's methods are based (viz., that the provision of a single ideology and social structure will produce therapeutic changes in individual patients) through an examination of the actual treatment careers of particular patients.[1] The points that will be made here will be drawn from materials of different quality taken from a variety of sources over the period of study.[2] Because of their fragmentary nature and uncertain reliability, the picture that we shall draw is to be construed as tentative, at best, and of greater value as a stimulus for further investigation than as a set of firm conclusions.

We shall first indicate how new patients actually react to the Unit, in terms of their impressions and ensuing behaviour. It is in the nature of the treatment that patients are likely to benefit most from it by overcoming whatever difficulties are encountered in their initial entry into the organization and becoming adjusted to its way of functioning—in

Unit parlance, to 'come into treatment', or to 'become part of the Unit', 'carriers of Unit culture'.[3] Those that remain in the Unit after having come through the initial problems of adjustment and have not been eliminated on diagnostic grounds or premature discharge will experience, then, the Unit's treatment. This consists in socialization to the therapeutic community and exposing oneself thereby to its putative treatment and rehabilitative benefits. We shall examine the effectiveness of these measures through studying a series of careers in terms of their 'improvement' within the Unit and their subsequent adjustment after discharge.

THE ABSORPTION OF NEW PATIENTS

As we have seen, new patients come to the Unit through a variety of referral channels. After having been screened for admission, they receive a note from the Unit director that explains a little about Unit life. This letter aims at alleviating some of their anxieties while awaiting admission and at channelling their fantasies about the Unit into realistic anticipation.[4]

From this point onward, it must be said that in general the impact of the Unit on new patients is an exceedingly complex matter. Patients react in a variety of ways, and undergo diverse experiences.

Some of the referred patients never actually appear at the Unit. Of a total of 121 patients accepted over one twelve-week period studied, only 83 actually arrived. No study was made of the persons who did not show up in this series, but the staff assign the following kinds of reasons to these defections, based on general experience: Some patients lose their symptoms when closely faced with the prospect of actual hospitalization and treatment. This is the familiar 'flight into health' even before exposure to treatment. Others cannot endure the delay and arrange to be referred elsewhere. Some patients experience changed social circumstances in the ordinary course of their lives (e.g., getting a job, having their wives return, etc.) and the new situation removes their wish for treatment. In some cases the information brochure which is sent to prospective patients to anticipate and alleviate their fears about hospitalization makes them more apprehensive or antagonistic.

Those referred cases who do come to the Unit are sent on arrival to the hospital's admission ward and information for hospital records is taken by the registration nurse. The nurse then introduces the new patient to the patient reception committee. This committee consists of one patient from each of the Unit wards—i.e., three men and one woman. The particular delegate from the new patient's own ward brings him over to the Unit and takes him to the central office, where he meets the staff nurse, and further information about him is recorded. The patient receptionist then takes him to his ward, introduces him to other patients, and to the social therapists on the ward. Ordinarily all patients arrive on a Monday, and the usual total number of admissions is six to eight per week, making the usual intake for each ward one to two new patients weekly.

During the first afternoon the new patients meet informally as a group over tea with the reception committee. The reception committee try to help with any problems that the new patients want to bring up. These range from practical things like, 'How will my wife get home?' or 'Where do I go for tea?' to complex problems related to their own psychopathology or to the Unit and its treatment.

At 2:00 p.m. the new patients and receptionists visit the medical director and Sister, who receive them in the director's office and assign them each to a doctor. During the afternoon each patient makes contact with his doctor, who conducts a medical examination. Aside from acute medical emergencies, this may be the only point at which a patient sees his doctor performing in the conventional manner and with the conventional paraphernalia of a physician.

The new patients are invited to join the Unit social activities as soon as they are able, but are not expected to go to workshops for a few days. The patient delegates on the reception committee remain, ideally, attentive to new patients' needs, assisting with any problems they may have.

On the second day, the new patients are expected to go to the community meeting and to doctors' groups. In the afternoon they are taken round to see the workshops by the reception committee. At 2:15 a group is held by Sister and the reception committee for the new patients. This is also attended by other staff members intermittently, but usually includes the PSW, DRO, and some social therapists. At this group, patients choose a workshop, and are encouraged to express initial reactions to the Unit. The actual details of individual problems, complaints, and interpersonal devices for gaining acceptance and support are legion. However, there are some recurrent reactions among the new patients based on features of the Unit that seem consistently to attract attention. These include the following:

a. The physical plant. Patients tend to expect the hospital to be clean, sanitary, efficient, and protective. They find in the Unit a comparatively untidy, somewhat ramshackle place that seems rather chaotic in its way of life.

Many patients comment negatively on the age and condition of the buildings. One hears such comments as, 'It looks like a workhouse.' 'It's depressing and gloomy.' 'The furniture is of poor quality.' 'The mattresses are hard.' Sometimes these comments bring in personal experience: 'It reminds me of the Army barracks.' 'It looks like the orphanage.'

Reactions are not always negative. Some patients express relief that there are no bars on the windows and no locked doors. Some who have come from prison are pleased with the absence of restraining walls and gates. Some patients who have been in mental hospitals are pleased with the freedom, and the lack of padded cells and restraints. Some of the latter are apprehensive about the 'hidden catch in it' or about their own ability to handle the relatively unrestrained situation.

The large communal patients' cafeteria is often felt to be a terrifying place. The long queues waiting to be served, the noise and crowds, make the shy or phobic patients so anxious that they sometimes refuse to go to meals.

b. Time. Patients become anxious about the indefinite length of time that treatment takes in the Unit, and how this will affect their own personal affairs. Some are shocked when they hear from other patients that they may be in the Unit up to a year. Others, welcoming institutionalization and mistaking the Units' permissive policies for being 'soft', look favourably on the chance to use the Unit indefinitely as a refuge or as a hideout from the law.

c. Finances. Most new patients are concerned in some way about money. Though there is no charge for treatment, patients usually need assistance in finding out about their eligibility for national insurance, family assistance, and other benefits. Some patients find it difficult to ask for money, some showing excessive pride, while others are obviously 'on the scrounge'. There is usually among the new patients at least one who is quite sophisticated from long experience with manipulating social agencies, and a good deal of advice is usually available about such subjects from the patients themselves.

Patients may sometimes need detailed assistance beyond what is available in the new patient's group. For example, a patient may require help with a complex insurance claim. Since their attitudes about these things often contain valuable treatment information, the staff attempt to divert discussions into groups rather than immediately referring them to the social worker. Some patients feel that they have been given a raw deal if they do not get unemployment compensation, even though they are ineligible because they have not worked prior to admission. The Unit has a fund for patients who are not eligible for such benefits to help them over the expenses of their initial hospitalization. Some feel resentful at having to ask for help in a group rather than in a private relationship with a social worker, doctor, or nurse. Sometimes the staff is seen as bad because they do not provide for everything that is needed without the patient having to ask, or because they subject them to the 'humiliation' of having to ask publicly.

In connexion with finances, patients are often concerned specifically with how their families can be helped while they are in the hospital; and they are also frequently concerned with how the hospital experience will affect their earning capacity. Many want occupational training Most are concerned about whether the stigma of hospitalization will affect their future employability.

d. Physical symptoms. Many patients have physical symptoms of one kind or another, and may get the initial impression from the lack of medication that the Unit cannot help these symptoms. Sometimes this arouses a great deal of anxiety, since many patients have a great emotional investment in their physical symptoms. The staff's deliberate refusal to focus on physical symptoms is sometimes taken to indicate their indifference or incompetence.

e. The staff. Patients tend to expect staff members to be authoritative, knowledgeable, and kind. They find themselves in a system where the differences in experience and status between themselves and the staff are 'submerged' and 'blurred'. Aside from the initial medical examination, even doctors do not behave, dress, or relate to others in the ways prevailing in the public image. The staff's informality, universal use of first names, etc., is sometimes reacted to negatively by patients. One patient told the DRO (who maintains a modicum of bureaucratic formality in his own office) that it was a pleasure to be addressed as 'Mr' for a change. Most patients are uncomfortable about calling the doctors by their first names, and a frequent compromise is to use the title plus the first name—e.g., 'Dr Max'. Some patients, of course, revel in it, and immediately and ostentatiously begin addressing the director as 'Maxie'. Sometimes patients feel that staff are not 'proper doctors' or a 'proper Sister'.

With regard to the social therapists, there are mixed reactions. Some patients like to talk to a young girl who is sympathetic, and who does not wear a nurse's uniform. Many find the fact that the social therapists are foreigners helpful and interesting in the same way as the ideal rationale for their role suggests. Others are more critical. One extreme statement of this position was embodied in the question, 'How can a young Scandinavian virgin understand my problems? (The speaker was a hardened psychopath in his forties with a chequered history of crime and social deviation.) Sometimes, when the therapists are regarded as sex objects, the initial response is favourable. However, in such cases complaints often come later in the patient's career from frustrated sexual stimulation and from rivalry.

f. Fellow patients. There are many kinds of reactions to fellow patients. Sometimes patients initially feel that everyone seems quite all right in the hospital, and they cannot tell who is staff and who is patient. Sometimes, however, new patients are impressed with how ill the other patients are and the idea that other patients will be responsible for much of their treatment comes as a shock. When they see patients expressing aggressive and egocentric feelings, they may feel that they will be at the mercy of the older patients, especially given the staff's comparatively passive role. On the other hand, some patients relate more easily to their peers and find it easier to make themselves at home in a situation that fosters such spontaneity.

Some patients envy the way old patients participate in groups and may feel that they can never do as well. For other patients the fact that older patients can participate in this sophisticated way acts as an incentive and the new patients use the skilful older patients as exemplars after whose behaviour they can model their own.

Some patients are distressed by what they see and hear among their fellow patients. They often think that they have been put among patients much sicker than they themselves are. On the other hand, some see that their problems are not unique, and derive reassurance from this. Patients who steal or who make sexual advances, or who are aggressive, arouse a variety of reactions. While some new patients are able to take the attitude that these others are simply showing their symptoms and need help, a frequent initial reaction is fear or disapproval. There is often a marked split between patients who are closer to the public stereotype of 'illness' (i.e., aches and pains, feelings of distress, etc.) and those who come closer to the public stereotype of 'badness' (i.e., stealing, etc.). Where such splits occur, neither group feels it belongs in a hospital with patients of the other type.

g. Specific activities. New patients react in a variety of ways to the Unit's regular activities. As we have already reported, what is most frequently criticized is the 8:30 meeting. Because the meeting deals with deviant behaviour within the Unit and a good deal of time is spent in the collection of evidence and analysis of motivation, it is frequently seen as similar to a courtroom. Some patients say that it is a place where people are brought up for trial and made to feel ashamed. The staff view that this is a place where certain kinds of understanding can be achieved is less frequently grasped among newer patients than among those who have been in the Unit for some time. The large size of the meeting, the expression of heightened affect, the apparent control over the meeting by patients who themselves have obvious difficulties, all contribute to producing anxious reactions in the early stages.

Even patients who easily take an active part in group discussions often find when they are new in the Unit that their remarks do not 'fit' in the same way as they would in comparable groups outside. For example, a new patient might respond positively to the directive to participate in an equalitarian way and react by being moralistic, giving advice, and other ways that are different from the more non-directive, analytic approach that constitutes approved 'U' participation. Thus, in their first attempts to contribute, they may be disillusioned by being told that they don't understand, or that they will think differently later, or they may simply not get a response of a kind they expected. These things may all contribute to new patients' negative reactions, especially to the 8:30 meeting. In doctors' therapeutic groups this tendency is present, but less marked, since patients have expectations of doctors' groups that are closer to what they find.

As we have indicated above, negative reactions are often directed at particular groups. Concrete activities like workshops and socials often come under criticism. These are activities, unlike the treatment groups, that have an outside counterpart, and that offer ready targets into which general critical reactions can be displaced. Sometimes workshops are seen as inadequate, unproductive, or boring, and socials as a farce which turns the treatment programme into nothing more than a glorified vacation camp.

The criticism of workshops, sometimes disparaging the whole work therapy programme as inefficient and unrealistic, and sometimes attacking elements of the particular workshop to which they have been assigned, offers a critical therapeutic problem. Here, as with all initial reactions, the treatment and rehabilitation problem is to distinguish between criticism that is 'realistic' and appropriate for the social context and aspirations of the patient, and criticism that is psychopathological in its basis. The staff seem more predisposed to regard such criticism as 'resistance to treatment', manifesting the patient's psycho-social difficulties. It seems, however, that at least from occupationally skilled or professional patients, there is often a realistic basis for these criticisms on sheer rehabilitation grounds. A jazz musician, a civil service engineer, a college professor of biology, an ex-Army Colonel, have all reacted in these terms. To have reacted more favourably to tailoring or cleaning as an occupation with direct rehabilitative benefit for them might have betokened a greater abnormality. To the extent that the staff explicitly present the workshops as *treatment* measures not closely linked with rehabilitation goals, the situation is different. But, as we have indicated, there are ambiguities in this that are sometimes troublesome.

h. Treatment methods. Each patient has certain expectations about the nature of the treatment. We have already indicated that these tend to be different from those of the staff. Patients tend to expect treatment to be 'given' to them—often to involve pain or loss of consciousness—but usually to mean an orderly efficient and disciplined régime in which the patient's role is a passive, receiving one. Patients with prior mental hospitalization may have developed specific attitudes towards psychiatric hospitals that affect their reactions to the Unit.

Many patients immediately request physical treatments. They feel that they need something drastic done to them, such as electro-shock treatment or surgery. In the Unit these wishes tend to be interpreted as expressions of needs to be punished. Often patients want drugs, and feel that 'All this talking gets you nowhere'. Many patients come into the Unit having taken sedatives for some time prior to admission. This practice may have been supported by the patient's general practitioner or other doctors. Such patients express anxiety about not receiving drugs. Patients say, 'I can't sleep without tablets', or 'I feel tense and depressed if I don't have them' (drugs). Some patients who do comply with the request to hand in their drugs, accepting the Unit ideology at least at an overt or intellectual level, have later emotional problems that arise from the unmasking of their tensions. Some who feel that they have 'nothing to fall back on' become anxious, aggressive, or depressed. Sometimes they say that their doctors outside know them best and that the hospital has no right to treat them in this way. In some cases patients actually leave the Unit on this account, or get their drugs clandestinely. The Unit doctors vary in policy towards drugs. One doctor practises abrupt, total withdrawal of drugs. Another doctor withdraws the drugs slowly and uses an intervening stage of administering luminol. In all cases one of the by-products of the general policy of renouncing physical treatments and withdrawing drugs is to stimulate a certain amount of imagery among the patients of the staff as harsh and depriving. Sometimes cliques form around this theme, often engaging in compensatory activities, like heavy drinking at the local pub.

At first there is an almost universal bewilderment with Unit methods. Even patients who have high scores on the ideological inventory and who subsequently adjust well in the Unit often find it difficult to understand Unit treatment initially. The *idea* of treatment is complex and abstract, difficult to communicate. The activities in which treatment presumably inheres are often disturbing to new patients. In the groups that the new patient attends he hears people talking rather freely and expressively about ordinarily taboo subjects, e.g., sexual perversions or anti-social experiences. Sometimes the discussion of these subjects is seen by the new patient (often correctly if the group is a moralistic or scapegoating one) as punitive in nature, and he may be distressed by this. On the other hand, even if the groups are going more according to the Unit ideal patterns and if the new patient does not particularly identify with the patient under discussion, he may be shocked and disturbed by the open way in which people discuss these things.

The permissiveness of the Unit allows not only for a great deal of spontaneous emotional expressiveness which may disturb some patients, but for untidiness. Some patients are distressed that no rapid and effective disciplinary action is taken to remedy untidiness in the wards.

The blurring of the hierarchy in the Unit may cause distress, and patients are often heard to express negative feelings about the lack of anyone to whom they can turn who is in authority and who will *do* something.

More specifically some patients react negatively to the Unit's conception of the doctor-patient relationship. The doctors are not only likely to express different views on diagnosis and treatment from those that had been expressed by prior medical contacts, but they are likely to behave differently. The tendency of doctors in the Unit is to channel patients' communications into group contexts rather than towards themselves, and there is sometimes anger at the doctors for not governing themselves according to what patients consider to be medically appropriate, viz. individual attention, intimate confidence, and authoritative action. Many patients fear that others in the group will be unsympathetic, ridiculing, or intimidating.

Another source of tension is the doctors' expectation that patients will be active in their own and other patients' treatment. Most patients feel that they have not been able to help themselves, certainly cannot help anyone else, and that they have their hands quite full enough with their own problems. Fear is also expressed about the capacity of other patients to treat them.

Some put their expectations that the doctors should do the work of treatment in terms of rights. It is felt that the doctors are paid by the Health Service to cure the patients, and it is difficult for such patients to understand that the doctors' attitude is not necessarily irresponsible.

The reactions described above emphasize deviations from the ideal norms for patient conduct. In the Unit context these are all seen, initially at least, as providing data for treating the patients' problems. In some cases there are positive reactions to the Unit which serve to promote adjustment to it. That is, some patients appreciate the relief from having to keep everything tidy, from having to behave deferentially to authority figures, and from restraining their feelings. In some cases patients might stay in the Unit to receive treatment where they would have withdrawn from a more conventionally organized hospital. Many take rapidly and positively to active participation in groups, friendly equalitarian relationships with senior staff, and the attention of attractive young social therapists.

An interesting problem that regularly arises is the case of patients who accept many of the Unit ideas on a superficial level, but then proceed to act in a way that runs counter to the Unit's intentions. Examples of this would be people who accept the idea of democratization, not because of its therapeutic potential, but because they hate authority figures and wish to see them debased; or those who accept the permissive standards with regard to tidiness, not so much because they wish to concentrate on motivation rather than symptom, but because they are habitually untidy; or the patient who accepts the idea that he can give treatment to others, and then proceeds to set up a private practice in the Unit or to dominate Unit groups in ways that are contrary to Unit ideals (e.g., being moralistic, controlling or punitive).

It is notable that the general tendency for patients is to react with a certain ambivalence. Even those who claim that everything is 'rosy' are considered by the staff to be hiding negative feelings on another level. They are often considered to present more difficult problems to work with than many overtly negative patients, because it is usually considered that massive defences of denial are at work.

In response to the initial and early stimuli provided by the Unit, patients make various adjustments. A substantial proportion meet the initial anxieties by physical withdrawal. About 15% take their own discharges in their first month of treatment. Some of these represent the 'flight into health' phenomenon, claiming to be completely cured after brief exposure to the Unit. They seem to re-evaluate their life situation and choose to 'have another go' at life outside. Where an improved adjustment ensues, exposure to the Unit may be said to be rehabilitative but not in the way intended, viz. through providing an 'ordinary' life situation for trial adjustment; but rather through providing an extraordinary experience with a powerful psychic impact in the direction of resuming one's prior life, perhaps on a new basis. Patients are heard, for example, to say such things as 'I didn't realize how well off I was'; or 'My problems are really small compared to X's, and I now feel that I can manage them.' In some cases, of course, this is erroneous, and the experience merely provides an interlude pending further treatment. Others are sent by the staff after more careful firsthand diagnosis to the more protected environments of mental hospitals.

It seems clear that the initial period, when many anxieties and misconceptions cloud the patient's evaluation of the treatment situation, is one of critical importance in determining whether or not the patient will successfully 'come into treatment'. In one study, Skellern found that about 15% of new patients (after their first few days in the Unit) felt that the Unit was good and could help them; about 43% felt that it was bad and could not help them; about 35% were mixed up and could not decide, and the rest gave no statements. These proportions vary a good deal according to the composition of the new patient group, the composition of the reception committee, and the overall state of organization of the Unit as a whole. Once they do decide to stay in the Unit, patients' reaction patterns to the conditions of life there vary according to a variety of factors.

FACTORS AFFECTING PATIENTS' ABSORPTION INTO THE UNIT

It is clear from what has been said that each patient must overcome certain hurdles in becoming socialized to the Unit. One of the most serious of these is overcoming a variety of discontinuities between his pre-Unit life and his experience in the Unit.

In entering the Unit the discontinuities involved for new patients are multiple. Anyone coming into a hospital must undergo the experience of separation from his connexions outside and absorption into a new kind of system. In most hospitals, relationships tend to be more formal than outside. In the Unit they tend to be more personal. In both cases there is a discontinuity.

Accepting the Unit's particular definition of oneself as psychiatrically ill may provide another form of discontinuity for new patients. In addition to the relational discontinuities, the fact that entrance into a hospital is occasioned by some kind of illness or trouble gives the situation a further anxiety-producing quality. Where the illness is a psychiatric one, the factor of stigma plays a part. Some patients do not define their 'trouble' as psychiatric illness; others place the locus of trouble in others; still others freely admit illness, but assign different causes and characteristics to it and expect different treatments from those offered by the Unit staff. All these perceptions of self in relation to psychiatric illness require revision if the patient is to receive Unit treatment.

In many institutions of this type, it is expected that novices in the role of patient will be at the bottom of a series of hierarchies. In the Unit, though these hierarchies in nursing, medical, and patient organization exist formally, the new patient in the Unit is told that these bases for organization are not binding in the situation and that he may find his own place in it as his personality prompts. Those who react negatively to formal and authoritarian systems may react positively to the Unit; while those who react negatively to a lack of clarity in formal social structure or to public participation may react negatively to the Unit situation. In every case the problem of discontinuity is one that must be handled somehow.

Thus, a problem area generally relevant to the situation of adult socialization, that of discontinuities, is particularly complex and acute in the Unit. In order to receive treatment, patients must overcome the problems posed by discontinuities in their experience. These discontinuities are of several kinds—the discontinuity involving separation from close relationships and the necessity for establishing a major new network of relationships; the discontinuity implied for some patients— particularly the first admission cases—of facing the concrete experience of being admitted to a psychiatric hospital and facing their definition as a psychiatric case; the discontinuity of reconciling their general ideas derived from the culture at large about what hospitals ought to be like with the ideas of the Unit as to what hospitals of this kind ought to be like; and finally, regardless of whether the patient accepts the 'U' views or not, reconciling himself to the actual pattern of living prevailing in the Unit (if he accepts the 'U' view, he must, as all pro-U members must, reconcile himself to ideal-real discrepancies; if he does not accept the 'U' view, he must reconcile himself to a régime that is likely to deviate from whatever standards he may have for hospital functioning). Each of these, of course, may or may not be operative for any particular patient, but they are all 'latent' in the situation, and all have been observed to be actuated.

Those already in the Unit must face the problem of absorbing newcomers into their midst. This, too, is a complex problem. Newcomers are part of a stream of transient members of the Unit, and the opportunity for the novices to enter is only made possible through the departure of someone prior to them. The way in which a novice is received partly depends on the social situation prevailing between his predecessor and the others. If he occupies the bed of a troublesome ex-patient and he himself is relatively sociable, he may be welcomed very warmly. On the other hand, if he takes the place of a patient who was important in a more positive way, he may be resented regardless of his own positive qualities. This resentment seems greatest when the loss of the prior patient was taken out of the hands of the community (e.g., if the prior patient were discharged by the director for disciplinary reasons).

The fact that every newcomer in the Unit is there because of his socially disruptive tendencies adds a note of apprehension to the anticipatory aspects of socialization. In the Unit, as in other institutions, there are some members of the group who look forward especially to the arrival of novices. Their motives may be of a positive, nurturant kind, or they may seek an opportunity for wielding power or for exploiting the novices' initial lack of orientation to the situation.

Learning the role of patient presents another set of problems to each novice. In entering any institution, one's level of skill in a prior social system is a factor that may not be directly relevant to the new system. In general, societies provide for meeting this problem in various ways —e.g., lowering initial expectations, providing a period of apprenticeship, and so on. One of the Unit's ways of handling this is to elevate the status of patients, partly by assigning explicit value to attributes that even neophytes may have. For example, Unit ideology stresses the importance of getting *ordinary* social reactions to people's symptomatic behaviour. But it is also clear that life in the Unit is different from participation in ordinary groups outside, and this requires adjustment. Talk about sex, for example, is to be reacted to neither in the framework of prudery nor in the framework of obscenity.

The Unit staff see the sublimation of many tendencies that had formerly been a source of difficulty for patients as valuable therapeutic potential. For example, patients who were physically aggressive on the outside and who got into trouble over this, may, if appropriately reoriented, become an effective force for social control in the Unit. Since the staff abstain as much as possible from the use of their power, controls over disruptive patients must come from within the patient group itself. This provides an opportunity for aggressive patients to learn constructive channels for their behavioural tendencies.

Incomplete sublimations may lead to difficulties, to which staff are alerted. A patient, for example, who was interrupted while behaving quite sadistically towards another, and said to the staff member, 'I was just trying to therapeut this bloke', may have been unsuccessfully attempting a 'constructive' (sublimative) solution to the problem of handling his aggression.

The staff's view of the meaning of patients' patterns of adjustment to the Unit is an important factor in determining the pattern itself. The staff see patients' behaviour and relationship patterns in terms of 'transference'. New patients are told that they can behave as they like in the Unit. This provides an undefined, anxiety-producing situation. They tend to set up in the new situations patterns with which they have dealt with anxiety in the past. These patterns are the ones in which their personal security tends to be invested. At the same time, they tend to be socially maladaptive patterns; hence their referral. 'Treatment consists partly in confrontation and interpretation of transference elements in these patterns. This may have a confusing, or even devastating, effect on patients who have weak defences. For example, patients who have always reacted to new or stressful situations by withdrawing may be told that they are reacting as they did when they were children in their early families. Patients who feel themselves to be frightened and anxious may be told on the basis of the social consequences of their behaviour that they are 'controlling' situations through the use of infantile patterns of passivity, manipulating through over-dependence, and so on. As patterns are manifested and problems redefined, even patients who stay and are receptive to the treatment often feel upset and confused as they reorient their images of themselves and others. A very common statement heard in the Unit is 'I came here with one problem, but now I have a hundred'.

The redefinition of one's therapeutic goals is another hurdle that is often necessary and difficult for patients to cross. New patients vary in the goals they hold out for themselves in treatment, from such global and abstract goals as 'happiness', 'salvation', etc., through such relatively mundane and specific goals as 'passing the university entrance examination', or 'holding a job'. The staff vary somewhat in the types of goals they formulate for particular patients, and this sometimes provides an additional source of complexity in the patient's field of influences. However, perhaps a more complex point for a patient to assimilate is that though the staff considers patients to suffer essentially from the same kind of disorder in different forms, and provide the same basic treatment régime for everyone, they implicitly recognize that the aims of treatment for patients vary. For one kind of patient 'improvement' may be taken to mean the alleviation of physical symptoms that stand in the way of role performance, while for another the show of symptoms is said to obscure the 'real' problems; for one patient, the goal of treatment may be the consolidation of a marital relationship, for another the dissolution of a relationship; for one it may mean the increase of controls over instinctual drives, for another the decrease of inhibitions.

Some institutions emphasize the definition of treatment goals for each individual and are relatively flexible about means for achieving these goals. In the Unit, the tendency is to blur the diversity of individual goals, and to emphasize the efficacy of common means for achieving all the goals.

UNIT PRACTICES AIMED AT ASSISTING THE SOCIALIZATION OF NEW PATIENTS

The ways in which the particular individuals handle the anxiety attendant on these initial 'hurdles' of entry will determine their pattern of adjustment to the system and consequently, in the Unit situation, their treatment. The following kinds of mechanisms are provided by the staff to help patients to overcome the anxiety generated by exposure to the Unit and to compensate for the attendant weakening of ego defences:

1. Anticipatory socialization—via the letter of introduction, reception, and orientation (see Appendix A).

2. Providing for some continuity by the use of the new patients' committee. This committee helps to bridge the gap between the patients' outside experiences and expectations and the Unit's. A few days are provided for this to occur.

3. The staff stress the fact that patients' participation is voluntary and they are welcome to leave any time they like. This removes the staff from coercive positions considered antithetical to therapeutic relations. It also tends to weed out patients who are not really motivated to participate. Those who come under court order provide a special case of 'unwilling patients', but from the Unit's point of view the restraining authorities are external to the treatment situation and so the staff can attempt to build non-coercive, therapeutic relations in the Unit.

4. However, the Unit staff stress the fact that if the individual is to achieve his aspirations, he must reconcile himself to absorption into the Unit. Absorption into the Unit or 'coming into treatment' is considered indispensable for improvement. If a patient states that he has no dissatisfaction with his life situation (i.e., says that there is nothing wrong with him and that he doesn't want anything from the Unit), he is told that he is 'denying' and '*really*' sick'. If a patient becomes concerned about his early discouragement and deterioration under the stress of new experience in the Unit, the aspiration potential is kept up by telling him that 'you've got to get worse before you get better'. The

problem of discriminating between 'progressive' deterioration that will eventually result in improvement and more devastating deterioration is a difficult clinical one. In general, however, the pressures are directed towards intense involvement in the Unit's social processes as a *sine qua non* for improvement.

5. The Unit's staff stress the positive skills which each patient has. Even the most inexperienced novice is seen as having something valuable to contribute to groups, since the response of ordinary persons from outside the hospital provides an element that is useful for re-habilitation.

6. By legitimating patient participation in the general therapeutic enterprise, the staff allow for the application of effect of potential therapeutic group support. As we note elsewhere, this is an important though variable factor.

Ordinarily any patient's entry into the system is preceded by a number of forces that commit him in some degree to taking treatment by the time he reaches the Unit. Given the stigma of mental illness and the hardships of prolonged unemployment and separation often required by hospitalization, entry to the Unit usually requires a good degree of motivation. But, nevertheless, the anxiety-producing elements in the situation may be so great for any particular patient that he will never really participate in treatment, but take his own early discharge. At the beginning especially, the forces keeping a patient in treatment and those impelling him to avoid hospitalization may be rather precariously balanced.

Once absorbed into Unit life, the field of forces changes somewhat and internal processes of Unit functioning play a different part in the individual patient's psychic economy. One of the problems that is particularly acute in the socialization process in the Unit, however, is that even after the initial anxieties attendant on entrance are overcome, additional anxieties are generated as a concomitant of participation that must be continually met and dealt with. The general outlines of these situations have been described in the chapters on the structure and process of the treatment régime.

In general, then, the Unit may be said to screen their patients through the referral processes so that the patient population will cluster in that grouping of the psychiatric spectrum that the Unit refers to as 'personality disorders'. The screening by this means, however, is not efficient, nor is the boundary line separating the category from the psychotic group of patients clear or fixed. Patients remain susceptible to the diagnosis of 'psychotic', or 'too ill for treatment in the Unit', throughout their stay, though these diagnoses and the attendant disposition of patients tend to cluster in the early period after entry to the Unit. Once the group is selected according to the Unit's diagnostic criteria, a single treatment régime is provided, applicable to all.

However, great variability of response to the Unit is found among new patients, and to some extent this persists among patients throughout their stay. These variations provide, of course, the individual materials for diagnosis and therapy. It must be noted, however, that they also provide reaction patterns of crystallized or persistent kinds that sometimes take forms divergent from those intended by the therapists.

In a very gross sense, these diversities of response types may be classified with reference to the goals of the Unit staff as 'improved' or 'not improved', which can, in turn, be divided into those that remained the same and those that got worse in consequence of treatment.

The concept of clinical improvement is an extraordinarily complex one. Patients do not simply get better, stay the same, or get worse. Being complex creatures, they tend to get better in some ways, remain the same in some ways, and get worse in others.[5] It is sometimes a problem to clinicians to decide whether it is better to improve a patient's individual comfort at the expense of his family relationships, better to improve his work productivity at the expense of his personal comfort or quality of social relationships, or better to assist him to see himself as he 'really' is at the expense of his occupational effectiveness (assuming all these things were so pliant). More usually, clinicians operate with a set of techniques which aim at producing certain immediate kinds of effects—such as insight, personal gratification and increase of comfort, social participation and training in effectiveness in handling relationships—and with the hope that these changes will produce a realignment of the patient's attributes that will be 'better'. Sometimes emphasis on one of the elements produces an anticipated temporary worsening of another element so that the first can produce its effects, with the ultimate goal in mind of improving both. For example, insight is sometimes aimed at with the knowledge that this is often accompanied in the short run by increased *dis*comfort and **social** ineffectiveness, but with the long-range goal of precipitating personality realignments that will improve comfort and effectiveness as well as self-awareness. In the Unit the favoured technique is to keep in immediate focus the goal of achieving greater effectiveness in patients' social adjustment, attempting to provide as much insight as necessary but subordinating this and personal comfort to secondary positions.

Thus, when a member of the Unit staff is asked the question in the crude form which we were able to employ, 'Did patient X improve a lot, get a little better, remain the same, or get worse?', they tend to answer in the strongly favourable category only if the patient improved on many scores or in a spectacular way, but always in terms of his capacity for social adjustment; and they tend to use the second category for cases of mixed or mild improvement. In most cases it was felt that a patient did not really improve very much unless his behaviour changed in the direction of better social adjustment, regardless of whether he was happier as a consequence of hospitalization or had a remission of symptoms or complaints.

In the section immediately to follow we must work with the global judgements of improvement that we were able to accumulate during the period of study. Some of the complexities that underlie or extend beyond this type of our analysis will become more apparent in the section on the family and treatment.

IMPROVEMENT IN THE UNIT

What factors make for improvement while the patients are under treatment in the Unit? When using judgements of global improvement there is a pronounced tendency for patients to view their improvement with an optimistic bias. Of those who rated their response to treatment, 77% felt they had improved, whereas the doctors felt that only 43% of them had shown any improvement under treatment. It may appear surprising that the doctors, who are leaders in an innovating method with such ideological overtones, show such conservatism. But conservatism is certainly the safer policy when making formal statements about such a problematic matter as improvement. While the doctors are the principal enthusiasts for the Unit method, they are also the most sophisticated in clinical experience. This is seen also in their value scores, which actually tended to be lower than those of many of the other staff, largely because of the qualifications they know to be appropriate in endorsing 'U' slogans. Accordingly, we shall rely on the doctors' rating of improvement rather than on the patients', which seem to be coloured with wishful thinking.[6]

As we might expect, demographic factors have only a slight connexion with improvement. The old seem to do slightly better than the young and women slightly better than men, but the differences are small. Neither variable becomes important when we control for the other, although among the younger people sex may have some importance because about two-thirds of the young women improve, compared with one-half of the young men (cf. *Table 9*).

TABLE 9   UNIT IMPROVEMENT BY AGE AND SEX

	*Age**				*Sex***			
	Young		*Old*		*Men*		*Women*	
	No.	%	No.	%	No.	%	No.	%
Imp.	55	53	39	60	65	53	29	63
Not. Imp.	48	47	26	40	57	47	17	37
Totals:	(103)	100	(65)	100	(122)	100	(46)	100

$* \chi^2 = \cdot4619$, 1 d.f., $p > \cdot05$
$** \chi^2 = \cdot9252$, 1 d.f., $p > \cdot05$

More interesting, perhaps, is the variation in improvement rate according to marital status (*Table 10*). Among single people the improved and unimproved are about equal in number, whereas among the married patients the improved outnumber the unimproved by almost two to one, with the divorced and separated in between. However, if we impose a control of sex on these data (*Table 11*), it becomes immediately apparent that the differential improvement rates according to marital status are accounted for solely by the men. Roughly five-eighths of the women improve regardless of their marital status, but among the men the differences noted in *Table 10* are amplified and though not statistically significant, the clear tendency is for progressively more men to improve as marital status shifts from single to married.

It is difficult to account for this finding, since role pressures should affect men and women of the same marital status with equal force. Thus, while married men may certainly be under some pressure to resume work and support their families, married women should be under similar pressure to return to work and/or the care of their families. And our data do indicate that married people respond in comparable ways. The larger differences centre on the single people, where the single women clearly show a greater improvement rate than the single men. The men may be more prone to violence, acts of aggression, or disruptive acting-out than single women and thereby run the greater risk of an unimproved rating. Similarly, it may be that the most disturbed and potentially most disruptive young women (such as the sexually promiscuous) may be more carefully filtered out of the referral channels than the disruptive young men. These possibilities, however, cannot be pursued in our data. Nonetheless, among the unmarried, women respond more favourably to treatment than men.

TABLE 10   ADJUSTED UNIT IMPROVEMENT
OF MARITAL GROUPS

	Single No.	%	Div.-Sep. No.	%	Married No.	%
Imp.	54	51	10	59	30	65
Not Imp.	51	49	7	41	16	35
Totals:	(105)	100	(17)	100	(46)	100

$$\chi^2 = 2\cdot5298,\ 2\ \text{d.f.},\ p > \cdot05$$

TABLE 11   ADJUSTED UNIT IMPROVEMENT OF MARITAL GROUPS BY SEX

	Men						Women					
	Single No.	%	Div.-Sep. No.	%	Married No.	%	Single No.	%	Div.-Sep. No.	%	Married No.	%
Imp.	36	47	8	57	21	66	18	62	2	67	9	64
Not Imp.	40	53	6	43	11	34	11	38	1	33	5	36
Totals:	(76)	100	(14)	100	(32)	100	(29)	100	(3)	100	(14)	100

$$\chi^2 = 4\cdot4700,\ 5\ \text{d.f.},\ p > \cdot05$$

Turning to personality factors, we find that frequency of improvement is not systematically related to the modes of behavioural defence, although the conformists improve more often (84%) and the withdrawers less often (30%) than the others. For purposes of improvement, withdrawal is clearly an ineffective way of coping with problems presented in the Unit. Given our earlier observation that the withdrawers were of disproportionately weak ego-strength, it would seem that this category of patients offers the most serious problems in the framework of the Unit's treatment through participation.

The importance of ego-strength for improvement is quite clearly shown in *Table 12*. About three-fourths of the stronger-ego group improve, compared with about 41% of the two weaker-ego groups combined. This supports general clinical experience that ego-weakness constitutes a definite therapeutic handicap and ego-strength a therapeutic resource.

TABLE 12   ADJUSTED UNIT IMPROVEMENT OF DIAGNOSTIC GROUPS

	Psychotic No.	Psychotic %	PD Weak No.	PD Weak %	PD Strong No.	PD Strong %	Neurotic No.	Neurotic %
Imp.	4	25	37	45	40	75	10	77
Not. Imp.	12	75	46	55	13	25	3	23
Totals:	(16)	100	(83)	100	(53)	100	(13)	100

$$\chi^2 = 20.1445, \text{ 3 d.f., } p < .0005$$

There seems to be a marked relationship between improvement in the Unit and initial values held (*Table 13*).[7] The data show that two-thirds of those with the most pro-Unit values improved, compared with only one-third of those with anti-Unit values.

TABLE 13   ADJUSTED UNIT IMPROVEMENT
                    ACCORDING TO INITIAL VALUES
                        (SERIES II ONLY)

	Initial Values Low No.	Low %	High No.	High %
Imp.	11	32	14	67
Not. Imp.	23	68	7	33
Totals:	(34)	100	(21)	100

$$\chi^2 = 4.8475, \text{ 1 d.f., } p < .05$$

This tends to echo the points already made that people with defences and beliefs which are initially the most compatible with Unit ideology are thereby the most susceptible to its influence. At the very least, then, nominal conformity to Unit ideology might increase their chances of being classified as improved.

Values, however, are not immutable, and the Unit, in keeping with its rehabilitation assumptions, would hold that patients can change their values to 'fit in' to the Unit system, and thereby gain an experience in social adjustment that will be of persisting value. Let us here examine the question of value shifts.

VALUE SHIFTS AND IMPROVEMENT

We might expect that patients whose values are most compatible with those of the Unit right from the start might show the greatest tendency to shift further in this direction, similarly to the reinforcement of existing values which is a common effect of propaganda. Conversely, one might expect the greater shift among those with initially low values on statistical grounds because this group has the greatest room for 'improvement'. Actually, however, those whose values do shift in the 'U' direction are not disproportionately selected from either the initially high or the initially low groups (*Table 14*).

TABLE 14   VALUE SHIFTS ACCORD-
ING TO INITIAL VALUES ON ARRIVAL
AT THE UNIT
(SERIES II ONLY)

Shifts	Initial Values			
	Low		High	
	No.	%	No.	%
Pro-Unit	21	53	9	60
Not Pro	19	47	6	40
Totals:	(40)	100	(15)	100

$$\chi^2 = \cdot0378, \text{ I d.f., } p > \cdot05$$

Value shifts basically do not depend upon the original values held on arrival.

Nor is there any tendency for value shifts to depend upon ego-strength (*Table 15*), or behavioural-defence, with all groups shifting in comparable proportions, except those who use invalidism as a defence

—this group showing a significant resistance to adopting Unit values. (*Table* 16).

TABLE 15   VALUE SHIFTS OF DIAG-
NOSTIC GROUPS
(SERIES II ONLY)

Value Shifts	Ego-Strength			
	Weaker		Stronger	
	No.	%	No.	%
Pro-Unit	17	53	13	59
Not Pro	15	47	9	41
Totals:	(32)	100	(22)	100

$\chi^2 = \cdot 0243$, 1 d.f., $p > \cdot 05$

TABLE 16   VALUE SHIFTS OF BEHAVIOURAL-DEFENCE TYPES
(SERIES II ONLY)

Value Shifts	Aggression		Emotional Insulation		Conformity		Illness		Withdrawal	
	No.	%	No.	%	No.	%	No.	%	No.	%
Pro-Unit	7	70	8	62	8	67	—	—	7	58
Not Pro	3	30	5	38	4	33	8	100	5	42
Totals:	(10)	100	(13)	100	(12)	100	(8)	100	(12)	100

$\chi^2 = 11 \cdot 5830$, 4 d.f., $p < \cdot 025$

The use of the total sample rather than of Series II alone does not appreciably clarify the picture. The only element of interest here is the high resistance to attitudinal change among those whose behavioural defence takes the form of illness. This group shows greater tenacity than any other in clinging to initial beliefs and resisting Unit influences. This would suggest that those using invalidism may feel less capable than others of coping with the real world and rely very strongly on their extreme dependence on others or on more regressive states. The aggressives and the conformists lead in the 'pro-U' shift, but, as we have stated, the margins are small.

Despite the lack of patterning, significant numbers of patients do show value changes which the Unit desires. In the sample as a whole, 45% shift in the direction of Unit ideology in the course of their stay.

The 45% who shifted in a pro-Unit direction do not tell the whole story. Forty-six per cent of the patients shifted *away* from Unit values and 9% showed no change from their original score on retesting. Further, the extent of the change was not very large. Forty-one per cent and 37% respectively showed medium pro- and anti-Unit shifts (with scores changing up to ± 10 points). Only a minority were extreme changers, but of these, more (9%) reacted strongly against the Unit values than strongly endorsed them (4%). The extreme changers involved gains or losses of over 10 points. Thus, while the bulk of the patients did shift their values, most of these shifts were fairly moderate and as many reacted against the Unit as responded favourably to it.

A perceptible, though not statistically significant, factor related to pro-Unit value shifts is length of stay, which is shown in *Table 17* for Series II patients.

TABLE 17 VALUE SHIFTS ACCORDING TO LENGTH OF STAY
(SERIES II ONLY)

Shifts	Number of Days							
	0–30		31–100		101–200		201+	
	No.	%	No.	%	No.	%	No.	%
Pro	6	43	5	42	14	64	5	71
Same, Anti	8	57	7	58	8	36	2	29
Totals:	(14)	100	(12)	100	(22)	100	(7)	100

$$\chi^2 = 3.1182, \text{3 d.f., } p > .05$$

Here the important breaking point in length of treatment appears to be about 100 days. Of those who leave the Unit within that time, some 42% show a pro-Unit shift, but of those who remain longer, more than half as many again (66%) change their values in the Unit direction. It is noteworthy that those who remain between one month and a little over three do not become any more favourable to the Unit than the so-called 'bouncers' who leave within a month.

Nor is it clear whether the overall differences disclosed in *Table 17* are a function of the sheer length of exposure to Unit influence, or whether there are selective forces at work which keep the more amenable and susceptible patients in treatment for a longer period of time. In other words, those people who find the Unit congenial and helpful may be more favourably disposed towards Unit ideology and may also be more inclined to stay on for longer treatment. We have no way of discriminating between the variables of influence and self-selection in remaining in treatment.

It is, however, quite clear that shifting values are significantly related to improvement in the Unit, as is shown in *Table 18*.

Of the Series II patients whose values shift in the Unit direction, 60% show improvement during their treatment, as compared with only 28% of those who do not shift in a more favourable direction. According to these data, then, the pro-Unit shifters are twice as likely to show improvement during their stay as the others.

TABLE 18 ADJUSTED UNIT IMPROVEMENT ACCORDING TO
VALUE SHIFTS
(SERIES II ONLY)

	Shifts			
	Pro-Unit No. %		Not Pro No. %	
Improved	18	60	7	28
Not Improved	12	40	18	72
Totals:	(30)	100	(25)	100

$\chi^2 = 4{\cdot}4069$, 1 d.f., $p < {\cdot}05$

We are somewhat constrained not to accept this relationship too literally. The verbal acceptance of Unit ideology and obeisance to it in behaviour would almost certainly increase the chances of a patient's being judged 'improved'. The pro-Unit shifters tend to harbour some 'chameleons'—people who conform to the expectations in the milieu, almost as a guise, but without the attendant internal emotional changes that will persist without the immediate supports of the hospital environment. Furthermore, *Table 18* shows that 40% of those who shifted their stated value position in the 'pro-U' direction did *not* improve; a slightly higher proportion than those who improved without becoming more favourable to the Unit. This simply documents the tendency towards verbal endorsement of the norms of the prevailing social order, the hallmark of the 'chameleon'. This does not gainsay the relation between favourable shift and improvement, but it highlights the importance of the deviant cases (over one-third of these patients) who fail to improve although they do conform, and who do improve despite their nonconformity. Further documentation will be provided in the section on post-hospital adjustment.

EXPERIENCES IN THE UNIT AND IMPROVEMENT

Without doubt, the most important single determinant of improvement within the Unit is duration of treatment, as is clearly demonstrated in *Table 19*. Here we see an unequivocal pattern in which improvement rates steadily increase with the length of stay. Only one-fifth (19%) of the 'bouncers' who leave the Unit within a month of their arrival are rated as improved, and substantial increments of improvement characterize the successive groups, until we find over four-fifths (82%) of the patients improved who were treated for over 200 days, or upwards of seven months. The Unit deals automatically with the hazard of achieving chronic institutional adjustments by limiting patients' stay to a maximum of one year.

TABLE 19 UNIT IMPROVEMENT ACCORDING TO LENGTH OF STAY

	0–30		*31–100*		*Number of days* *101–200*		*201+*	
	No.	*%*	*No.*	*%*	*No.*	*%*	*No.*	*%*
Imp.	5	19	11	37	42	62	36	82
Not Imp.	21	81	19	63	26	38	8	18
Totals:	(26)	100	(30)	100	(68)	100	(44)	100

$$\chi^2 = 31 \cdot 6416, \ 3 \ \text{d.f.}, \ p < \cdot 0005$$

Although the patients receiving such lengthy treatment represent about one-fourth of the total sample, they tend to be the exceptions. Unit policy is geared to a fairly high turnover of patients who receive intensive short-term therapy for about three or four months. These particular data call the benefits of such a policy into sharp question. It is true, of course, that *Table 19* does not settle the dilemma of whether improvement is essentially a function of self-selection or of exposure. But in the long run this may be immaterial. Even if self-selection factors are operative, those patients are apparently receiving treatment who can best benefit from it. If exposure is the determinant variable, then it might be more economical to treat fewer patients over a longer period of time than to process many more at only a fraction of the same effectiveness. This is a strategic policy decision to be faced: whether it is preferable to put a thin patina of improvement on a large number of patients which may quickly wear off, or to devote longer attention to a more select group with a better chance to retain the benefits. We shall subsequently see that longer treatment does have more durable benefits after discharge than short treatment, but that its relative advantages tend to diminish with time.

The foregoing contributes an additional support to the theme running through most of our data, implying that improvement is inversely related to severity of illness. The interaction among degree of disorder, therapeutic resources of the patient (e.g. ego-strength), and length of treatment, will largely determine the patient's improvement. Unfortunately, our measures are not sensitive enough to discriminate between the relative importance of these three major variables. Length of treatment (*Table* 19) and ego-strength (*Table* 12) are positively related to improvement in the Unit. For the third variable, severity of disorder, we have only the crudest index. Patients were classified according to whether they had difficulties of four specific kinds: work, criminality, alcoholism or addiction, and relationship to friends. Each patient was then scored according to the number of these areas in which he was incapacitated. All patients were incapacitated in one area or another, and some in all four. On this basis, patients were arranged in three groups: those incapacitated in only one area (23%), an intermediate group of two or three areas of incapacity (37%), and those 'totally' incapacitated in all four areas (40%). This is admittedly a very crude and most unsatisfactory index of severity of illness, since it simply reflects pervasiveness of trouble in these four discrete areas, which encompass at best an important, but limited, range. Actually, the factor of intensity of disorder is not tapped at all.

Nonetheless, despite the limitations of this index, we do find a small but regular relationship between severity of disorder and improvement in the Unit (*Table 20*).

TABLE 20 UNIT IMPROVEMENT ACCORDING TO SEVERITY
OF DISORDER

	Total No.	%	Severity of Incapacity Moderate No.	%	Single Area No.	%
Imp.	32	48	35	56	27	66
Not Imp.	35	52	27	44	12	34
Totals:	(67)	100	(62)	100	(39)	100

$$\chi^2 = 4.6232, 2 \text{ d.f.}, p > .05$$

Here about one-half (48%) of the totally incapacitated improved, com-pared with two-thirds (66%) of those with a disturbance in only one area. This relatively small range of difference (as compared, for example with the range of difference in improvement according to length of stay shown in *Table 19*) would itself cast suspicion on our index of severity. A 50% improvement rate among patients who are ostensibly *totally* incapacitated should be viewed with caution and scepticism, if not alarm. For our purposes, however, the important thing is that these differences, though not statistically significant, run in the right direction and are consistent with our previous data on the variables of length of stay and therapeutic potential.

We shall now examine the association between improvement and different modes of participation in the Unit.

One set of data has implications for the Unit's assumptions about 'transference'. According to Unit ideology, special relations between individual patients and individual staff members are strongly dis-couraged. Instead of highly-charged emotions between patient and therapist based on a psychoanalytic model, the Unit encourages the diffusion of such affect to the community as a whole on the assumption that the distrust which patients feel towards humanity generally can best be handled on a global level with the total resources of the com-munity. Rather than individual staff members becoming highly salient transference figures who carry the bulk of the patients' therapeutic in-vestment, the Unit wants patients to set up viable relationships, per-haps of less intensity, with many more people in the Unit. Thus, the staff would discourage many of the concomitants of highly concen-trated transference relationships—privileged communications, private therapeutic interviews, claims for personal attention, etc. In fact, Dr B has gone to extremes in discouraging patient-therapist involvement by giving up his private office, discontinuing individual interviews, and generally making himself inaccessible for private attention except in medical emergencies.

Our data throw the value of these assumptions into question. We find that, whether they like it or not, senior staff members are the most significant people in the Unit to the patients and that those patients who establish a strong identification with the senior staff improve at a higher rate than those whose primary identification lies elsewhere. For example, of those people who regard a core staff member as the most admirable model for themselves, a significantly greater proportion improve than patients who locate their personal exemplars among other patients, with those patients who admire peripheral staff members occupying an intermediate position (*Table 21*).

TABLE 2I ADJUSTED UNIT IMPROVEMENT ACCORDING TO MOST ADMIRED PERSON

Improvement	Core Staff No.	%	Other Staff No.	%	Other Patient No.	%
Improved	55	72	8	61	5	64
Not Improved	21	28	5	39	9	36
Totals:	(76)	100	(13)	100	(14)	100

$\chi^2 = 5.5819$, 1 d.f., $p > .025$

Furthermore, the people who set up an identification with their own doctor do significantly better than those who regard another doctor as an admirable model (*Table 22*).

TABLE 22 ADJUSTED UNIT IMPROVEMENT ACCORDING TO IDENTIFICATION WITH OWN DOCTOR OR OTHER DOCTOR

Improvement	Exemplar Own Doctor No.	%	Other Doctor No.	%
Improved	34	83	17	59
Not Improved	7	17	12	41
Totals:	(41)	100	(29)	100

$\chi^2 = 3.9229$, 1 d.f., $p < .05$

About five-sixths (83%) of the former patients improve, compared with about three-fifths (59%) of the latter. Thus, the Unit's efforts to establish barriers to individual doctor-patient relationships may be seriously questioned insofar as the patient who has the most positive attitude towards his own doctor improves more frequently than do those whose feelings centre on other figures.

Incidentally, the sex of the patient makes no difference in his choice of models. Women do not especially identify with the senior staff women or the junior therapists. Insofar as such women are assumed to be readily available ego-models for female patients (as well as maternal figures and adumbrated sex objects for the males), they are not appreciably serving this function. The women's preferences in ego-models does not differ from those of the men.

The Unit staff try to minimize and de-emphasize the importance of objective status differences within the Unit. But our evidence shows that patients basically do not accept this definition. On the contrary, they are sensitive and positively responsive to such status differentials. In *Table 21*, for example, almost three-fourths of the patients chose a core staff person as their model, quite apart here from the effect of such choice on improvement. And the higher up in the status hierarchy the patients were able to locate the sources of their help, the more likely they were to improve. Here the data are clear-cut and the differences statistically significant. *Table 23* shows that when patients chose doctors and other core staff as the most helpful people in the Unit, 84% of them improved. However, as the most helpful people were selected from successively lower status levels, fewer and fewer of the patients improved—only 68% of those who chose other staff members and 52% of those who named another patient. Even fewer improved when nobody was found helpful.

TABLE 23   ADJUSTED UNIT IMPROVEMENT ACCORDING TO PERSON
FOUND MOST HELPFUL

Improvement	Senior Staff No. %		Junior Staff No. %		Other Patient No. %		Nobody No. %	
Improved	38	84	13	68	15	52	2	33
Not Improved	7	16	6	32	15	48	4	67
Totals:	(45)	100	(19)	100	(29)	100	(6)	100

$\chi^2 = 12 \cdot 5698$, 3 d.f., $p < \cdot 01$

The overall pattern is reasonably straightforward. Unit ideology tries to submerge status differentials as anti-therapeutic, while the patients cling to them. Furthermore, the emotional identification with people in different status levels seems directly related to improvement. If this is the case, then Unit ideology may be weakening a positive therapeutic resource in favour of a value commitment which limits therapeutic gains. Alternatively, a more qualified acceptance of Unit ideology may be in order if it can be demonstrated that positive identifications with high status individuals can be achieved in patients of this type only if the individuals in authority deliberately refuse to behave authoritatively. Controlled experiment on these lines should help to clarify this point.

Aside from such evidence of the effects of identification patterns, there are data on the therapeutic value of group integration in the Unit. We find a striking relationship between having friends and improvement (*Table 24*). Only about one-fourth of those who were not chosen as someone's friend improved, compared to over 80% of those who did receive such choices. While improvement prospects increase with increased popularity, the critical difference lies between being isolated without friends or having some friends.

TABLE 24   ADJUSTED UNIT IMPROVEMENT ACCORDING
TO POPULARITY

Improve-ment	None No.	%	1-2 No.	%	3+ No.	%
Improved	5	28	33	80	20	95
Not Improved	13	72	8	20	1	5
Totals:	(18)	100	(41)	100	(21)	100

Friendship Choices Received

$\chi^2 = 24 \cdot 8101$, 2 d.f., $p < \cdot 0005$

Further, the probability of improvement increases significantly if one's chosen friends reciprocate the friendship (*Table 25*). Almost 90% of those with reciprocal friendships improved, compared with about two-thirds of those whose friends did not reciprocate.

There is also some indication that friendships do not form haphazardly, but tend to be highly selective. One aspect of this selectivity is that patients seem to group themselves according to similar probabilities of improvement. In other words, patients with a better prospect of improvement tend to cluster together, while those with poorer prospects also cluster together (*Table 26*).

These data show that three-fourths (74%) of the patients whose best friend improved also improved themselves, compared with only one-half (48%) of those whose best friend did not improve, and only one-fifth (21%) of those who were without friends, differences that are highly significant.

TABLE 25 ADJUSTED UNIT IMPROVEMENT ACCORDING TO RECIPROCATION OF FRIENDSHIP

Improvement	Reciprocated Choice			
	No.		Yes	
	No.	%	No.	%
Improved	34	64	24	89
Not Improved	19	36	3	11
Totals:	(53)	100	(27)	100

$\chi^2 = 4.3326$, 1 d.f., $p < .05$

TABLE 26 ADJUSTED UNIT IMPROVEMENT ACCORDING TO IMPROVEMENT OF BEST FRIEND

Respondent's Improvement	Best Friend's Improvement					
	Improved		Not Improved		No Best Friend	
	No.	%	No.	%	No.	%
Improved	55	74	15	48	6	21
Not Improved	19	26	16	52	23	79
Totals:	(74)	100	(31)	100	(29)	100

$\chi^2 = 25.5604$, 2 d.f., $p < .0005$

Such inclusive friendship patterns may reinforce prevailing group norms which facilitate or impede improvement. They may give support by integrating patients into friendship groups. Furthermore, the friendships themselves may give substance to the Unit's contention that, under favourable conditions, people do care about each other and accept mutual responsibility for each other.

A critical aspect of these selective friendship patterns is that those people with the greater therapeutic potential and the greatest likelihood of improvement are precisely those who have the greatest capacity to enter into and sustain personal relationships. Hence, those who are most capable of making friends are the ones with the best chances of improvement and these chances are increased by the support of their friends.

We also have data which bear on the Unit's assumptions about permissiveness. The patients' problems are presumably bound up with at least one major pathology of perception. They commonly see the world as essentially punitive, and can gratify their impulses only at the risk of punishment. There are two polar types of reaction to this perception. One is severe inhibition, in which the person contains his impulses and lives in a frightened state of semi-paralysis. This is especially typical of the 'inadequate psychopaths'. The other reaction is one in which people confirm their image of a punitive world by aggressive behaviour which systematically evokes punishment from society. This typifies the 'aggressive psychopaths'. The Unit's answer to these perceptual distortions is to foster a permissive environment which will encourage the acting-out of impulses and assimilate the consequences. The basic idea is to disrupt the punitive expectation. Inhibited patients are encouraged to 'behave as they feel' so that they may learn that punishment is not an inevitable consequence. Hopefully they may thus lean to greater freedom and less fear in the future. The tolerance of the aggressive's disruption is also intended to challenge his image of a malevolent, punitive world. He is not met by punishment, but rather by efforts to give him insight into the foundations of his aggressive motives, and to wean him from them where possible. There would be little possibility of his gaining insight before his picture of the world is unstructured.

Against this background, then, what is the therapeutic value of such permissiveness? Our data contain four gross indices of acting-out disturbances. These include: psychological disturbance, social disruption, the more passive acting-out in the form of illness, and absence or tardiness. The patients were classified according to the average number of incidents per month recorded in the nursing records for each of the four types of disturbance. *Table 27* shows the proportion of patients improved according to the frequency of involvement in each type of acting-out disorder.

From these data it is evident that the extreme actors-out are not in the majority. But, most significantly, improvement is not proportionate to the degree of acting-out. Without exception, in each type of disturbance, the highest improvement rate is found among the moderate actors-out, those who are involved in *some* disturbance, but less than

TABLE 27 ADJUSTED UNIT IMPROVEMENT ACCORDING TO
FREQUENCY OF ACTING-OUT DISORDERS

| | Percentage Improved among Disturbances Reported per Month | | | | | |
| | None | | One | | One+ | |
Disturbance	No.	%	No.	%	No.	%
Psychological	57	49	74	65	37	49
Social*	126	53	42	64	*	
Illness	52	54	52	60	64	55
Absence-Tardiness**	54	50	65	77	48	35

* Because of few cases, social disturbances are simply dichotomized as None or Some.
** For this variable only, the size as well as the patterning of differences is statistically significant. $\chi^2 = 20.6158$, 2 d.f., $p < .0005$

once a month. Extreme disturbers and those who do not act out at all improve less often than the moderates. The size of the differences is less important than their consistency (though in the case of absence—tardiness the size of the differences is also significant), for in seven possible comparisons not a single reversal occurs. In other words, those people who fail to take any advantage of the Unit's permissiveness, and conform too closely to behavioural expectations, or whose inhibitions are not appreciably loosened, will not improve as often as those people who act out a little bit. Similarly, the 'excessive' actors-out seem less capable on the whole than the moderates of achieving behaviour which will be judged 'improved'. The excessive and the deficients may represent patients with defences too amorphous to be easily managed or, on the other hand, too rigid to be loosened by reassurance, at least within the time limits of the typical course of treatment.

The permissiveness doctrine is important in another respect: the handling of sexual impulses and sexual problems. The permissive Unit atmosphere creates opportunities for patients with sexual difficulties to begin straightening them out. This does not mean that the Unit is a hotbed of sex and promiscuity, but rather that sexual opportunities are available and the permissiveness allows patients to take advantage of them. As we have indicated in the section on 'pairing off', not all sexual activities and experimentation is approved, but individual experimentation may be encouraged for some therapeutic problems and needs. These needs are fairly important among the Unit patients, of whom fully 40% are either sexually inhibited or perverted, and another 55% have seriously troubled sex lives. None of the perverts and only 7% of the sexually inhibited are married; while 44% of the sexually normal are married.

To what extent, then, do patients take advantage of the Unit's permissiveness about sexual opportunities to establish relations with members of the opposite sex? We obviously cannot answer this question definitely, but only on a probability basis. Our sociometric data include the sex of the patient's best friend. Patients were classified into those with no best friend, best friend of the same sex, and best friend of the opposite sex. It goes without saying that these friendships do *not* necessarily indicate sexual relationships. But we simply assume here that patients with best friends of the opposite sex will have a greater incidence of heterosexual experience in the Unit than patients whose friends are of the same sex.[8]

Friendship selection is patterned according to the patient's sexual functioning (*Table 28*). These data show that one-half (51%) of the sexually 'normal' choose friends of the opposite sex, or with up to three times the frequency of the inhibited and perverted groups. Conversely, friendships with members of the same sex increase as we move from the 'normal' (37%) through the inhibited (44%) to the perverts (58%). It is noteworthy that almost three out of five perverts establish homosexual relationships in the Unit. For this group, too, the Unit's permissiveness may be functional from a rehabilitation point of view. If a pervert cannot be converted to a normal heterosexual life, the Unit is interested in reducing his guilt and anxiety and promoting as favourable an adjustment as possible to his homosexuality. In this sense, the sexual freedom may be therapeutic for this group if it allows the sexual problems to be faced with much less stigma and public censure than is customary outside.

TABLE 28   SEX OF BEST FRIEND ACCORDING TO SEXUAL FUNCTIONING

Friend's Sex	'Normal' No.	'Normal' %	Sexual Adjustment Inhibited No.	Sexual Adjustment Inhibited %	Perverted No.	Perverted %
Opposite	50	51	10	23	2	17
Same	37	37	19	44	7	58
No Friend	12	12	14	33	3	25
Totals:	(99)	100	(43)	100	(12)	100

$\chi^2 = 15 \cdot 5349$, 4 d.f., $p < \cdot 005$

It is germane to ask whether the heterosexual relationships have any discernible therapeutic value. The question is somewhat complicated by the patient's marital status. Clearly, for single people the permissiveness provides a fairly sheltered environment for heterosexual experience, and may give them practice and confidence in heterosexual association. The situation for married people, however, is not so simple. Although 92% of them are classified as sexually normal, this does not mean that they are free of sexual problems. Both positive and negative effects might be expected from their heterosexual friendships. If they have sexual affairs while they are in the Unit, guilt is one obvious possible consequence. Falling in love and becoming alienated from one's spouse is another possible hazard. Harming the other person through entering a relationship that must be terminated abruptly is another. On the other hand, if these consequences can be avoided, then sexual affairs in the Unit might help patients to work through and overcome certain sexual problems so that they can return to married life as more adequate sexual partners. Similarly, heterosexual friendships without sexual relations might give married people the sympathetic perspective of someone of the opposite sex in working through other personal problems which threaten a marriage.

On this basis, how do heterosexual friendships affect the rate of improvement in the Unit? These data for people of different marital status are shown in *Table 29* (where the few cases of divorced and separated people are included with the single patients).

TABLE 29 PROPORTIONS IMPROVED IN THE
UNIT ACCORDING TO MARITAL STATUS AND
SEX OF BEST FRIEND

Friend's Sex	Marital Status			
	Single		Married	
	No.	% Imp.	No.	% Imp.
Opposite	30		12	
		84		83
Same	42		21	
		57		67
No Friend	24		5	
		17		40

$\chi^2 = 16.840$, 5 d.f., $p < .005$

These data show fairly clearly that heterosexual friendships are significantly related to improvement. Of the patients who had friends of the opposite sex, five out of six improved, while proportionately fewer with friends of the same sex got better. Furthermore, we see that heterosexual friendships have no adverse effects on the improvement rates of married people. Thus, marital status is apparently not a limiting condition of the therapeutic value of heterosexual friendships.

Of additional interest, perhaps, is the fact that such friendships have similar value for both men and women. Controls imposed on the sex of the patient reveal that the heterosexual friendship patterns resulted in similar improvement rates for both sexes.

We must bear in mind that we may here be facing a halo effect. The patients with greater ego-strength and greater therapeutic potential are both more likely to improve and more able to sustain heterosexual friendships. Therefore, to assess the value of heterosexual friendships more carefully, it is necessary to control for ego-strength. The improvement rates of patients with different friendship patterns and similar ego strength appears in *Table 30*.

TABLE 30 PROPORTIONS IMPROVED IN THE
UNIT ACCORDING TO EGO STRENGTH AND SEX
OF BEST FRIEND

Friend's	Ego Strength		
Sex	Weaker		Stronger
	No.	% Imp.	No.	% Imp.
Opposite	20		20	
		75		85
Same	34		28	
		35		82
No Friend	21		8	
		10		50

$$\chi^2 = 41\cdot8916,\ 5\ \text{d.f.},\ p < \cdot0005$$

From these data it is apparent that heterosexual friendships make a significantly greater difference to people with weaker than to those with stronger egos. Among stronger ego patients who do name a best friend, the same proportion show improvement regardless of the friend's sex. However, among people with weaker egos, those with friends of the opposite sex have twice as high an improvement rate (75%) as those with friends of the same sex (35%). But, although ego strength may represent the primary set of improvement determinants, heterosexual friendships do exert an independent influence, notably among patients with lower therapeutic resources. In this respect, as with the data on 'acting out', permissiveness policy seems to receive some vindication.

IMPROVEMENT AFTER DISCHARGE

In this final section we will try to assess the effects of treatment on 70 patients in our sample who were seen in the course of a follow-up study. All 70 were seen six months after their discharge and 64 of them were re-visited a year after treatment. On these visits, the research workers compared the patient's condition with what it was before treatment. On each occasion, the patients were classified as Improved, the Same, or Worse than when they entered the Unit.

This mode of evaluation is far from satisfactory. One set of judges (the doctors and therapists) assessed the patient's response to treatment while he was in the Unit. A second set of judges (research sociologist and research social worker) estimated the patient's condition six months and a year after treatment. We cannot be certain that both sets of judges are using the same criteria of evaluation, or the same referents of the patient's original condition. Even though self-conscious efforts were made to obtain as full clinical notes as possible and to discuss criteria of judgement, the case notes and the Unit records are uneven and incomplete, making it uncertain to what extent common base points for comparison were taken by all the judges. Consequently, the follow-up assessments may be weak from the standpoint of reliability. Consequently, the follow-up data must be viewed with extreme caution. Nonetheless, they are the only data at our disposal and are valuable insofar as they can be related to treatment careers and other variables which we have already examined. Hence we will use these data, but with full recognition that they may conceal many hazards and pitfalls for the unwary.

What, then, were the apparent effects of treatment and rehabilitation in the Unit on this sub-sample? *Table 31* summarizes their profiles at the time of discharge and on the two follow-up visits.

Table 31 gives a very instructive summary and exposes a pattern which will constantly recur in the remaining data. We are immediately

Condition	At Discharge		After Six Months		After One Year	
	No.	%	No.	%	No.	%
Improved*	43	61	22	31	26	41
Same	20	29	32	46	18	28
Worse	7	10	16	23	20	31
Totals:	(70)	100	(70)	100	(64)	100

$\chi^2 = 18.7354$, 4 d.f., $p < .001$

* The follow-up sample has a somewhat higher rate of improvement in the Unit (61%) than the remainder of the sample (52%), but this bias will not compromise the interaction of the variables in the ensuing analysis.

struck by the significant difference in condition of the patients at the three time periods, and, most strikingly, with the degree of relapse during the first six months after leaving the Unit. Only one-half as many patients are Improved six months after treatment (31%) as at discharge (61%). In other words, almost one-third of the sub-sample are in worse shape than when they left the Unit. And this one-third is about equally divided between patients who relapsed to their pre-treatment condition and those who get worse. From this, two probable interpretations suggest themselves. First, the interlude of treatment apparently delays the collapse of the most seriously disturbed patients who were originally headed downhill. This can be seen in the steady increase of the proportion of patients classified as Worse at these three points in time, rising from 10% of those at the conclusion of treatment to almost one-fourth (23%) six months later, and one-third (31%) after the first year. Consistent with this is the observation that the Unit's permissive and sheltered environment was salutary for the majority of this sub-sample who showed improvement during treatment. Thus, a substantial number of these patients could respond favourably when relieved from the pressing demands of the outside world.

Secondly, it is apparent that release from the Unit itself constitutes a trauma for which the patients are inadequately prepared. The transition from a sheltered environment to an open one must be quite severe to cause half of the Improved patients to relapse. This implies drastically different sets of demands and adjustments to treatment in the Unit compared with adjustment afterwards. The whole question of effective rehabilitation measures in the Unit is once again raised.

A comparison of the follow-up profiles at six months and one year indicates perhaps our most important post-treatment finding. The second six months after treatment represent a new critical phase in which the reality pressures and supports are heavily brought to bear upon the patient. The remission trend of the first six months is modified in the second half-year and a polarization of patients tends to take place. The proportions of patients who decline into a worse condition and those who recover an improved state both tend to increase, at the expense of those who remain unchanged. In other words, it becomes increasingly clear that, away from the sheltering Unit, a large group of patients are simply inadequate to cope with the demands of adult life, while another, larger group successfully mobilizes its resources to meet the demands. Such resources may be both internal and external to the patient, drawn not only from insights he has gained in treatment but also from the possible support of family members and others around him.[9]

Primarily, though, we observe here a greater number of people improved at the end of a year than after the first six months, and this pattern consistently repeats itself in our follow-up data.

Our raw follow-up materials add further perspectives on the resettlement process. Here is sharper evidence that the second six months after treatment continues to be a period of dynamic adjustment. While the condition of a majority of the patients is judged to be the same after one year as it was at six months, others have experienced changes during this time. The nature of this shift between the six-month and one-year follow-up has been condensed in summary form in *Table 32*, which omits the six cases for whom there are no data at one year.

TABLE 32   CONDITION AFTER ONE YEAR
COMPARED WITH CONDITION AT SIX MONTHS

One Year (v. Six Mths.)	No.	%
Better	10	16
Same	42	65
Worse	12	19
Totals:	(64)	100

This information shows that the condition of about two-thirds (65%) of the patients remains stable between six months and one year. This includes all the cases rated as Improved, Same, or Worse on both follow-ups. But slightly more than one-third of the assessments have changed. Roughly equal numbers of patients have a Better or a Worse rating after a year than they had at six months. To the extent that the forces outside the Unit from which the patients have been insulated during treatment played an effective part in producing this pattern of post-treatment adjustment, they seem to have about equal degrees of positive and negative rehabilitative value.

What attributes of the patients, or experiences during treatment, are related to the persistence of improvement after discharge? Are major correlates of improvement in the Unit equally important variables for improvement afterwards? Our first observation is that follow-up condition is significantly related to improvement in the Unit, both at six months and at one year following discharge (*Table 33*).

TABLE 33   FOLLOW-UP CONDITION ACCORD-
ING TO IMPROVEMENT IN THE UNIT

Unit	% Improved in Six Months*		Follow-Up One Year**	
	No.	%	No.	%
Improved	43		38	
		46		55
Not Improved	27		26	
		7		19

* $\chi^2 = 9.9959$, 1 d.f., $p < .005$
** $\chi^2 = 6.8761$, 1 d.f., $p < .01$

Of the people who improved during treatment, 46% were rated as improved after six months and 55% after one year. The non-improvers showed only small fractions of these levels who were judged improved during the follow-up. Three times as many improvers (55%) as non-improvers (19%) were better a year later than they were before treatment. We should note, however, that the non-improvers made as great absolute gains as the improvers in the period between six months and one year. Each group showed roughly 10% more who were improved after a year than were improved at six months. One possible interpretation is that patients do have or use therapeutic potential which the

Unit does not exploit. Our data do not allow us to disentangle this from the hypothetical possibility of a 'sleeper effect'—i.e., where patients show delayed effects of treatment which are not apparent while they were actually in the Unit.

As we might expect, patients with stronger egos made significantly greater gains in the post-hospital period than those with weaker egos (*Table* 34).

TABLE 34 FOLLOW-UP CONDITION ACCORD-
ING TO EGO STRENGTH

Ego Strength	% Improved in Six Months*		Follow-Up One Year**	
	No.	%	No.	%
Weaker	40		37	
		20		27
Stronger	30		27	
		47		59

* $\chi^2 = 4.4836$, 1 d.f., $p < .05$
** $\chi^2 = 5.4501$, 1 d.f., $p < .025$

The patients with stronger egos have twice the improvement rate of the weaker in both follow-up periods. Again, however, even some of the weaker people—the worse therapeutic risks—make gains during the second six months after treatment.

In general, of the behavioural-defence types, the conformists and illness group do relatively well and the aggressives quite poorly after treatment (*Table* 35) with the relationship between defence-type and adjustment becoming statistically significant after a year out of hospital. We must warn, however, against the specially small bases of these percentages.

Except for the aggressives, all groups show slight gains in the second six months after treatment. The data indicate fairly clearly that the more passive modes of behavioural-defence (illness and withdrawal) are more conducive to satisfactory follow-up adjustment than active aggression. But this was notably not the case for improvement in the Unit where the aggressives showed a higher rate of improvement during treatment than either of the passive groups. The defences of the more passive people may not be strongly approved either in the Unit or in the world outside. But as modes of adaptation, they are not terribly disruptive and, hence, tend to be relatively more tolerable than aggression to people outside the hospital.

TABLE 35 FOLLOW-UP CONDITION OF
BEHAVIOURAL-DEFENCE TYPES

Ego Defence	% Improved in Follow-Up			
	Six Months*		One Year**	
	No.	%	No.	%
Aggression	12		11	
		8		9
Emotional Insulation	23		21	
		30		38
Conformity	15		13	
		47		62
Illness	6		5	
		50		80
Withdrawal	14		14	
		29		36

$* \chi^2 = 5\cdot6061$, 4 d.f., $p > \cdot05$
$** \chi^2 = 10\cdot312$, 4 d.f., $p < \cdot05$

The Unit encourages aggressives to act-out with a permissiveness not commonly found outside. During treatment, aggression is viewed as a symptom and is responded to with therapeutic efforts. Hence, within limits, aggression is functional in treatment and may be conducive to a substantial level of improvement within the Unit's sheltering walls. But outside, the situation changes. The tolerance of aggression is drastically lowered, its consequences are correspondingly more disruptive than in the Unit, and aggression typically evokes responses of control, punishment, or counter-aggression. Therefore, for the aggressives, there is a severe discontinuity between the Unit and the outside, between the behavioural adjustment in treatment and in rehabilitation. For the aggressives, the treatment period may be an encapsulated interlude immersed in a stream of worldly intolerance. What may help them to improve in the Unit may afterwards promote relapse if treatment does not fundamentally affect the basic personality determinants of active aggression.

A similar contrast between functional adjustment in treatment and afterwards is echoed in the relationship between trouble in the Unit and follow-up improvement (*Table 36*).

TABLE 36 ONE-YEAR IMPROVEMENT RATES ACCORDING TO DISRUPTIVE
ACTING-OUT IN THE UNIT

Monthly Frequency of Acting-Out Reported	% Improved in Follow-Up Type of Acting-Out*							
	Psychological		Illness		Absence, Tardiness		Social**	
	No.	%	No.	%	No.	%	No.	%
None	18		16		17		48	
		50		56		41		44
One	32		23		39		16	
		41		39		41		31
One+	14		5		18		—	
		28		40		39		—

* Chi-squares were computed for each 'acting-out' variable, and no statistically significant relationship was found with follow-up condition.
** Dichotomizes between None and Some reported.

It will be recalled (*Table 27*) that a moderate amount of disruptive acting-out was more conducive to improvement in the Unit than either a great deal or no acting out on four available measures of recorded trouble-making. The direct behavioural expression of personal problems was helpful to the patient in the Unit so long as it was kept within bounds. The limits of these bounds were, of course, much more liberal in the Unit than outside. Nonetheless, the people who were ostensibly most inhibited and were not reported in acting-out incidents did not improve in the Unit as much as those who showed a moderate degree of trouble. But our follow-up data show that, on the whole, people who did *not* get into trouble in the Unit have a higher improvement rate after a year than those who did. The tendencies reported, though not statistically significant, are regular in occurrence. The non-troublemakers may or may not have had lower levels of tension to erupt into nonconforming behaviour in the liberal atmosphere of the Unit. But afterwards they apparently showed a superior capacity to fill conventional roles and function normally. Hence, while the disruptive acting-out in the Unit seems to have had some cathartic value in treatment, it did not have as much carry-over value for rehabilitation as the sustained controls of those who were not disruptive.

Certain variables related to Unit improvement are also conducive to sustained improvement after discharge. We noted earlier (*Table 10*) a positive relationship between marital status and improvement during treatment, especially for the men. This pattern persists in our follow-up data as well, as can be seen in *Table 37*, where a small number of divorced and separated people are grouped with the single because their profiles are similar. According to these data, the transition from the Unit to the outside is about as difficult and has as great impact on the married as on the unmarried. But after the first six months, the married patients show a relatively greater gain in improvement than the unmarried. The gain is marked, though not statistically significant. They apparently benefit from pressures of role responsibilities, possible guilt from defaulting on these obligations, sympathetic support from other family members, and even changes in the functioning of the family as an adaptive response to the patient's illness. The family may also provide an arena where insights and therapeutic gains made in the Unit may be immediately applied to the working through of very important interpersonal relationships. Some of these points will be elaborated in Chapter 8.

As a group, the unmarried people may not benefit as much from such situational forces. They may not have as effective supports or as compelling responsibilities. Nor, as a group, are they as likely to be thrown into as intimate contact with people who are highly significant to them. In other words, despite all its stresses, the family represents a weighty set of constructive forces. For one thing it confronts the married person immediately upon discharge with reality pressures which he cannot avoid as effectively as an unmarried person. On balance, the family of procreation seems to operate as a stabilizing force, at least for individuals of the kind treated in the Unit.

TABLE 37   FOLLOW-UP IMPROVEMENT OF
MARITAL GROUPS

Marital Status	% Improved in Follow–Up***	
	Six Months* No. %	One Year** No. %
Married	17	15
	35	53
Unmarried	53	49
	30	37

* $\chi^2 = 0.0092$, 1 d.f., $p > .05$
** $\chi^2 = 0.7178$, 1 d.f., $p > .05$
*** Chi-squares were also computed to determine whether a relationship existed between marital status and degree of change in improvement condition as between six months and one year following discharge. The relationships found were not statistically significant at the ·05 level.

Marital status, incidentally, is the only demographic factor which bears any relationship to follow-up condition. Age, sex, and similar variables, have no influence on a patient's improvement after treatment.

But an interesting result appears with the crude measure of severity of illness previously used in *Table 20*. Follow-up improvement according to severity of disorder is shown in *Table 38*. Though the tendencies shown are not statistically significant, they are clear in outline.

TABLE 38 FOLLOW-UP CONDITION ACCORD-
ING TO SEVERITY OF ILLNESS

Severity of Incapacity	% Improved in Follow-Up***			
	Six Months*		One Year**	
	No.	%	No.	%
Total	29		25	
		31		32
Moderate or Single Area	41		39	
		35		47

* $\chi^2 = 0.0002$, 1 d.f., $p > .05$
** $\chi^2 = 0.7499$, 1 d.f., $p > .05$
*** Chi-squares were also computed to determine whether a relationship existed between severity of incapacity and degree of change in condition as between six months and one year following discharge. The relationships found were not statistically significant at the .05 level.

The one-year follow-up shows that the more severe the disorder, the less resiliency in post-hospital gains. Of those classified with a nominal total incapacity, just under one-third (31%) were judged to be improved six months after treatment and almost the same proportion (32%) after a year. On the other hand, those who were less severely disordered showed a comparable level of improvement after six months, but a greater gain after a year.

Further analysis of the data according to this three-category breakdown indicates that the greatest change occurs in the moderately incapacitated group. Both the severely and the relatively slightly incapacitated hold after a year to their respective levels of adjustment at the six-month point. The moderately incapacitated, however, make the bulk of gain shown by the less incapacitated groups.

The moderately incapacitated register the lowest improvement rate of the three at the six-month follow-up (23%). But, between six months and one year, their improvement rate doubles and reaches the level of the least disturbed group. The moderately disturbed, then, tend

H   215

to be the most problematic group in rehabilitation insofar as they show the greatest capacity for change after treatment. Presumably this is the group whose prognosis on discharge would be the most uncertain and most qualified, who have the greatest potential for improvement or deterioration. Accordingly, we might expect them to be disproportionately senstive and vulnerable to situational pressures which would heavily influence the course of their adjustment after treatment.

Previously we have seen that improvement in the Unit is related to pro-Unit value shifts (*Table 18*). But the failure to assimilate Unit values and shift to a more favourable stance during treatment apparently imposes no lasting handicap to adjustment in the world outside the hospital. Those patients whose values did not shift in a pro-Unit direction showed a steady increase in improvement rates, gradually erasing the statistically significant relationship that had existed between value-shift and improvement. They had one half the improvement rate of the pro-Unit shifters at discharge, three fourths the improvement at six months, and fully caught up after a year (*Table 39*). On the other hand, the pro-U shifters showed fairly stable improvement rates between six months (42%) and a year (45%) after discharge.

TABLE 39   FOLLOW-UP CONDITION ACCORD-
ING TO VALUE SHIFTS DURING TREATMENT

Value Shifts	% Improved in Follow-Up***			
	Six Months*		One Year**	
	No.	%	No.	%
Pro-Unit	24		22	
		42		45
Not Pro-Unit	32		28	
		31		46

* $\chi^2 = 0.2747$, 1 d.f., $p > .05$
** $\chi^2 = 0$, 1 d.f., $p > .05$
*** Chi-squares were also computed to determine the relationship between value-shifts in the Unit and change in improvement condition as between six months and one year following discharge. The relationships found were not statistically significant at the ·05 level.

Thus it is a moot point whether the acceptance of the Unit ideology significantly eases rehabilitation after the early transitional stage. The assimilation of Unit values is clearly helpful in the adaptation to the treatment situation and to improvement at discharge. But the ideology is so different from outside values and expectations that it poses a conflict between treatment and rehabilitation needs. However, post-hospital situational forces impose the outside reality so that those who have not accepted the Unit values are not significantly more handicapped than those who have in long-range rehabilitation.

We can also examine some of the more extended results of heterosexual friendships in the Unit which we discussed previously (*Tables 29 and 30*). Unfortunately, some of our follow-up data on this problem are so sparse that they cannot be meaningfully tabulated. But a few points may be reviewed.

In terms of carry-over value, we have observed that married people fare better than single people, and those who have heterosexual friendships benefit more during treatment than those who do not. Among the unmarried people, the gains from association with members of the opposite sex in the Unit may include increased recourse to sexual gratification, positive effects of role-practice in courtship, perhaps less awkwardness and self-consciousness, greater ease and self-confidence, and similar evidence of personal growth that comes from effective therapy. We might expect problems of heterosexual relations to be more salient for the unmarried than the married people in our sample. Accordingly, one might expect that the lasting benefits of heterosexual association are even more important for the single patients than for the married.

But our data show that these benefits have only a short life for the unmarried people after treatment (*Table 40*).

These patterns indicate that improvement rates during the first six months vary markedly, though not statistically significant given the small numbers, with the type of friendship which people establish in the Unit. Forty per cent of those with heterosexual associations improved, as compared with 30% of those with friends of the same sex, and only one person in seven who had no friend. Thus, heterosexual association seems to ease the process of transition from the treatment setting to life outside. But the one-year follow-up data indicate that these early rehabilitative benefits soon began to wear off. The improvement rate among those with heterosexual friendships dropped off to about 25%, while it rose by a comparable increment for those with friends of the same sex. Thus, heterosexual association seems to carry people through a period of 'after-glow' which loses its sustaining power and wanes during the second six months after treatment.

While these people apparently benefited from this type of experience

TABLE 40 FOLLOW-UP CONDITION OF UN-
MARRIED PATIENTS ACCORDING TO SEX OF
BEST FRIEND DURING TREATMENT

Friend's Sex	% Improved in Follow-Up***			
	Six Months*		One Year**	
	No.	%	No.	%
Opposite	17		15	
		41		27
Same	23		23	
		30		43
None	7		6	
		14		17

* $\chi^2 = 2.9756$, 2 d.f., $p > .05$
** $\chi^2 = 2.0855$, 2 d.f., $p > .05$
*** Chi-squares were also computed to determine whether a significant relationship existed between friendship pattern and change in improvement condition as between six months and one year following discharge. The relationships found were not statistically significant at the .05 level.

while in treatment, the benefits might have depended upon the special conditions which the Unit provided. In the relations between the sexes, the Unit was, after all, a sheltered environment. The norms favoured liaisons between people who had sexual problems or were shy. Furthermore, extensive opportunities to establish and develop these friendships were available in the nightly socials, free time, and other occasions. In such a sheltered, encouraging atmosphere, the burden of initiative on the patient was rather minimal. Under these conditions, heterosexual friendships had good results in the treatment situation. But such sheltered conditions do not necessarily prevail in the world at large. Friendships, dating, and courtship may require considerably more effort and initiative. People's defences in situations of potential involvement may not always leave them sympathetic and sensitively responsive to one another's needs. They may be more given than in the Unit to the ritualized dalliance and game-playing of dating and seduction. They may not search for serious personal involvement with the conscious purposiveness or grim earnestness in courtship with which neurotics sometimes advance and then defensively recoil if they meet rejection or conflict. In other words, in the association between the sexes, the sheltered conditions of the Unit provide different norms from those prevailing outside. Insofar as the situational supports and protection in the Unit are not duplicated outside, the ex-patient is thrown almost exclusively on his personal resources. While these may be adequate within the Unit, they may not be adequate for the heterosexual give-and-take of the rehabilitation period, so that benefits gained in the Unit might not last long.

We can turn now to evaluate the effect of length of treatment upon adjustment afterwards. It will be recalled that period of treatment was the most crucial single determinant of improvement at the time of discharge (*Table 19*). *Table 41* presents the follow-up data according to length of stay.

TABLE 41   FOLLOW-UP CONDITION ACCORD-
ING TO LENGTH OF TREATMENT

Days in Treatment	% Improved in Follow-Up***			
	Six Months*		One Year**	
	No.	%	No.	%
0–30	8		8	
		25		37
31–100	7		6	
		14		33
101–200	32		29	
		31		34
201+	23		21	
		39		52

* $\chi^2 = 1.7381$, 3 d.f., $p > .05$
** $\chi^2 = 1.8235$, 3 d.f., $p > .05$
*** Chi-squares were also computed to determine whether a significant relationship existed between number of days in treatment and change in improvement condition as between six months and one year following discharge. The relationships found were not significant at the .05 level.

These materials indicate several things. First, they show little association between length of treatment and rehabilitative improvement in contrast to the striking relationship shown in *Table 19* for improvement in the Unit. Also, they suggest that the very-short-stay people—the so-called 'bouncers'—do not significantly suffer for their intolerance of the Unit. One year after they leave, as many of them are improved as people who stayed six months. This may only be a manifestation of the 'flight into health' which is precipitated by the anxieties which the Unit may arouse. None the less, the 'bouncers' function as well a year after discharge as others who have been in treatment for a considerably longer time. To this extent, their low improvement rate in the Unit may be specious. They may not have changed appreciably in the short time that they spent there, but their designation as 'unimproved' may only be an indication of staff disapproval of their rapid departure and, of course, their lack of opportunity to observe the effects of the treatment stimuli.

It is perhaps significant that, after a year has gone by, the only group that distinguishes itself is that which was in treatment for almost seven months or longer. One-half (52%) of these people are improved a year later, compared with roughly one-third of all the others. This group also seemed to handle the early transitional state somewhat better than the rest of the patients. Thus, there is additional evidence that short-term therapy, however intensive, does not have the rehabilitative value of longer treatment. If treatment runs under six months, then length of stay is immaterial to the patient's adjustment a year after discharge. Patients who stayed six months were no better off than those who left after two weeks. This raises the possibility that intensive community therapy offers few rehabilitative advantages over no therapy at all unless patients can be treated for more than half a year.

SUMMARY

In this chapter we have examined the diversity of patients' responses to the Unit. We have tried to isolate factors related to improvement during treatment and afterwards, and have tentatively evaluated those assumptions of Unit ideology which were amenable to our limited data.

The data impose very severe restrictions. The small sample size, critical for many sub-groups examined, and the crudity of available operational indices necessarily limit the nature of our conclusions. We can only offer our findings as suggestive rather than definitive, and their validation or qualification must await further research. With this clear *caveat*, however, what do our data indicate about the effectiveness of the Unit's programme?

In general, demographic factors (age, sex, education, class) are not important in distinguishing among patients' responses. However, the Unit is more successful with less disturbed patients who have greater personality resources than with others. Patients with relatively greater ego-strength improve during and after treatment significantly more often than those with weaker egos. Those with relatively milder illnesses adjust better in the Unit and afterwards than the severely disturbed, although the moderately ill are an extremely problematic group in rehabilitation because their uncertain equilibrium makes them highly vulnerable to situational forces. The marital relationship apparently offers a predominantly stabilizing force. The married people do better in treatment and after discharge than those with broken marriages or those who have never tried marriage, although this factor is more important during treatment for men than for women. The lack of supportive out-patient services (especially for the moderately ill group who are not married) to ease the transition to normal life may be a critical factor for rehabilitation. The importance of personal relationships is underlined by the finding that patients who have a greater capacity to enter into friendships in the Unit respond more favourably to treatment than those who are more limited. Thus, in overall outline, the Unit is most effective when dealing with cases of less psychic disability and greater personal resources. Its marked interest, however, is in patients with inadequate personality development. While we cannot evaluate the relative success of the Unit and other institutions with such cases, it is clear that within the Unit itself the principal rewards of therapeutic success come from the patients with relatively stronger and well integrated personalities.

The factors resting on ego strength and personality resources show a marked association with both improvement in the Unit and adjustment afterwards. To this extent they can be said to delineate comparable responses to treatment and to rehabilitation. But areas of major discrepancy remain in which variables functional for the patient in treatment are of negligible value or positively dysfunctional for his subsequent rehabilitation. Skills or characteristics which facilitate his success during treatment may prove of minor or even negative importance outside. Thus, there is evidence which casts doubt on some of the staff assumptions about therapy and their equation of treatment needs with rehabilitation needs. For example, we have shown that the democratization and communalism themes might be reassessed in view of the disproportionate improvement in the Unit by patients with marked positive orientation to salient staff members, especially high-status staff. Such emotional investments seem to be associated with greater therapeutic success in the Unit than diffuse emotional involvement with groups, though the latter mode is the preferred one according to Unit ideology. Similarly, discrepancies between adjustment during and after treatment may call other staff assumptions into question. The most problematic areas concern the long-range importance of permissiveness and of the assimilation of Unit values.

Holding initial values similar to Unit ideology and shifting one's values closer to Unit beliefs are both conducive to improvement during treatment. But such conformity has only transitory significance insofar as nonconformists are as successfully rehabilitated following discharge as the conformists. The assimilation of Unit beliefs may cushion the transition to normal life after treatment, but this can probably be accounted for to the extent that any adoption of a positive set of beliefs or a faith may increase confidence and furnish ego support, regardless of its substance. Both the converts and the non-converts move into the outside world where drastically different norms and expectations prevail. These impose a new reality to which they both ultimately adjust in similar fashion. But for the nonconformists the ideology may create problems early in rehabilitation. This may be due to the fact that they feel guilt or anxiety and their confidence is undermined because of their ideological deviance in the Unit. Or it may be due to the fact that ideological nonconformists tend not to receive whatever supportive assistance the Unit does offer, providing at least an interruption of the trend toward confirmed social maladjustment.

Another manifestation of the problematic aspect of the Unit's equation between treatment and rehabilitation is seen in reference to aggression. The aggressives do better in the Unit than those with more passive forms of behavioural defence. Yet the aggressives are conspicuously less successful in rehabilitation than the passive groups. This pattern is echoed in the actual records of disruptive acting-out. The moderate acters-out in the Unit improve more than the extremists or those who get into no trouble, but those who do not act-out disruptively at all are still better adjusted in post hospital rehabilitation. Here the dissimilarity of prevailing values becomes crucial. Fundamentally the Unit encourages and rewards disruptive participation, so long as certain limits are observed and the disruptive tendencies of any given patient tend to decline over time. Correspondingly, the Unit frowns on passivity and regards the quiet observance of expectations with some suspicion, as if the patient were not properly manifesting his anxiety, hostility, or fear for 'treatment'. However, the outside world distributes its premiums otherwise. Simple role fulfilment without disruption and acting-out will satisfy the demands of most situations. The follow-up evidence shows that those who were most disruptive in the Unit are not sufficiently weaned from acting-out before their discharge. While the Unit gives them an opportunity to blow off considerable steam, this seldom equips them for a stable social role outside. But the docility of the passive groups which constitutes a treatment problem in the Unit becomes a good deal less problematic later on.

Another implicit problem of permissiveness is revealed by the interesting data on heterosexual friendships and activity. The Unit's encouragement of heterosexual association and even tacit approval of the development of interpersonal intimacies, though not at the expense of group participation, are apparently conducive to improvement during treatment, especially of unmarried patients and those of weaker ego structure. But such sexual experimentation and interaction do not affect the long-term rehabilitation of the unmarried. Presumably, the sheltered environment of the Unit does not approximate to the give-and-take of the courtship arena outside. Without the environmental supports, these patients apparently cannot function adequately on their own resources. The problem of applicability and persistence of treatment effects to the rehabilitation situation is thus raised once more.

Finally, we may contrast the progressive relationship between length of treatment and improvement at discharge with the necessity to have over six months' treatment before incremental rehabilitative benefits appear. While improvement in the Unit increased steadily with length of stay, a year later those who had been treated for six months showed no better adjustment than those treated for two weeks. Only patients with more than six months' treatment seemed better rehabilitated. This underscores the necessity to exercise caution in accepting what seems to be the Unit's tendency to equate improvement with conformity to Unit norms rather than with capacity to meet conventional problems outside.

This array of factors emphasizes the central point of the book. The Unit staff, while overtly stressing their subscription to rehabilitation goals and the attempt to make the hospital more like an ordinary community outside, have in fact developed a specialized therapeutic programme geared to their ideas of the treatment requirements of patients with socially disruptive personality disorders. Their notion that treatment and rehabilitation are being simultaneously and conjointly pursued blurs the actual continuities and discontinuities between treatment programme and compelling rehabilitative needs. They are sensitively aware of the treatment world in which they are immersed, but take less account of the outside world. These worlds are willy-nilly different and function according to drastically different norms. The failure to distinguish between these conceptually different sets of goals leads to an insufficient attention to the problems of differentiating treatment stages, grading experiences, and providing for adequate transitions between one stage and the next.

The fragmentary data reviewed on the impact of the Unit may be extended and given depth by qualitative data from our intensive studies of patients' families before, during, and after treatment. These materials are the subject of the next chapter.

NOTES AND REFERENCES

1. The term 'careers' has come into increasing use to describe the sequences of life experiences and adaptations an individual makes in connexion with having assumed at some point the role of psychiatric patient. Cf., for example, Goffman, Erving: The moral career of the mental patient.' *Psychiatry*, **22**: 123–42, 1959.

2. The materials presented on the absorption of new patients into the Unit are largely drawn from an unpublished report by Eileen Skellern. The collection of data on patient careers was made by Robert N. Rapoport, but a major part of the form in which its analysis appears draws on an unpublished report by Irving Rosow, 'The Patient and Treatment' (1958). Coefficients of correlation were computed by Miles Davis. The judgements about the condition of patients in our series after their discharge from the hospital were made by Terence and Pauline Morris. More detailed analysis of the bearing of treatment on patients' family adjustments outside the Unit will be presented in Chapter 8.

3. Jones, Maxwell, *et al.*; *Social Psychiatry*. London, Tavistock Publications; under the title *The Therapeutic Community*. New York, Basic Books, 1953.

4. Cf. Appendix A.

5. Kelman, Herbert C., and Parloff, Morris, B.: 'Interrelations among three criteria of improvement in group therapy: comfort, effectiveness, and self-awareness.' *J. abnorm. soc. Psychol.*, **54**: 281–8, 1957.

6. Unfortunately, the doctors' ratings present other difficulties. According to the doctor's rating, Dr B's patients were significantly less improved than the cases of other doctors. Roughly one-half to two-thirds of the other doctors' patients got rated better, as compared with only 14% of Dr B's. This is a significant difference. However, social therapist ratings agreed with Drs A, C, and D 86% of the time, while they disagreed with Dr B's ratings on individual patients' improvement about half of the time. Furthermore, despite the systematic bias in the patients' self-assessment, B's patients rate their improvement as no different from the patients of other doctors. Thus, we have a picture in which B systematically underrates improvement, for which some adjustment must be made.

In view of the high agreement between the therapists and the other doctors, we can substitute the therapist's rating of B's patients for his ratings. This will not completely eliminate error, but it will minimize it and reduce this source of bias to a negligible level. Accordingly, the remaining analysis will use this adjusted rating of improvement in the Unit.

7. This is despite the rather weak relationship between 'U' values and ego-strength, noted above.

8. Our data immediately reflect the imbalanced sex ratio of the patients, in which men outnumber women by almost three to one. On this basis, we would immediately expect proportionately more women than men to have friends of the opposite sex. Of those persons who do name a best friend, this is precisely what happens. Women are three times as likely as men to have best friends of the opposite sex. Three-fourths (77%) of the women have men friends and one-fourth (25%) of the men have women friends. Thus, the scarcity of women immediately increases their sexual opportunities and the available choice of men reduces the necessity to compete for male attention.

Furthermore, patients with greater ego-strength are better equipped to take therapeutic advantage of the opportunities presented and, accordingly, are more likely to have friends of the opposite sex. The data show a progressive incidence of heterosexual friendships from the weakest to the strongest ego groups. The neurotics (40%) are twice as likely as the psychotics (20%) to have such friend-ships, and the intermediate groups have frequencies between these extremes.

9. The Unit operates an ex-patients' club in a down-town London hospital one evening a week. This is not used systematically, but on a self-selected basis. We have no data on what part it may have played in producing our findings.

CHAPTER 8

The Family in Treatment and Rehabilitation

In previous chapters we have analysed the functioning of the Unit in some detail, and examined a cross-section of patients' careers. We found, with reference to families, that on the whole married patients, especially males, did better in the Unit than did others. However, we noted that 'improvement' as rated in the Unit is not necessarily correlated with 'improvement' six months following discharge: there was a decrease in the percentages of people helped in any discernible way by their Unit experience. Assuming a reasonable degree of observer reliability in the two sets of ratings, we are still left with the question as to whether post-discharge setbacks were due to the irrelevance of socialization in the Unit ('improvement') for life outside, to the temporary remission of illness in the Unit's sheltered circumstances, or to factors in the family (or elsewhere) that worked to undo any benefit from the experience in the Unit. However that may be, it was also found that married patients managed after a year to recover their improved level of functioning in larger proportions than other patients, suggesting either superior regenerative powers in family relations, or alternatively superior personal adaptive capacity in patients who had married. (On the whole the married group contained large proportions of patients categorized with strong-ego, who in any case tended to do well). In the present chapter we shall examine some of the characteristics of the family life of patients so that a deeper understanding can be derived of the therapeutic implications of a patient's being 'married' or 'living with parents'.

We shall describe the Unit's ideals and ideas about the place of the family in treatment and rehabilitation and the practices they employ to implement these ideals. We shall then examine some of the kinds of difficulties they run into as they seek to develop these new therapeutic dimensions, and discuss how the clarification of certain crucial conceptual points might facilitate the further development of these dimensions.[1]

IDEOLOGY AND RATIONALES FOR 'FAMILY TREATMENT'

The Unit staff are concerned with patients' families as a part of their general interest in taking socio-environmental factors into account when treating and rehabilitating patients. In some ways, 'bringing the family into the treatment' seems to epitomize for them the approach that blends treatment with rehabilitation, in that the people who become involved and to whom the patient must learn to adjust are probably those with whom he will relate following discharge (rather than merely people in 'comparable' types of relationships).

A set of ideas about the place of families in treatment and rehabilitation has become increasingly important in the Unit's treatment programme. Staff members talk of 'bringing the family into treatment', 'treating the patient in his family context' or, 'with reference to his total family constellation', or, 'treating the family as a unit'. Patients are sometimes told that continuation of their treatment depends on bringing in their family members, or that there is no use treating them as individuals since the family as a whole needs treatment. It is frequently stated among the staff that the patient may be the current casualty of the family, but that he need not be seen as the sickest one or the one most in need of treatment.[2]

Though these statements and ideas actually represent a variety of standpoints and assumptions, they are usually voiced in the Unit as though they were of a more or less unitary nature. The prevailing tendency is to see it as a 'good thing' to involve family members in the hospital situation in much the same way as it is generally considered a good thing to be democratic, permissive, and so on.

While the Unit staff do not explicitly systematize the variety of goals they have in dealing with patients' family members, they seem to use the following considerations most frequently:

Seeing family members may help to derive information about the patient that will be valuable in understanding the aetiology of the patient's disorder and in making a diagnosis.

Seeing family members may be useful in treating the patient because additional information can be added to the patient's own account of his familial relationships for the task of correcting his reality distortions. It is considered that in work with personality disorders, where perceptual distortions are less evident than among other kinds of psychiatrically ill, supplementary data of this kind are especially valuable.

Furthermore, the Unit staff consider it valuable to see patients' families because it is recognized that in the relationships between the patient and his family members there lie vital forces that not only have contributed to the patient's illness, but that might affect his actual career in the Unit. Where they see these forces as assets for the patient's treatment the Unit staff hope to harness forces as therapeutic 'allies'. If they see them as liabilities the staff would aim at neutralizing or transforming them so as to enhance their therapeutic effort.

Seeing the family members may, in this connexion, give the Unit staff some impression about the field of forces into which the patient is likely to return on discharge. The carry-over value of Unit experience is considered to have greater potentialities if the family environment is favourable. In unfavourable circumstances it is considered that a family can undo what benefit the Unit is able to achieve for the patient. The hope in working with such families is to mitigate these unfavourable circumstances, and improving the overall balance of assets and liabilities in the patient's network of relationships following discharge.

A final consideration sometimes mentioned is that seeing the family may make evident loci of disorder as severe as or more severe than those seen in the individual who happened to be referred as the patient. The primary aim of the Unit staff in locating these problems is to deal with them as potential sources of difficulty for the patient in his rehabilitation. However, there is also the feeling that members of the patient's family may also need treatment for their own psychological health. It is recognized that treating the patient may not only leave untouched other foci of pathology in a family, but that the treatment may actually aggravate old problems or give rise to new problems for others in the family.

All the above considerations are used on occasion. They tend not to be used as a systematic set against which the requirements of a particular case are evaluated, but rather as a collection of available ideas that are used eclectically in response to a variety of pressures and preferences.

It should be noted that although it is sometimes said in

the Unit that 'the family is the unit of treatment', we can see from the specific rationales (and as we shall indicate in describing the practices) that the family is not actually used as the unit of treatment. The rationales aim at bringing in family members to help the original patient. Sometimes the family member may, after this contact, come into the Unit for treatment for himself. Even in the latter, rarer case, the family population being seen as the extended limit of responsibility for the physician is quite a different idea from seeing the family as an integrated system of relationships which is to be treated *as a system*.

UNIT'S MODES OF INVOLVING PATIENTS' FAMILIES IN THE TREATMENT PROCESS

In general the Unit uses four techniques in attempting to work with family relationships of patients.

1. The 'family group', which meets weekly in the patients' 'free time' under the leadership of Dr B, is open to any of the Unit's staff or patients, with or without family members. This is the most 'U' method of dealing with families in its resemblance to meetings like the community meeting. At the same time it is the one towards which some staff members entertain greatest reservations because of the uncontrolled follow-through on family members, who are only transients and who do not have the group supports following the session that inpatients have, say, after a community meeting.

2. The induction of a relative into the Unit as a patient, and consequent treatment of original patient and relative (usually spouse), together in the same doctor's group. This technique, favoured by Drs C and D, has the advantage of examining both partners in the relationship in a round of activities, and then applying this additional information to their joint treatment. A disadvantage seems to lie in the abnormality of the hospital and Unit's living arrangements. The spouses must sleep in separate wards and participate in organized activities that are almost certainly atypical of the structure of their relationship outside.

3. Dr A prefers to receive relatives in his office, usually with the patient, often forming a small group discussion drawing in the appropriate nursing and other personnel. This maximizes control and the application of technical expertise, but differs most from the valued 'U' modes.

4. The social worker sometimes visits the family of a patient—on the impetus of his, their, the doctor's, or her own concern for some element in the relationship. While her visits are often occasioned by practical considerations such as securing money or housing, there is often a direct therapeutic component in her interest, and by feeding information back into the Unit she acts as liaison in an attempt to 'work with the family constellation'. Where she considers it relevant and possible, she attempts to bring about the family's use of one of the above three methods of participating in the therapy.

In the sections to follow in this chapter we shall present a picture of the problems that seem characteristically to arise in the Unit's handling of families in treatment and rehabilitation. In order to arrive at this picture, we studied a series of families in an exploratory though systematic way. We shall present the conceptual framework that we developed to make the study, and then discuss the problems observed in families of patients receiving treatment and rehabilitation.

A CONCEPTUAL FRAMEWORK FOR STUDYING FAMILIES IN TREATMENT AND REHABILITATION

In order to study systematically the problems of treating and rehabilitating patients with reference to their family contexts we developed a conceptual framework. We chose concepts that seem adapted to the Unit's ideas and approaches as well as being useful for the development of general theoretical ideas about family relationships.

In keeping with the Unit's orientation, we discuss a patient's 'improvement' in terms of his role performance. Since our focus is on family relations, we give greatest explicit attention to these, keeping other relevant arenas, e.g., occupational and recreational, peripheral. The patients on which we base our observations in this chapter are all males living with their families. Two kinds of families are represented, families of orientation and families of procreation. In the families of orientation the primary role relationships with which we are concerned are the parent-son relationships, where the patient is the son. With the families of procreation, the relationship in primary focus is the husband-wife relationship. Our discussion, then, centres on the role performances of *adult sons* and *husbands*.

It seems that the expectations in British society about what behaviour is required for individuals in these roles is fairly broad and non-specific. A husband, for example, may be very domineering with his wife, or he may be equalitarian and 'companionate' or very submissive. In some households husbands help with cooking and washing up, while in others this would betoken a 'feminization' or fall in status of the 'head of the household'. In one family it might be considered acceptable or even desirable for the wife to work, while in another it might be considered disgraceful.

If we think of the criteria for judging role performance we cannot profitably confine ourselves to *general* ideas of what is acceptable for a 'husband', or 'grown-up son'. There are a great many patterns that are acceptable for husbands or sons in different kinds of families. One approach to refining ideas about normative patterns of role performance is to consider sub-cultural groups as providing systematic differences in normative standards. Thus, it has been argued, while one cannot state with precision what is expected of 'husbands', one can become more precise if one knows the characteristic expectations prevailing among certain class or ethnic groups within society,[3] like second generation Italian-Americans, or working-class Yankees. These distinctions may be useful as a first approximation, particularly if patients of contrasting backgrounds are being dealt with. In a situation like that of the Unit, where most of the patients come from the more working-class sectors of society, intraclass distinctions become more relevant. Some of the important variations in family structure seem to cut across class lines.[4] However this may be, we are concerned with these variations from two standpoints:

Firstly, from the standpoint of therapeutic goals, the variations in family structure, even within a single social class in the larger population, provide different socio-environmental contexts to which patients return following hospitalization. It therefore would seem valuable in attempting rehabilitation to distinguish between *general rehabilitation* (i.e., activities aimed at fitting the patient into a social role conceived in a very general way), and *specific rehabilitation* (i.e., activities aimed at fitting the patient into the specific social role that is given form and substance by the expectations of the particular members of his family).

Secondly, from the standpoint of therapeutic *methods*, it is important to isolate elements within the family that contribute to role performance of an individual. Our preliminary investigations clarified the point that role performance could not be seen simply as a matter of the individual's personality, since people with similar personality structures were found to behave in a variety of ways in their familial roles. Furthermore, the individual's norms did not seem satisfactorily to 'explain' role performance, since we found that people with similar ideas of what constitutes right and proper behaviour in their social circles actually behaved in different patterned ways.

We therefore concluded that a profitable way of understanding how particular individuals came to be performing in their roles as they were could be arrived at only through seeing their role performances as emergent patterns of adjustment according to which they achieved some kind of a 'fit' between their own needs and orientations in the situation and those of the others with whom they had relationships.[5]

Looking at this 'fit' concept a bit more closely, it is clear that the unit of analysis becomes the relationship rather than the individual and his own set of norms or personality needs. Each family is composed of a number of role relationships, and these are combined in various groupings of relationships with different degrees of importance and different characteristic alignments in each family. Within any given relationships, the performance of the individual in his role is determined, hypothetically by:

a. the 'fit' between his personality and the personality of the other person in the role relationship;

b. the 'fit' in norms between the two individuals, and

c. the 'emotional toning' of the relationships, a qualitative factor that builds up as an emergent semi-autonomous factor in determining how the individual will behave in the relationship.

These concepts are schematically presented in *Figure 15*.

While this figure delineates a framework for a relational analysis, it does not specify particular variables within each category, i.e., of norms, personality, emotional toning. These can be varied according to different problems. For example, psychoanalytically derived categories of sexuality, aggression, and ego-defence mechanisms might be useful for typing personality dynamics. To localize therapeutic problem areas with reference to norms, it might be valuable to begin by distinguishing between people's ideas as to what is right and proper and the ideas held by their social group. Emotional toning might be described initially in terms of such gross differentiae as 'tension levels'. Role performance might be expressed in terms of various prerogatives and responsibilities. The most useful sub-categories in each of these dimensions will depend on the nature of a particular research or clinical problem.

FIGURE 15   *MODEL OF RELATIONAL ANALYSIS*

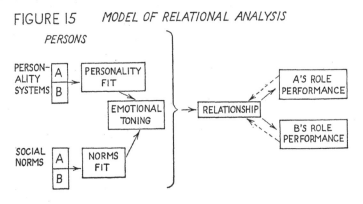

'The determinants of role performance and the actual emergent pattern of behaviour in the role, then, form a system in which successive adjustments are made to change in any element within the system. For example, if a husband and his wife were to disagree as to whether she should work and the disagreement were strong enough to keep her at home despite her own needs to be active occupationally, or if she went to work despite her husband's strong convictions, psychiatric difficulties might develop in one of the pair. If this individual were to become a psychiatric patient, the poor norms-fit in the relationship might be seen as a therapeutic liability that had to be dealt with. Changes in the pattern of role performance may come about through changes in the fit of norms, of personality, or of the emotional toning associated with particular behavioural patterns. By working towards such changes, liabilities can be minimized or even transformed into assets. In any given relationship, it may be expected that some elements are more amenable to change than others, and therefore there may be more than one 'solution' to the therapeutic problem of maximizing the assets in the patient's family. In most cases it is necessary to clarify the different perspectives from which elements are seen as assets or liabilities (the therapist's may differ from the patient's and/or those of his family members). Only after this has been done can consensus be reached and a shared therapeutic plan made.

With these concepts and orientations in mind, we shall present some tentative observations about the Unit's treatment and rehabilitation of the actual study series of patients with reference to their family contexts. We shall first present some characteristic problems noted in the families we observed. Secondly, we shall present some of the difficulties that the Unit staff seem to run into in applying their ideas and techniques. Thirdly, we shall indicate how we think that the use of a conceptual framework like the one we have described above could be used systematically for planning and implementing treatment and rehabilitation programme like that of the Unit.

For our first two purposes we shall draw on illustrations from all the cases studied. For the third, we shall present only a single case from the series to demonstrate in a more detailed way the use of the framework in taking into account some of the problems and difficulties described.

SOME CHARACTERISTIC FAMILY PROBLEMS OF MALE PATIENTS

The patients in the family study present the total range of variation in psychiatric characteristics described in the chapter on the Unit's patients. Most of the patients studied were diagnosed by the Unit staff as personality disorders; the two or three cases diagnosed as psychotic were among the younger unmarried patients. The personality disorder group, however, as already noted, were very heterogeneous in individual clinical terms. At one extreme—closer to the psychotics—were individuals with very weak egos, such that their fantasies verged on the bizarre and their affectual reactions were inappropriate. At the other extreme, also diagnosed as personality disorders, were individuals who might easily in another institution be diagnosed as neurotics.

Sociologically the patients studied were heavily clustered in working class groups. In the organization of their role relationships, however, they showed a very wide range of variation. From the point of view of internal organization, some of the families organized the division of labour—e.g., between husband and wife—along lines of strict segregation and rigid differentiation of who did what; some of the families showed an organization of great 'jointness' in role performance, with the husband and wife doing many of the same tasks together; some showed great 'interchangeability' in who performed the various tasks they faced. In external relationships, some families showed a very 'tight-knit' network (many of the people the husband knew were known to the people the wife knew), while others showed a rather 'loose-knit' network. They varied very markedly in actual numbers of people involved, with some having many external relationships while others have few.[6]

With reference to these overall patterns of organization in the family, two types of change were noted as the illness developed—*intensification* and *transformation*. Intensification involves the continuation in a more extreme form of a type of organization that was 'normal' (i.e., prior to the development of difficulties), while transformation involves change from one form to another as illness develops. Families show these tendencies in a variety of ways; some show them sequentially, some variably in different selected aspects of their overall organization, some in a fairly global way, but the striking thing among this series of patients was the way in which their developing psychodynamic problems were reflected in family organizational changes. This is not surprising, in the light of the Unit's emphasis on the interpersonal manifestations of their patients' disorders. However, relatively little attention has been given to the way in which these interpersonal aspects of the problem are linked to social systems like the family which function to some extent in response to systematic forces larger than those contained in particular relationships. An illustration of the intensification tendency is seen in one family, for example, where the husband had always tended to have relationships apart from those of his wife; as the illness progressed the tendency became increased to the point where he actually moved out and into the all-male residence of a monastic order, where women were allowed only as visitors. Another example of this intensification is seen in a family that had always had a small number of rather tenuous external relationships. As the illness developed, a process of attrition was noted, in which the terminal state at time of referral was that the family was almost completely isolated, save for the absolutely essential excursions for national assistance benefit and food shopping. The reverse trend, still exemplifying the intensification process, was seen in one family where the number of the husband's external relationships was found to mount as internal dissatisfactions between the marital pair increased. In such situations the most frequent pattern was for the spouses' network to become separated, with the husband seeking compensatory relationships with his friends in the public house or neighbourhood.[7] When this happens the wife often sees her husband's friends as 'rough' or 'a bad influence', and feels excluded. A parallel set of patterns can be seen with the son-patients.

Some increased their separate external relationships (e.g., visits to prostitutes), and others retreated almost entirely into the bosom of the family (e.g., staying at home all the time, discussing their problems with 'mum').

The social structural concomitants of illness, however, are not always in the direction of intensification of the family's pre-morbid patterns. The alternative pattern of *transformation* is seen in some families where types of internal organization and external relationship very different from their ordinary patterns emerge as the illness progresses. One family, for example, with strong segregation of functions by sex-role and a 'tightly knit' and extensive network of external relationships changed to a highly interchangeable internal and atrophied external structure as the husband's illness mounted.

It would seem that the intensification or transformation of certain aspects of family activity affecting the organization as a whole reflects the psychodynamic problems of the ill member(s) and those relating to him. Assessing a *family's* type and degree of disorder would seem important for social psychiatry for at least two reasons. From a therapeutic point of view where intervention occurs in the social relations network, it would be important to know which aspects of the network are 'normal', and which are reflections of psychopathological processes of the family members. If a family shows an extreme degree of segregation in their task performance in the family, it would be important to know whether this is merely an intensification of their 'normal' pattern of segregated role performance, or a transformation from their preferred pattern of joint activity that has emerged concomitantly with the illness of one or more of the family members. Different therapeutic strategies might be effective in the two situations. The second consideration is that of rehabilitation. It cannot be assumed, for example, that either more jointness or more segregation is better for the ultimate rehabilitation of any patient in his family context without reference to the family's normal (and normative) patterns. The Unit's stress on jointness as a therapeutic technique might not be appropriate in the ultimate rehabilitation of a particular individual.

An approach to assessing these processes of degrees of family breakdown has been suggested by Elles.[8] She argues on the basis of observing several such cases that the overall organization of the family shows states of breakdown that can be characterized in sociological terms comparable to the clinician's gradations of severity of illness and that a useful criterion for severity of illness would be degree of discrepancy between long-term norms and present behaviour. A family can be seen as least ill, having comparatively few disturbances in its system of role relationships, when each of the individuals is behaving in a way acceptable to his own sets of norms and expectations and those of the others in the family. The individual may be considered psychiatrically ill but the system may still function fairly well (e.g., if the illness is psychosomatic; or if the norms and expectations allow a wide variation; or if the signs of illness are kept outside the system. Some of the patients, particularly the single males, showed their psychopathology by 'acting out' quite outside the family system, so that the parents were surprised to learn of their symptomatology). The degree of family disorganization mounts as individuals perform in their roles contrarily to the needs and expectations of members of the system. Intermediate stages are noted where individuals may behave in ways that are disruptive, but the others in the family react in 'normal' (valued) ways so that to some extent integrity of the system is maintained (e.g., the husband gets drunk, but the wife does not *reject* him). More extreme stages are to be found where individuals not only behave contrary to norms and expectations, but the reactions of others are contrary to their own norms and expectations (e.g., husband gets drunk, wife has become so fed up that she no longer accepts him as a person, a state of chronic interpersonal rejection, retaliation, and warfare becomes crystallized).

While these degrees of social disorganization are related to the degrees of clinical illness of individuals, the relationship is not a simple one. It is a familiar enough pattern in clinical experience to find an aggregate of individuals, each of them seriously disturbed psychiatrically, living together fairly amicably (e.g., through insulation or collusions of various kinds). Similarly, families in which the individuals are not particularly disturbed psychiatrically can get themselves into crystallized states of disorganization and discord that require skilled intervention to sort out.

Actual problem situations, particularly among the types of patients treated in the Unit, embody an interplay between psychological and sociological factors. The more detailed patterning of the relationships between personality disorders and social structural changes in families is an important area deserving further research. We can indicate here illustrations of how some of the problems of disordered individuals get

237

played out in family situations. In presenting illustrations of problems frequently found in each of our family types studied (i.e., where the patient was an unmarried male living with his parents, and where the patient was a married male living with his wife), we claim neither novelty of research findings nor exhaustiveness of analysis of our data. As stated above, we seek only to call explicit professional attention to family factors affecting treatment and rehabilitation.

The illustrative 'type' problem to be discussed for the unmarried males focuses on the intense involvement of the patient with his mother, coupled with a complex relationship with the father. In such cases it was noted that the early intense relationship with the mother seems to have been at the root of the son's restlessness and later unsatisfying attempts to relate to women (e.g., through the use of prostitutes, through seeking an attachment with an inaccessible or forbidden partner, or seeking to make a relationship with the use of techniques that antagonize and alienate the girl, or simply through making it psychologically difficult to consummate a relationship).

In these families the part played by the father is usually very significant. In one case, for example, the father was idealized while he was absent during the war. When he returned, the mother experienced a severe disillusionment in him and turned her attention to the substitute relationship with the son. The son, who had been brought up with an idealized picture of his father, was now subjected to the mother's feeling of contempt for father and solicitousness for the son. It is not surprising that on referral this son presented a picture of extreme confusion over his own identity, capacities, and life goals. The general tendency in these families for the mother to see the father as a tyrannical, ineffectual, or otherwise contemptible person tended to be reflected in the sons' attitudes. On the one hand they seemed gratified by their special relationship with mother, but on the other hand they felt overwhelmed by the implications of this, angry at the mother's rejecting the father, identifying with, yet sharing mother's contempt for the father.

Where the patient lives with his family of procreation, our data indicate that a very prevalent type of problem is that of mutual disparagement between the spouses.[9] There was a great deal of jealousy, quarrelling (often accompanied by violence) and withdrawal of affection (sometimes expressed in frigidity or impotence in actual sexual relationships). These marital relationships tended to be described by the clinical staff as sado-masochistic. Sometimes in such relationships the husband would look outside the family for compensatory involvements—heterosexual affairs or involvements with other men. In one case, for example, the husband became more and more involved in the life of a monastic order of Anglican priests; in another case the husband got involved in business deals with shady men whom he really despised, in most cases to be ultimately cheated and deserted by them. Two of our patients sought escape in alcohol or drugs, usually with male companions. By the time most of these patients were referred to the Unit, the marital relationship had deteriorated to the point where primary motivation for entering therapy was not to be sought in the wish to repair the marital relationship, but in the concern for the effects of the bad relationship on young children in the family. Several of the patients mentioned this as the main consideration prompting them to get treatment. In at least two cases even this motivation had to be bolstered by external pressures like the law or family agencies called in by neighbours. To the extent that the patient is motivated to change relationships in his family along the lines that would be consistent with therapeutic goals, the family members in these relationships may be enlisted (if they are accessible) as assets to the therapeutic effort.

THERAPEUTIC PROBLEMS

In providing treatment and rehabilitation for patients representing these various problems, the Unit ran into a series of difficulties. We shall illustrate these by choosing two problem areas that seem both important in the clinical situation and germane to some of the central arguments of this book: first, the problems implicit in Unit ideology of family treatment; and second, the problems stemming from the ambiguities of boundaries and limits to Unit responsibility in the matter of family treatment.

As we noted above in discussing the staff's ideology on family treatment and rehabilitation, it is increasingly considered a 'good thing', or even a necessary thing, to get family members to come into the treatment situation. While 'treating the family as a whole' is considered desirable, there is no prescribed way for doing this, and each doctor is allowed considerable autonomy in his choice of techniques and rationales. This situation gives rise to several problems on the level of ideology.

While the staff refer to contacts with patients' families uniformly as 'bringing the family into treatment', various agenda seem to be at work in actual attempts to involve family members. Sometimes, for example, a doctor wishes to have a relative visit the Unit in order to get information about a patient so as to treat the individual patient's psychodynamic problems. In other cases the principal aim may be to assess family assets and liabilities so as to make an estimate about the probable consequences when the patient leaves the hospital and returns to his family. In still other cases the focal concern might be in changing the attitudes of the relative so as to shift the balance of family assets and liabilities in a favourable direction.

Family members, too, come for a variety of reasons. One might be primarily motivated by curiosity about the Unit; another by a desire to help the patient; some come out of guilt and the desire to be vindicated; some for self-help, and so on. The relation between the staff goals and the family members' goals are not always close to start with and they are not always reconcilable.

They may have different perspectives on what elements in the family relationships constitute assets and what elements constitute liabilities to the patient. In some instances, where a family member comes in ostensibly to help his relative who is the patient and then has his own motivations and relationships subjected to close scrutiny and re-evaluation, the feeling of being attacked is acutely experienced, with consequent antagonism toward the Unit and its methods.

An example of these different perspectives is seen in the Simpson case:

> Young John Simpson, a patient afflicted with a severe and long-standing personality disorder with limited prognosis, had a father who was highly successful and ambitious for his son. Both the father and son saw the father's high status and record of achievement as assets in setting up conditions for the son's career, but the therapist tended to interpret them as liabilities in that they provided impossibly high standards and pressures for the son which might exert a crippling effect after his return from the hospital.

> John and his father had a good norms fit about how John should perform in a work role. They both aspired to John having a successful career like his father. However, John's personality did not fit well with his father's ambitious drive and ability; he was relatively ungifted and lacked persistence and drive. Thus John's personality did not articulate well with either his own norms or those held by his

father. John's prognosis was poor and the therapeutic goal for him was limited. The work role considered realistic for him was as an unskilled labourer. It is with reference to this goal that the norms of *both* John and his father can be evaluated as liabilities (their concurrence making the situation worse), and the poor personality fit as constituting a further liability.

Put in its most general way, it would seem that the maximization of therapeutic gain to be had through involving families' members would be achieved by distinguishing among the different rationales for involving family members. By so doing a more careful consideration could be given to the purpose of any particular family member's entry. This consideration could then affect the timing and strategy of the entry, and ultimately the achievement of the goal itself. The Howe case illustrates this:

Jack Howe, whose violent episodes with his wife and family had got to the point of involving the police, had been in the Unit for three months and learned to use its language and to conduct himself in groups. He had become something of a group leader, and though he had not shown his own problems behaviourally in the Unit, he seemed to fit in well enough to be regarded as 'in treatment'. His doctor, however, left at this point, and before leaving told him that he would not be likely to receive more help in the Unit unless his wife came in too, so that the problem between them could be dealt with. In his new group he felt abandoned by his doctor, a drop in status among the patients as a result of being in a group who did not regard him as a leader, and his tendencies to run away were strongly mobilized. At this point he sought to take his prior doctor's advice and bring in his wife.

Mrs Howe was a person who had great difficulties in verbalizing, and when faced with a therapeutic group that demanded free communication and the expression of intimate feelings, she tended to withdraw and become passive. Jack used this reaction to mobilize his own defences against the treatment, and promptly left the Unit, stating that his doctor had said that he could not be helped more unless his wife came into treatment. His wife had come but had shown herself incapable of facing her problems and benefiting by the Unit, so he decided to leave.

It was the consensus of all concerned (including Howe himself on later follow-up) that his departure was premature. If Howe's family problem had been considered in more specific terms than simply the advisability of getting his wife into the Unit, it may be that more could have been done for him. It seemed clear that her presence stimulated his uncontrolled behaviour; this having been the principal therapeutic rationale for involving her in the first place. However, this also implied that bringing her on to the scene would require special precautions. The blanket prescription under which she was brought in tended to obscure this. Furthermore, with a person like Mrs Howe, whose difficulties in verbalization and participating in a group made the situation a rather awkward one, it might have been better if the participants had had a clearer idea of what she was there for. Neither she, nor her husband, nor the members of the new doctor's group had a clear idea of what the purposes of the visit were or what part the group might play in helping the family. The Unit assumption that the problems in any particular case would be discovered and worked out in the groups did not work out well in this case. The couple involved did not share this assumption and the varieties of motives at work were neither brought out nor reconciled.

Another instance of this problem can be seen among the unmarried patients illustrated in the Castle case.

Castle, a restless, suspicious lad of 22, claimed that nothing was wrong with him aside from a certain self-consciousness that made girls dislike him. He was the only case in the series studies in which the doctor felt that it was a 'bad' idea to have the family involved in the case. Castle had been the recipient of an inordinate amount of attention from his mother, who despised his father. The Unit psychiatrist felt that Mrs Castle had an enormous emotional investment in infantilizing Castle, and that she could not bear to see him grow up and become self-sufficient. The relationship between Mrs Castle and her husband was so bad (this being at the root of young Castle's problems) that she would have lost a major source of strength if Castle became well. She aligned herself against the Unit, and worked to get Castle out of the hospital. The situation was complicated by Castle's developing a strong negative transference for his doctor, accompanied by 'falling in love' with one of the social therapists. He saw the staff as hypocritical and snobbish since they would see one another socially outside the Unit hours, but would not date patients. This became something of an *idée fixe* with him, and he finally took his own discharge. When he realized that this was unwise and applied for readmission, he was refused as not suitable for treatment in the Unit.

This case illustrates the kind of situation in which the Unit staff frequently reason that *specific* rehabilitation (particularly in the mother-son relationship) is either an unfeasible goal or one that does not contribute to the *general* rehabilitation and/or treatment of the patient. An improved 'fit' in the particular relationship may be impossible with the methods at hand or undesirable. However, in this case there was a lack of clarity about the grounds of Castle's rejection. His diagnostic category placed him in the eligible group; his familial situation might have provided an unfavourable context for either rehabilitating him or treating his parents, but his own treatment and rehabilitation into another context might have been possible had all the issues been made explicit and dealt with on that level. The lack of clarity allowed him to perceive his rejection as retaliation for his interest in a social therapist.

The other rationale associated with the staff's apparent reluctance to deal with Castle's 'family problem' centres on the personal problems of the mother. Helping Castle seemed to entail harming his mother. We see here the second kind of problem coming into focus—viz., the problem of limits and boundaries of the Unit's therapeutic responsibilities. This aspect of the problem involves the degree of interpersonal extension to be dealt with. The recognition that changes in the patient have complex effects on others with whom he is involved does not necessarily imply a professional responsibility for these ramifications. Many forms of therapy explicitly restrict themselves to the patient himself. While the Unit takes an explicit interest in the broader ramifications, it does not clearly define the limits and conditions under which intervention in these extended realms will be attempted.

The problem of handling ramifications of the Unit experience has a temporal as well as an interpersonal dimension. In almost every case studied, problems were noted in the handling of after-effects of exposure to the Unit. The Unit is, in its present form, best equipped to deal with short-term effects of its treatment methods. Observation indicates that distinctions should be made between short-term and long-term consequences. In one case the Unit's group discussion methods stimulated a mother to disclose long-hidden family secrets including the fact of her own illegitimacy. In this case, though the short-term results were disturbing, the unmasking—which led to a chain-effect of unmasking of many elements in the relational system of a family that used a great deal of concealment and denial—created a new situation that seemed more favourable to the patient's ultimate healthy functioning.

We have considerable indications on both sides of the issue that reaction within the Unit does not necessarily predetermine reaction later. The Pyle case further illustrates that a negative reaction to the family group was followed subsequently by a constructive realignment outside afterwards. In the Knight case a positive reaction in the Unit only shielded certain negative after-effects of the family group:

> Mrs Pyle visited the family group with her husband and her son, who was the patient. In the group it came out that she was an illegitimate child, and this proved rather shattering for her—with much weeping and upset. Mrs Pyle steadfastly refused to visit the Unit again. However, this was the beginning of a good deal of unmasking of secrets in a family where there was a great deal of shielding and deception. As a consequence of this the family faced up to the severity of their son's illness—something that had been denied before —and so changed their expectations of him and their way of relating to him. While these changes did not, in the time of observation, change him in terms of his psychopathology, they did seem to affect the emotional toning of the family life as a whole, and ultimately there may be changes in Pyle's personality structure as well.

The obverse illustration:

> Mrs Knight visited the Unit and attended a family group. Both she and Mr Knight performed well, in that they discussed their problems in the light of their earlier lives and current problems and seemed to derive some new understanding. However, following discharge Knight used the idea that his wife bossed him too much (as had his mother) to assert himself inappropriately—determined to be the boss and apply the knowledge of the Unit experience. He used psychiatric interpretations of his wife's motivation as a weapon, and the net result was increased discord.

Another typical problem of delayed effects is when the patient has derived in the Unit a new awareness of the nature of his personality problems but as yet no new ways of handling them. Jack Howe, for example, recognized himself as a much more aggressive person than his self-image had allowed prior to hospitalization. However, his retreat to a monastery only served to bolster the defences against the expression of his aggression while no new channels were provided for discharge of these impulses. At a year after discharge from the Unit, Howe was showing psychosomatic symptoms and suicidal ideas while he kept a tight control on his aggressive feelings.

In most of the families studied, the patients at some point following discharge had a flare-up of their old difficulties in which the entire pre-hospital problem situation was repeated. In some cases there was an attempt to turn this re-enactment of the family problem to therapeutic benefit by 'having a group' and analysing it in the family in the Unit way. The ostensible aim in doing this was to try to understand the acting out so that the net gain might be a situation in which the problem was better worked through than ever before. In many cases, however, the use of Unit language and interpersonal techniques was abortive and the analysis of motivation took the form of epithet and mutual disparagement.

In several cases it seemed clear that the presence in the family of a disinterested professional person during these periods of recurrence of the old family problems helped to turn these episodes in a therapeutic direction. In one family, a social worker from a family agency visited periodically. While his pre-treatment visits had not been sufficient to stem the tide of family disorganization, his visits after treatment seemed more effective in keeping the therapeutic balance in the family. In another family a similar sequence was seen with visits by psycho-therapy-oriented probation officers. In four other families an impressive tendency in this direction was noted in association with very intensive research visits. While most of our research families were visited only about three times in the year following discharge, the intensively studied families were visited at least a dozen times. As an indication of the importance of the relationship with the research visitor we noted that in two of the families where earlier recurrences of the problem situation were constructively handled there were serious flare-ups just at the point when the research worker was about to terminate her visits. In one case the ex-patient lost his job as a result of knocking out his boss, and in another case the ex-patient was sent to prison for a recurrence of his characteristic pattern of swindling some money from the place where he worked.[10] It is impossible, of course, from our data to tell whether these flare-ups were the result of situational determinants unknown to us, to the usual recurrent pattern of the disorder, or to the withdrawal of the domiciliary visitor's support. The impressions in favour of the last explanation are very strong, but this remains an important problem area for further research. Whatever the determinants of these post-hospitalization difficulties, it seems clear that there is a marked and frequently disturbing discontinuity between hospital care and post-hospital experience. While the provision of after-care is a complex and controversial problem area, it is one that deserves more systematic attention. The present situation in the Unit is one in which the problems are recognized but the responsibilities are vague and the measures are rudimentary and haphazard.

In the section that follows we shall present in some detail a case analysis of a Unit patient studied before, during, and after treatment in his family context. In presenting the case we wish not only to illustrate how the conceptual framework outlined above may be applied to concrete data, but also to show how the use of such a framework can help to clarify issues like those implied in the ideological and jurisdictional ambiguities already described. We have, throughout the book, been concerned with the particular issue of the relationship between the concepts of treatment and of rehabilitation. The case presented provides an especially good illustration of how the retention of the conceptual distinction might have yielded therapeutic advantages.

THE FISHER CASE[11]

Don Fisher was a married man of twenty-seven who lived with his wife, Joan, and six-year-old child, Jerry, in his parents' home in a working-class neighbourhood in London. At the time of referral the relationship between Joan and her mother-in-law was strained, and the young couple ran their own household within the larger one. They could not afford their own housing at that time and had low eligibility for subsidized housing because of the number of rooms Don's parents made available in their home. In addition, Don preferred living with his parents, so made no great attempt to change their situation.

Previous to his breakdown, Don had been working for about six years in a garage, servicing and washing cars. He did well on the job, although it had been obtained for him by a brother as he always had difficulty in getting work on his own. At various times in the past when he had been expected to be out looking for a job he preferred to be sitting about at home, doing odd chores for his mother or making toys for his child.

Don always had a close, protected relationship with his mother, but a pervasive fear of his father whom he tended to avoid. His mother fostered the childlike attachment to her by not providing opportunities for his growing away from her. Even after he was married she always made facilities available in her own home for him and his family so that they could remain with her.

Although Don had shown various phobic and psychosomatic symptoms for some years, he had continued working until two of his fellow workers suddenly died. At that point he became unable to leave the house and go to work every day. When he was seen in the research he appeared more like an immature adolescent than a male adult. He displayed a syndrome of stereotypically non-masculine attributes, being dependent, having to stay close to his mother and wife, being easily frightened, indecisive, and unable to take appropriate action and initiative.

After psychiatric consultation he was referred for treatment in the Belmont Social Rehabilitation Unit and was clinically described as: 'an immature personality who has adjusted himself inadequately to the responsibilities of marriage and is still mother-fixated and homebound. The emotional dilemma is resolved by acute attacks of anxiety of which agoraphobia, a fear of insanity, and fears of illness are prominent features.'

He was first seen while at home waiting for entry to the hospital. At that time his wife, Joan, was also at home, having stopped working when Don could no longer go to work. Their son, Jerry, went to school daily and the household revolved round his timetable. They got up when it was time for Jerry to be got ready for school; while he was away Don made toys for him, Joan did the household work and prepared lunch for Jerry's return. After lunch they again got him off to school and then waited for his return. They had little contact with the outside world apart from Joan's daily shopping and contacts with social agencies, which she handled. Don did not like to be with people and resented it if Joan left him for long even to go and visit her own parental family. Don, too, put great pressure on Jerry to remain at home with him rather than play outdoors with his school friends. All in all, at the time Don was accepted for treatment, the household was pretty isolated and everyone in it was upset and afraid about what was happening. Don's mother took Don's illness badly and tended to blame Joan for it, while Joan saw Don's mother as the cause of his illness. Though Don and the family hated him to leave the house, by the time he entered the hospital there was little else that could be done as the household had almost come to a standstill.

With regard to the personality fit between the Fishers, it seems that Don came to the marriage wanting and expecting a replica of his mother in his wife. He expected a constant flow of gratification, love, and indulgence from her. He expected his wife to withdraw her attention from her previous friends and her family and be always available for him. He wanted this in addition to the gratification from his actual mother. By marrying he became responsible for other people, and from a reality point of view he could no longer depend on continual gratification of this kind. This created many problems for him. He pressed his wife to live with his parents and was continuously disappointed with her inability to indulge him constantly. He tended to see others as need-gratifying objects or as threats. Thus he had few links outside his immediate family, had a few close friendships which were not maintained, and did not seem to want to develop external relations.

While what Don wanted in a wife did not exist, what Joan wanted was also not realistic. She was looking for the affection, security, and understanding that she felt she had not had in her home. Don and his mother were, in some sense, parental substitutes for her. But they, too, did not come up to expectations. Not only did Don's mother reject her in many ways (she felt that Joan had taken her son away from her and that she had made him ill) but Don could not 'father' her. In addition, she was further frustrated when she found herself expected to be a 'mother' to Don.

Don and Joan experienced each other as unsatisfying in many ways and each felt the other was making burdensome demands. They both showed exaggerated dependence needs. Joan's anxiety about her own father's rejection of her was paralleled by a constant fear that her husband would leave her. This led her to attempt to control Don's movements so that he was away from her as little as possible, playing right into Don's own dependency needs. Don, too, needed to control things and people around him. However, their *modes of control* conflicted and generally led to frustration for at least one of them. Don used the passive mastery technique of the omnipotent child—by being very passive he would get others to do what he wanted. Joan, on the other hand, had to plan actively for her security. Don's passive mode of control reinforced Joan's need to control actively. She thus took on more initiative and responsibility than she might have otherwise have done. On the face of it, this seemed like a 'good fit' with the frustration for Joan taking place only at a deeper level. Since Don would not do the planning and make the decisions, she tried to take over these functions. But she could not be successful in this without the active cooperation of Don as the chief wage-earner in the family. Eventually she found it almost intolerable to allow their lives to drift on in an unplanned way. An instance of how they reached impasses that became intolerable for her can be seen in the whole problem of housing. Though having a separate home of their own was immensely important to Joan, the young couple did not have sufficient money to live on their own. Joan urged Don to save money and make some concrete plans for the future, but he could not do this. Don's avoidance of the ordinary restrictions of everyday life, of the problems of long-term planning and the anxiety they caused filled some psychic needs for him while Joan's frustration mounted. When Don was *no longer able to work* because of his symptoms, this frustration reached such a point that, coupled with the norms of all the people involved in the situation, some critical action was called for. The definition of Don as a psychiatric patient and his acceptance of this role legitimized his passivity and, at the same time, his willingness to accept treatment, and the very definition of his illness meant that Don's dependency needs took precedence over Joan's.

As far as norms about *conjugal roles* are concerned, it is relevant that Joan and Don both come from families in which the husband did steady jobs and so guaranteed economic stability in their families; and in which the wives played a more active part in decision-making and in taking initiative in other spheres of the family organization. There was a marked segregation of activities with the husband giving the wife a fixed amount of money and the wife not knowing the actual earnings of her husband. We may assume that Joan's and Don's original perceptions of how husbands and wives ordinarily behave originated in their families of orientation. The norms of both held that it was the duty of husbands to work and provide for the family, while the wife had primary responsibility for the management of the household. Don's default in this major area of responsibility could only be tolerated while he was defined as sick; even in the sick role, however, it was difficult to avoid the tensions and conflicts that arose specifically from the deviation from these norms (not simply from the economic and similar consequences of his illness).

In some areas, Joan had developed a set of conscious personal norms different from those of her parents. She felt that affection should be shown overtly between husband and wife and *towards children*. Don, however, seemed to accept his own parents' behaviour in this matter, and they did not make shows of affection. Joan's personal norm that the nuclear family should be united and separate from parental families conflicted with that of Don, who did not feel it was necessary to live separately from parents after marriage. According to Joan's norms, Don should have been stronger and more assertive as a husband and more prepared to share with her the household responsibilities and planning for their future. She felt that he participated too much with Jerry, their son, and usurped some of her mothering functions, while at the same time he was not sufficiently united with her against his mother. Don, on the other hand, felt that Joan was too active, that she should never have gone out to work as she did after the marriage, and that she should have been less concerned with her own mother and siblings. He felt that he should be her main preoccupation.

In general, then, Joan came to regard Don as an unsatisfactory husband and father, while Don came to perceive Joan as an unsatisfactory wife, mother, and daughter-in-law.

The *emotional toning* in the couple's relationship developed from their sustained interaction with each other. The way the personality fit and norms fit operated in the relationship affected the emotional toning and in turn was affected by it. As the frustrations for both Don and Joan mounted and their needs became demands on each other rather than their being able to gratify each other, the tension between them increased and they began to view each other rather

as enemies than supports. This fed back into the way they were dealing with their anxieties and they increased their demands on each
other. This only contributed further to their feelings of disappointment when these needs were not fulfilled.

The Treatment Phase

While both Joan and Don's mother were eager for him to receive
treatment, they were apprehensive about his going to the Unit,
which involved an indefinite absence from home and the necessity
for Don to live with 'unpleasant' types that might have a poor influence on him. Also, Joan was six months pregnant and the uncertainty
of his period of absence and the necessity for her to rely directly on
Don's mother whom she disliked were difficult for her to bear.
When he came home for weekends she tended to cry and to become
ill and panic just as he was about to leave. She was anxious to have
him return to help her, which tended to arouse Don's guilt more and
more each weekend he returned home.

During the weekdays when Don was away in the Unit, the actual
relationships in the home improved. To the extent that Don had
been instrumental in playing the two women off against one another,
their relationship improved with his absence. Jerry, who had been
kept at home through the attentiveness of his passive, phobic father,
was now 'liberated' to normal relationships with the children in the
neighbourhood, and partly through these contacts the family's
general isolation was somewhat diminished.

In the Unit, Don was a model workman in his workshop. He was
punctual and regular in attendance, got on well with the instructor,
did not waste time, and was reported as performing on the job like
an ordinary working-man in a shop.

He had little contact with other staff members—being a bit shy
with social therapists, talking to them only when he had their private
and exclusive attention—and he had a strong negative feeling towards his doctor. He resented being dealt with in groups, and rarely
used the groups actively. He desired, but did not get, more private
attention from Dr D, who, Don said, talked to patients 'not for their
sake, but for the sake of the Unit'.

During his off-hours in the Unit, Don tended to avoid women,
but to spend his time with two or three male friends. One was a
ward neighbour, an attentive homosexual towards whom Don was

initially friendly but less so later on when he heard that this man had told a social therapist that he thought Don had homosexual tendencies. Another was a rather aggressive, violent man.

Throughout Don's stay, he felt that the Unit was not coming to grips with his problems, which he defined as an inability to go out to work or to mix with people. Though his psychosomatic complaints multiplied in the Unit, neither he nor the staff focused on these as integral to his problems. He was obviously performing well in the Unit work role, which did not necessitate leaving 'home'. Yet he could not speak up in groups—showing such symptoms as palpitations or breathlessness at the critical points—and for the first time in his life he felt an inclination to smash things. These problems were interpreted as related to his underlying, unrecognized feelings of aggression. He showed recurrent disturbance as the topic of homosexuality came up, and began to express the view that this type of treatment was a waste of time for him, his problems being so different from the people he was 'lumped' together with. He tended to use the research interviews as places where he could express his feelings of antagonism toward his doctor and the Unit.

Don asked Joan to come to family group, and she came on one occasion. She was terrified by the Unit, resisting all attempts to draw her into discussion in the family group, and refused to return. She felt that the Unit was grim and depressing, and she didn't like Don's friends with whom she became increasingly reluctant to leave him all the week.

When Don, spurred on by his wife's mounting anxiety, raised the problem of her pregnancy, a few weeks before the delivery, in the group and his desire to return home to help her in the crisis, his gesture was interpreted as an attempt to run away from treatment. It was felt that to achieve his own defensive ends in this regard, he had raised his wife's anxieties and was now presenting this as an excuse to leave the Unit. It was felt that the pressure exerted on him by his family hindered his treatment.

Don's doctor left on vacation at about this time and Don brought up his domestic situation with greater clarity and vigour once the doctor was not present in the group. The members of the group were reluctant to act to let Don take leave of the Unit because of what the doctor had said prior to leaving on vacation. Meanwhile the time for Joan's delivery was drawing near and she put more pressure on him to come home to help with the housework. About two weeks before the delivery Don took his own discharge. He had come home for the week-end to find his mother and father ill in bed and Joan unable to do any of the heavy housework. He responded to this crisis by taking over control of the household work and insisting that it be done his way.

Don's new assertiveness at home was, interestingly enough, both a defiance of the Unit's position and a fulfilment of it. That is, Don was leaving treatment at a time where it was pointed out that unconscious acting-out processes were at work, with a strong implication that he should stay to work these through; but at the same time he was able to meet the new situation with a kind of resourcefulness that was partly due to insights he experienced in the Unit. He had realized that his moodiness and inability to be assertive in situations where other people 'stepped on him' stemmed from a basic confusion about his sex role and his consequent ambivalence about his desire to take the male role. On the one hand he seemed to submit to 'female' definitions, while on the other he reacted with resentment at not being manly enough. While he had rejected many aspects of the male role as being 'tough' or 'unkind', and his own preferred modality of behaviour as being 'kind', 'sincere', etc., he came to see in the Unit that often people who behave very aggressively may do so because of problems similar to those of other people who behave in a more 'soft' way. He was thus able to act within a less extremely polarized set of stereotypes about the meaning of active mastery as against passivity. Furthermore, he defined his wife's problem somewhat differently. Rather than seeing her as a person who was possessive and bound to have trouble with his mother, he came to see her as a person with certain insecurities stemming from her childhood situation where she was given insufficient love in her family.

Thus while Don left the hospital in direct opposition to his doctor, he did so with a set of attitudes that represented 'improvement' within the framework of the Unit's treatment and rehabilitation goals.

When Don flouted the authority of his doctor and took leave of the Unit, he did so with the explicit understanding that this act meant that he would not be readmitted. Curiously, the norms in the hospital about Don's participation in the treatment situation were so sharply discrepant from the norms about what was expected of him at home in the role of husband and father that he was jolted into clarifying his family responsibilities in a way that might have been less spectacular if the Unit had been operating more closely to its own ideals of rehabilitation. According to the latter, patients are meant to govern their behaviour in the hospital according to norms similar to those prevailing outside. In Don's case a set of treatment principles were in conflict with the rehabilitation principles and the Unit was acting in compliance with the treatment directives. By overriding these in the interests of 'ordinary' norms, Don actually accomplished his own rehabilitation, at least in the short run.

Post-Hospital Phase

After the baby was born and Joan returned from the hospital Don made it clear that the household was to be organized according to a sex-linked division of labour. Joan was to do 'women's work' and he was to do the breadwinning and to help her in the household only in an emergency. He got a job as a mechanic in a local garage that was so close by that he could bicycle home for lunch, thus re-assuring his wife about his absence and satisfying his own needs for home cooking. Don and Joan seemed to understand one another's needs better, and the emotional toning of the relationship was now characterized by a kind of resignation and acceptance of the feeling that they could not realize all their ideals in one another. Another factor affecting the emotional tone at that time was that Joan found a great deal of gratification in looking after her second child. The first child had been largely looked after by Don's mother while Joan was out working, and Don's mother had become rather pro-prietorial about Jerry.

The family was visited 18 months after Don's discharge. Don felt that though his job paid well, it was a 'dead-end' one. He vaguely felt that he should do something about getting a better job, but he had not stirred out of his old passive pattern to do much about it. There seemed little idea of getting a separate house, and Joan was suffering an increase in psychosomatic symptoms. However, she was clearly happy with her second child and her relationship with Don's mother had improved. The latter had been firmly put in her place at the birth of the second child and related to Joan subsequently more as a helper than as a competitor. While Don and Jerry were still very close, Jerry had a 'normal' pattern of relationships with his peers in close, Garry had a 'normal' pattern of relationships with his peers in the neighbourhood. Some of Don's phobias remained—e.g., against going into crowded places like cinemas—but he could now visit relatives. Don and Joan felt it less necessary to conceal their hostile feelings toward one another and expressed them in a joking way.

Thus this family was left with a sense of definite improvement, though only partly achieved in the ways intended by the Unit; but also a definite feeling of residual unhappiness, aimlessness, and resigned dissatisfaction.

Analysis

We would like to make several points on the general implications of the consideration of an individual's family functioning for his treatment and rehabilitation. When we consider the *fit* between the personality, norms, emotional toning, and role performance, in the familial relationships, certain points become clear that are not always seen if such conceptualization is absent.

First, *the way Don became defined in his family as a psychiatric patient* had implications for his treatment in the Unit.

For two to three years Don had shown various symptoms—fears of death, psychosomatic symptoms, and phobias about being in crowded places and open spaces. This led slowly to a more and more restricted life for himself and his family. Previous to these symptoms he had shown certain role deficiencies when looked at from his wife's point of view. That is, he had been unable to provide her with a home of their own and his passivity in this and other matters was a source of tension between the pair. Don's mother and brothers had helped a great deal to keep the family going by providing a home and finding jobs for Don. But as the stress on him increased, his role deficiencies became more pervasive. The patterns resulting from the personality fit, norms fit, and emotional toning in the couple's relationship were played out in the various areas of household organization. When the dysfunctions in the economic region became very severe, Don was defined as a patient. This was primarily because he was expected by all in the system to work and be the chief wage-earner. While many deficiencies could be carried by Joan, Don's mother, and others, once he was unable to go to work the family almost became paralysed. There were various situational supports—e.g., from the parents, but these could only be regarded as palliative. Don had come to a standstill, and at this point Joan could no longer take up all the role deficiencies Don displayed.

The recognition of Don as a psychiatric patient was delayed by a number of factors. Amongst these were:

(*i*) The fit between Don's passitivity and Joan's activity: Joan could make up for Don's deficiencies in many external contacts; also, she liked Don being at home so that she knew what he was doing; she could accept the demands that accompanied this pattern while the money for running the household was available.

(*ii*) Don's mother's need to have Don close to her, and his dependence on her, resulted in her making up for many of his role deficiencies, e.g., by supplying housing for Don and his family and increasing this as the family grew.

(*iii*) Don's norms about young married couples living with parents enabled him to avoid accepting Joan's definition of this as a role deficiency connected with his inability to grow up and become a man.

Other factors contributing to his definition were that, as a patient, he could draw unemployment insurance and sickness benefits, and his parents could help for a while. The only other alternative was for Joan to leave him and return to her family until the baby was born and she could work again. This was clearly less favoured than his definition as a patient. However, when Don's role deficiencies increased to such an extent that, according to the norms of everyone in the family, he was failing as a husband and father, the conditions were present for his definition as a psychiatric patient and for his acceptance of the sick role. The *delay*, however, may have affected his response to treatment, as it is frequently held that the earlier the illness is treated the better.

Usually, the definition of a person as emotionally ill, or as a 'mental patient', is thought of as having marked disrupting effects on the patient's family. In this case we see that the definition of Don as 'sick' had many positive effects for the family. This definition made his behaviour more acceptable in the short term and thus less likely to provoke anger, bewilderment, and disappointment. Defining him as a patient was preferable to seeing him as a neglectful husband. By assuming the sick role, Don accepted an obligation to get well and change some of his behaviour patterns. This was accompanied by a resurgence of hopefulness in the family, which was given a respite by his physical absence.

Explicit recognition of the social and psychological factors that moved him into the patient role might have aided the Unit to see how he would move out of it and what being a patient meant to him and the family.

Secondly, the *pervasiveness of the behaviour patterns and of the disorder in the family is of interest* in planning treatment and rehabilitation.

In the detailed analysis of this case, it was clear that Don's personality patterns and their *fit* with those of his wife played themselves out in a very similar way in each region of family activity. At the point where he was defined as 'sick', his role breakdown was pervasive—the manifestations being similar in each region. He became more and more passive in each area, until he did very little at all. As we have indicated in preceding chapters, this pervasiveness is not a universal pattern. Some people break down in one area and not in another; compensation in one area may make up for the deficiency experienced in another area. A knowledge of the loci of breakdown outside the Unit is important in relating role performance and its revisions in the Unit to problems outside. In the long run, it is important in gearing hospital treatment to post-hospital adjustment to be aware also of the family's changes during the patient's hospitalization.

Where the breakdown is partial it is more nearly possible for other people in the system to take up the role default. For instance, if it is only in the household organization that a man is unable to perform well, his wife may cover up this deficiency. If he is unable to work consistently, his wife may complement his earnings; but the more pervasive and total his deficiencies become, the less she is able to do this. In addition, in this case, Don did not like his wife going out to work and she was about to have a second baby; these circumstances combined to make it very difficult for her to take over Don's role obligations in the economic sphere, though she had worked for many years. Thus, if the family was to remain financially solvent, something had to be done to get Don back to work. The only apparent workable solution was to define him as a patient and get him to accept help. This permitted the family to reorganize themselves without his constantly demoralizing presence. Don's removal to the hospital, although disapproved of by his family, actually led to a reorganization which mobilized them once more. During the period Don was away, both Joan and Jerry seemed to take the opportunity to 'grow' emotionally. The relief occasioned by his absence enabled them to take stock and act more 'normally' again. The family thus developed potentials that enabled them to deal better with Don's emotional demands on them.

Facilitating such resilience in the family system so that a less strained balance can be regained is probably of great importance in helping the patient when he returns from the hospital provided that the new balance is not so consolidated that it does not allow for the easy accommodation of the returned patient. Changes in patients may, however, conflict with the family reorganization, so it becomes relevant to understand the areas in which the problems are displayed and to know where the *fit* is flexible enough to tolerate changes.

The *third point* is that *different social roles in this family supported different behaviour as 'non-sick'*. The 'sickest' individual (by clinical standards) in the family may not be referred as the patient because he may be in a social role that supports rather than highlights his pathology.

In the Fisher case it may be that Joan or Don's mother could, by clinical standards alone, be regarded as 'sicker' than Don himself. However, their familial roles and the fit in the elements affecting their role performance supported their behaviour sufficiently for this never to become a reality. Don, as husband and father, was expected to provide for his family. However flexible the norms that govern behaviour for fathers and children in Western type societies, contravention of this aspect is generally not tolerated. Thus, when Don got to the point of not being able to go to work, something had to be done. Although he had exhibited psychiatric symptoms for some time, his behaviour did not deviate so much from what was expected of him as a husband and father for any crucial action to be taken. Even his general practitioner, who was aware of his 'nervous' symptoms, did not refer him for psychiatric investigation until he broke down in his job.

On the other hand, Joan had many psychosomatic symptoms, was tense, irritable, bad-tempered, and depressed. She continued, however, to perform her minimum obligations as a mother to her child and as a wife. She cooked, shopped, cared for Jerry, and generally looked after the household. She cried frequently, and her doctor gave her 'something for her nerves' at one time, but never did she become defined as a psychiatric patient.

In this particular case, there probably was a real difference in the pathologies of Don and Joan. It seems that under stress Joan did not regress to such infantile behaviour patterns as did Don. In many ways, too, she seemed more adaptable to real life situations than Don, who needed a constant 'sheltered' life arrangement. But even if Joan could be defined as 'just as sick' as Don, her behaviour was such that the feminine role she was involved in supported rather than created strains on her. Even much of her obsessionalism, tidiness, need to plan, and so on, were constructively used in her household activities and duties. Don's passive, indecisive, clinging behaviour was, on the contrary, not supported by the social roles he had to fill.

The *fit* between the actors did not result in Joan's being defined as sick. Nor did she participate in the treatment situation to help her husband. Both these factors have implications for his treatment.

When Don came home from the hospital neither he nor the family defined him as sick any more. In addition, during hospitalization, he changed his orientation about his role in the family. He returned home determined not to be 'sat on' by his wife or mother. He desired to be more active in the control of the household. The opportunity was available because he returned home when his mother and father were ill in bed and Joan was waiting to go to the hospital for her confinement. He handled the situation very well, and when the immediate crisis was over he stopped his involvement with household activities, saying they were 'women's work' except in times of crisis, and he set about getting himself a job. He thus behaved in a way expected of him as husband and father, though this occasioned some surprise within the family.

The original definitions of Don's role deficiencies and the conditions in the family got him defined as a patient, while the new conditions and definition of him as non-sick operated to reinforce his desire to avoid further contact with the hospital.

In terms of treatment and rehabilitation goals, it would seem important to be aware of the ways in which an individual's social role support or bring out his 'sick' behaviour, since social roles in any family are partly a function of the expectations and behaviour of the other family members. To the extent that the goal is to fit the patient back into the same system, an understanding must be achieved of the specific characteristics of the system.

The fourth point is that the articulation between *familial norms* and the *norms of the treatment institution* was not in this case very good. This disjunction affected the *patient's response to treatment*.

In general, the manner in which familial norms articulate with the norms prevailing in the treatment system may have significant effects on the course of a patient's treatment.

As we indicated, the essential duality of the Unit's treatment goals and rehabilitation goals became highlighted in the Fisher case, where the Unit used norms antithetical to the family's norms. This confronted Don with a vivid contrast at a time when he was sufficiently 'treated' to be able to choose and implement the family norms even though this meant contravening the Unit's norms. In acting in this way he was actually serving the Unit's goals of rehabilitation.

Though some of Don's troubles were obviously still with him, when it was later relayed to him that he could return to the hospital if he wanted to, he was unable to, saying that his doctor did not really want him. If the norms in the treatment system had been better articulated with the familial norms, it is conceivable that some way could have been found for Don to be encouraged to fulfil both sets. For example, he might have been specifically told he could go home for a while and been actively encouraged to return. This might have facilitated further progress in the treatment situation and even given him a sort of trial at home. As the situation was eighteen months after treatment, he was still in a job, but resignedly, and still with his original psychiatric symptoms, sufficiently under control for him to be able to continue working in favourable circumstances. Subjected to undue stress, he might easily revert to the pattern he exhibited during his breakdown.

Here it becomes increasingly apparent that there are important implications of the family and hospital being interconnected social systems in that what goes on in the one affects the other. The explicit recognition of these articulations in a systematic form might improve the scope and effectiveness of treatment and administrative decisions. The two systems met, through the patient, when he broke down and was unable to continue working. At that point, the family's norms, the norms of the general practitioner, and the norms of the hospital coincided and Don's behaviour was judged as of such a kind that he was defined as a person needing psychiatric treatment. At that point too, Don's own personality needs were such that he 'wanted' treatment. This convergence led to treatment. The divergence of norms at the end, combined with some alteration in Don's immediate personality needs, led to the discontinuance of treatment.

With reference to the overall procedure of appraising and working with the family's assets and liabilities, initially, the perspectives of therapist, patient, and family members were fairly discrepant. The therapist saw Don's wife's demandingness as a liability that coincided with the liability of Don's mother's tendency to infantilize him. It was only after some therapy that Don came to see these aspects of his mother and wife as liabilities.

When he had been in the hospital for several weeks and his wife put pressure on him to come home, the psychiatrist, viewing the wife's demand in terms of the long-standing pattern, interpreted this as a therapeutic liability and Don's tendency to succumb to the demand as a resistance to treatment. Don, on the other hand, defined the demand and his own tendency to respond to it in this situation as normal and positive. He left the hospital, but with a re-definition of his participation in the household work as a temporary crisis expedient, a definition he was able in part to sustain.

The Fisher case further illustrated that the therapist and all the family members concerned need not bring their assessment of assets and liabilities completely into congruence for some improvement to occur. However, it would seem that, in the long run, Fisher would have benefited more had explicit attention been given by the therapist to the family situation. Had he returned to the hospital after the crisis of his wife's delivery, and received further therapy, he might have capitalized more on the assets uncovered in the crisis situation.

It would seem that therapy that aims at maximizing family support both during and after hospitalization involves not only working towards the establishment of collective therapeutic goals and definition of intervening stages along which movement is pressed, but also the alertness for changes in the overall situation that might require reappraisal of the therapeutic and rehabilitation plan. Situational changes may occur in the family whereby liabilities quite suddenly become assets. For instance, Mrs Fisher's demandingness, perceived as a liability by the therapist both in the precipitation of the disorder and in the context of the treatment relationship, became an asset in the new situation. Alertness to such changes enables the therapist to utilize them, or at least not to block them where favourable to the therapeutic goals. Thus, rehabilitation planning should begin in early stages of therapy; the goals to be kept clearly in mind if the family assets are to be maximally used in relation to them; and finally, sufficient flexibility should be maintained for changes in the situation to be incorporated in the treatment and re-habilitation plan.

The Fisher case thus illustrates many issues in the problem area of involving families in treatment. It is clear that others besides the patient may be 'ill' at different points in the process. The traditional focus of treatment has been on the patient; another viewpoint suggests focusing on the most 'ill', or alternatively the most 'pathogenic' individuals in the family; and still a third requires concentration on the overall family system without reference to the concept of illness but with re-cognition of the fact that different role definitions can be managed by different personalities with greater or less difficulty.

Perhaps the most crucial issue highlighted by this case from the point of view of our focal interests in this book is that of how the norms of the treatment system should articulate with the norms of the family and other systems external to the Unit. As we have seen, the Unit operates with twin sets of normative rationales—one geared to the aims of 'treatment' and often implying a kind of participation that is highly 'abnormal' in ordinary terms, and the other geared to 're-habilitation' and implying (in their terms) a kind of participation that is considered 'normal' in outside systems. Don's behaviour in the Unit seemed to the staff so 'overdetermined' by motivations that they con-sidered to need treatment that they acted on treatment rationales to the point of being diverted from the potential rehabilitation advantages to be gained by Don's at least temporary leave of absence. Whatever the psychological meaning for Don of his 'manipulation' of a 'withdrawal' from the treatment situation, such a withdrawal was in reality an appropriate thing. It was consistent with ordinary norms for a husband to return home to deal with a crisis. The Unit's construing this move as manipulative, and not providing any way for it to be worked through in Don's doctor's absence, actually provided such a discrepancy be-tween the requirements of the external life situation as to force the rejection of the former for the latter. Don's psychic health allowed him to achieve this, and it seems that his period of treatment contributed to this capacity. Subsequent events, however, raised the question whether a more effective level of rehabilitation might not have been achieved if Don could have been given a leave of absence to help at home and then reabsorbed into the Unit for a further period of treatment, perhaps helped by the home experience.

SUMMARY AND CONCLUSIONS

In this chapter we have described the Unit's ideas relative to the family and treatment and rehabilitation, the techniques they employ to implement these ideas, the typical family problems found in male patients, characteristic difficulties encountered in applying their ideas and techniques to these problem situations, and finally a case demonstration of how the use of a more explicit and systematic conceptual framework can not only highlight family problems but can also clarify possible ways of dealing with them.

We have indicated that the general ideology of 'bringing the family into treatment' subsumes a very complex set of therapeutic problems and practices. In some cases the physician's aim may be to improve the treatment of the patient, in other cases to assist with his rehabilitation (general and/or specific), or in other cases to help other family members in the situation. The perspectives of the others may or may not correspond with those of the physician. This discordance may create difficulties that interfere with treatment and rehabilitation, and an important initial task is to work towards goals that can be shared by therapist, patient, and family if possible. This entails an assessment of assets and liabilities in the family situation and a plan for enlisting effective supports and eliminating or changing liabilities for the actual therapy.

The actual choice of therapeutic techniques is based on the general preference of the physician rather than the specific and rational application of a technique to its relevant problem. The rationales tend to be expressed in blanket terms with a tendency to focus on cases that respond favourably to the method and give less attention to those that do not.

We have indicated some of the difficulties that these ideas and techniques seem to generate. Some patients, who could be helped by having their families come in, do not receive this help because their family members are not absorbed successfully in the Unit groups. There is no necessary correlation between the capacity of a patient to use a group and that of his spouse. Even where the patient is an active functioning member of the Unit community, his spouse may be unable to participate on sudden brief exposure and without supports external to the group. Cases like this might be better helped by more careful clarification of the specific purposes for drawing the family members into the treatment situation and more careful attention to the particular treatment technique that would be appropriate to the specific case.

A patient's transition from the hospital to the community is affected by the assets and liabilities to be found in his family. Assets and liabilities, however, are relative and evaluative terms—subject to reclassification according to goals and to redefinition according to the situation. A framework was suggested to examine systematically the determinants of role performance; this framework was also used for assessing family assets and liabilities relative to the goals of therapy.

One aim of making appraisals of assets and liabilities was taken to be the development of a plan for treatment and rehabilitation. Guidance can thus be obtained in making shifts in the asset-liability balance. Beneficial shifts may take the form of changes in norms fits, changes in personality fits, and direct reduction of tension in specific behaviour patterns.

The family provides only part of the assets and liabilities affecting an individual's post-hospital adjustment, and even these are affected by extra-familial influences. However, the assets and liabilities in a family which are relevant to the patient's transitions to the community can be best utilized if given explicit and systematic attention throughout the therapeutic programme.

In the cases we studied, the most acute problem noted was that of the absence of follow-up procedures. This is the problem of the ambiguity as to the Unit's sphere of therapeutic responsibility. The Unit staff provide some post-hospital support for patients in the London area by operating an ex-patients' club in downtown London once a week. Aside from the limited number of home visits made by the social worker, all contacts with anyone other than the patient anywhere except in the Unit, at any time besides the actual period of the patient's enrolment on the hospital books, is a departure from conventional practice and formal role prescriptions.

As the awareness of the Unit staff has grown that other individuals beside the patient may need help, that the greatest and most persisting help for any member of the family may be achieved by treating the family as a whole, and that there is a serious need for post-discharge aftercare, gestures have been made in the direction of filling these gaps. They have all been to some extent unsatisfactory, however, not only because of the lack of conceptual clarity but because of this disjunction between the ideals generally and the dictates of the conventional and formal system.

The question of the distinction between treating the family as a unit and treating members of the family as an aggregate of individuals has been raised. The Unit's tendency is in the direction of seeing its treatment goals in terms of treating the family as a unit. Its methods, however, are still geared to individual treatment. Primarily their responsibility and efforts focus on the individual who is referred as a patient. Most involvements of other family members pertain to helping the originally referred individual either in his treatment or in his general or specific rehabilitation. Under some circumstances another family member may come into focus and be handled as a patient in his own right. These instances, however, are exceptional and occur only under certain kinds of duress. The aim of rehabilitation can be seen in some ways as intermediate between individual treatment and treatment of the family as a unit. When the rehabilitation framework is taken as the conceptual orientation for action, the emphasis is on fitting an individual into his social context. When one takes the orientation of treating the family as a whole, the focus is on taking whatever steps are necessary to make the system as a whole function well, without particular allegiances or responsibilities to any individual within the system. While there is much discussion of this point in current psychiatry, its systematic implementation is rudimentary.

Ultimately some of the questions of treatment, rehabilitation, and system therapy are problems of values. Our essential position is neutral in this regard in that we do not advocate *per se* adopting more of a treatment orientation, more of a rehabilitation orientation, or more of a system therapy orientation. We do, however, advocate that the distinctions among these orientations be kept clear, so that when choices of activities are made to implement any of the orientations, they may be made on an increasingly rational basis. In the case of the Unit, we have indicated how some of its own goals and values could be better implemented through the use of more systematic conceptualization of their activities.

NOTES AND REFERENCES

1. The observations in this chapter are drawn from general data derived from studying the Unit, but more especially from the family study that was conducted under the direction of Dr Rhona Rapoport for the explicit purpose of exploring factors affecting patients' role performance. The family study consisted of a sample of 20 families of male patients living in the London area, of which 14 were

families of procreation and 6 were patients' families of orientation. Research workers included Miss Gillian Elles, Mrs Pauline Morris, and Miss Joy Tuxford. Occasional family visits were also made by Dr T. Morris.

Preliminary reports on the findings of the family study include: Rapoport, Rhona, and Irving Rosow, 'An approach to family relationships and role performance', *Hum. Relations*, **10**: 209–21, 1957; Rapoport, Rhona, 'The family and psychiatric treatment: a conceptual approach', *Psychiatry*, 23, No. 1, Feb. 1960; Morris, Pauline, 'Some disturbances of family functioning associated with psychiatric illness', *Brit. J. med. Psychol.*, **31**: 104–16, 1958; Elles, Gillian, 'The post-hospital care of the family', paper presented to the British Medical Psychological Association, 1957; Rapoport, Rhona, 'Patients' families; assets and liabilities', paper read before the Boston Research Conference, Massachusetts Mental Health Center, March 1960.

The present chapter is not a full report of the family study, but draws illustrative materials from it.

2. Most of the ideas presented in this chapter—both with reference to the Unit ideology and with reference to research findings—are not new. The work of Lidz (e.g., Lidz, R. W. and T., 'The family environment of schizophrenic patients', *Amer. J. Psychiat.*, **106**: 332–5, 1949), Spiegel (e.g., Spiegel, John P. 'The resolution of role conflict in the family', *Psychiatry*, **20**: 1–16, 1957), Alexander Thomas (e.g., 'Simultaneous psychotherapy with marital partners', *Amer. J. Psychother.*, **10**: 716–27, 1956), and Nathan W. Ackerman (e.g., *Psychodynamics of Family Life*, New York, Basic Books, 1958), and others have already covered the same ground and much more. Our main interest here is in relating these views and findings to the enterprise of providing treatment and rehabilitation in the context of a therapeutic community.

3. Cf. Opler, Marvin K., and Singer, J. L.: 'Ethnic differences in behavior and psychopathology: Italian and Irish', *Int. J. soc. Psychiat.*, **2**: 11–22, 1956; Kluckhohn, Florence R., 'Family diagnosis', *Social Case Work*, Feb.–March, 1958 (deals with Italian and Irish Americans and native Americans); Spiegel, John P., 'Cultural aspects of transference and countertransference' in press (Irish-American working class and American middle class); and Hollingshead, August B., and Redlich, F. C., *Social Class and Mental Illness*, New York, Wiley, 1958.

4. Cf. Herbst, P. G., 'The measurement of family relationships', *Hum. Relations*, **5**: 3–35, 1952; Winch, Robert F., *The Modern Family*, New York, Holt, 1952; and Bott, Elizabeth, *Family and Social Network*, London, Tavistock, 1957.

5. Rapoport, Rhona, *Psychiatry, op. cit.*

6. Bott, Elizabeth, *op. cit.*

7. It is interesting, as an aside here, that the English working-class term for male friends is 'mate', which in other usages implies the marital tie.

8. Elles, Gillian: 'The process of valuing and stages of family breakdown' (unpublished ms.).

9. Cleveland, Eric J., and Longaker W. D.: 'Neurotic Patterns in the Family' in Leighton, A. H., *et al.*, *Explorations in Social Psychiatry*, New York, Basic Books, 1957, noted a similar pattern in a rural township. Eisenstein, Victor W., *Neurotic*

Interaction in Marriage, New York, Basic Books, 1956, contains a wide coverage of types of problem in this area.

10. In the latter case some signs of progress were seen in that the ex-patient went off with the firm's secretary for two weeks with the stolen money, instead of, as his earlier, more infantile pattern had been, exposing himself to elderly ladies.

11. This section is based on a paper by Rhona Rapoport, 'The family and psychiatric treatment', *Psychiatry* (*op. cit.*).

CHAPTER 9

Summary and Implications

The Social Rehabilitation Unit at Belmont Hospital is an experiment in milieu therapy. Its work is part of the larger movement sometimes termed the 'third revolution in psychiatry'. The Unit developed in response to the convergence of a number of favourable forces during and after the Second World War in England.[1] These included the increasing awareness of the inadequacies of the conventional 'custodial' system of hospital care for the psychically ill, the growth of a national sense of responsibility for dealing with pervasive health problems, and the influence of psychoanalytic and social scientific ideas in psychiatry generally.

Experimentation with therapeutic milieux has taken different forms, the particular form in each hospital being governed by the type of patient being treated, the position of the hospital or unit in the larger psychiatric context, the orientation of the staff, and the personality of the director. It has been pointed out that innovating directors tend to have certain personal qualities in common—their dedication, optimism, and enthusiasm in keynoting conspicuous change.[2] Now that the therapeutic milieu approach is more widely acknowledged as relevant to the general treatment of psychiatric patients and an interest in its principles is becoming increasingly modish, it is perceived as germane to the work of a wider range of psychiatrists.

In this chapter we shall examine the implications of the Unit study for 'live' and controversial issues in the contemporary field of milieu therapy.[3] We use our Belmont observations in this chapter to derive general principles for the development of therapeutic milieux in other contexts.

We shall divide our discussion of issues into five categories that reflect problems in the field of milieu therapy generally. In each case we shall discuss the general problem and principles involved, state the Unit's position, and indicate the implications of the Unit study for the development of a milieu therapy programme. The problems are concerned with: (1) the formation of a treatment ideology, (2) the organization of staff roles, (3) the organization of the patient role, (4) the involvement of individuals external to the hospital in treatment, and (5) the conceptualization of treatment and rehabilitation as goals.[4]

THE FORMATION OF A TREATMENT IDEOLOGY

Ideologies are formal systems of ideas or beliefs that are held with great tenacity and emotional investment, that have self-confirming features, and that are resistant to change from objective rational reappraisal. Ideologues not only perceive and interpret the world around them in terms of the precepts of their own system of beliefs, but they tend to be especially convinced of the moral worth and special importance of their own particular orientations.[5] Ideology welds observable aspects of the environment into a kind of unity by filling in gaps in knowledge with various projections that ultimately supply a coherent belief system on which action can be based and justified.

The beliefs of the Unit staff showed many features characteristic of ideology. The staff have taken ideas from a variety of sources and added some of their own to integrate a nominally logical system for the active treatment of problems about which there was incomplete knowledge, considerable professional controversy, and few precedents or technical skills. After a formative period, their system of belief and action was presented as a unified group product shared by all members of the Unit and as an effective approach to the problems at hand.

The fundamental position on which the Unit treatment ideology is based is that socio-environmental influences are themselves capable of effectively changing individual patterns of social behaviour. Aetiologically, patients with no clear organic defect are seen as having personalities malformed by pathogenic social influences in their early lives. The Unit staff conceptualize this malformation of personality in terms of anomalous ego growth. These abnormal ego-structures are presumably manifested in defective performance of social roles. The Unit holds that faulty performance in social roles is a reliable index of psychiatric disorder, particularly for patients diagnosed as personality disorders. But the staff consider that therapeutic socio-environmental influences can be mobilized to reduce or modify the effects of harmful early experience. The most effective harnessing of socio-environmental forces for this purpose is the creation of a therapeutic community.

The deliberate choice of milieu therapy is thus *focal* within the Unit. This is in contrast to some other hospitals, where it may be ancillary, perhaps supplementing other forms of treatment which are considered the principal therapeutic agents—e.g., chemotherapy or individual psychotherapy. In the Unit, the use of milieu influences is not only focal but is also *total*. This means that every aspect of hospital life is regarded as relevant and potentially therapeutic. Hence the term 'therapeutic community' is used to denote the total hospital (Unit) involvement in the treatment enterprise.

As with many innovations, the Unit's ideas are based in large part on a reaction against the 'evils' of custodial hospital and punitive prison régimes. Many of the staff's ideas are derived from attempts to avoid some of the problems of the conventional mental hospital system. We have abstracted four major themes as comprising the core of the Unit ideology—rehabilitation through reality confrontation; democratization; permissiveness; and communalism. Each of these themes embodied a protest against perceived shortcomings of the conventional hospital system.

Patients in conventional mental hospitals were seen as becoming 'institutionalized' through adaptation to the special conditions of a closed, impersonal, controlled, and bureaucratic social system. Rehabilitation ideals were initiated to counteract the effects of a prison-like environment. In the Unit, the theme of 'rehabilitation through reality confrontation' is intended to make the hospital as much like the ordinary world as possible, and the adjustment of patients to this microcosm is assumed to prepare them to adjust to society outside.

The Unit staff saw many characteristics of conventional mental hospitals as inimical to the goals of rehabilitation. Patients were handled in custodial hospitals in an impersonal, standardized way. This tended to reduce their participation in, and ultimately their capacity for, forming ordinary social relationships; and it encouraged a passive, dependent relationship to the hospital authorities.

The Unit staff consider this process to be perpetuated in the training of individuals for conventional psychiatric hospital roles. In consequence, they emphasize the value of 'untrained', 'natural' persons, particularly in nursing roles, to form personal relationships with patients. Thereby they hope to eliminate impersonal, bureaucratic hierarchies, and to replace 'bad' relationships in patients' significant interaction networks with 'ordinary', 'good' relationships.

Under the conventional hospital system there was not only a chronic shortage of trained personnel, but presumably the definition of roles within the hospital system did not allow for the most effective use of what talent did exist. This was largely attributed to the medical staff's narrow conception of what therapy comprised and who was qualified to administer it. Conventionally, only physicians were authorized to give therapy, and therapy was considered to cover a limited range of transactions between the physician and the patient. The theme of *democratization* in the Unit aims at increasing patients' authority and participation in the therapeutic process. The Unit's position holds that everyone should be involved in both clinical administration of the hospital and in the administration of therapy; that *each member of the Unit* should have an equal voice in conducting these affairs; and that every experience is potentially therapeutic and every relationship potentially a channel of therapeutic influence.

The suppressive régime in the old-fashioned mental hospitals and prisons tended, it was felt, to reinforce patients' resentment of and anger against the established authorities. This is considered especially true of patients with 'psychopathic' personality disorders. Disciplinary situations induce in these patients either rebellious withdrawal or other forms of expressing negative attitudes towards authority, all of which are unfavourable for psychotherapy. The Unit theme of *permissiveness* is intended to foster a more positive attitude towards authorities and to permit freer behaviour that could be studied by staff and patients in order to help offenders to improve their social adjustment. The Unit theme of *communalism*—according to which a quasi-familistic environment relatedly provides patients with a supportive group acceptance—was developed to prevent the bureaucratic hospital's depersonalization and isolation of its patients.

The development of these ideological themes within the Unit serves several valuable functions. For one thing, a collection of staff and patients with diverse social and cultural backgrounds can be integrated into an organization about a minimum set of shared values and beliefs. Furthermore, the ideology helps members of the Unit to choose among alternative courses of action in complex problematic situations, thus improving morale, flexibility, and effectiveness. The ideology can also be seen as a loose body of theory whose development aids the quest for scientific psychiatric and sociological knowledge.

There is a tendency for the Unit staff to state its tenets in absolute terms (such as 'free all communications') which may raise problems. Such slogans are rooted in opposition to features of the old-fashioned mental hospital system. Slogans may lend a clarity and cogency that qualified statements would vitiate. For example, the *ex cathedra* simplicity of the slogan, 'We favour free communications', gains neither clarity nor elegance with the added proviso that 'We favour more open communication, particularly in authorized groups or with members of the staff'. Similarly, a psychiatrist and a hardened psychopath might agree that 'Most doctors don't know enough about the emotional problems of working-class people', and still establish a relationship. But if all the implicit qualifications of this statement were immediately made explicit, they might not be able to find a basis for even beginning the relationship. Thus, to leave many qualifications implicit allows for increased consensus when there are possible grounds for dissensus and where solidarity is necessary to achieve the group's goals.

However, if taken literally, slogans are not fully attainable. It is neither possible, nor in practice always desirable for communication, for example, to be absolutely free or for any staff member to be completely permissive. Ideological tenets are ideals which function with numerous implicit qualifications. Taken too literally they suffer from the discrepancy between ideal policies and real necessities, imposing a sense of 'contradiction' or inconsistency, as when a staff member behaves non-permissively because of incompatible or conflicting pressures in the situation.

One factor tending to keep qualifications implicit is the great gap in level of abstraction between the statement of ideals and the concrete situations to which they nominally refer. Everyone is willing to agree that permissiveness is a desirable thing. But the therapeutic value of permissiveness in a particular situation depends on the careful assessment of motivation and subjective and objective consequences of behaviour for the patient and for others. The decision may rest on the relative importance assigned in the circumstances to permissiveness, communalism, or reality confrontation. The principles themselves furnish no *a priori* basis of judgement. Particular acts are capable of being rationalized in terms of different ideals, and often it is not clear how any particular deal is to be implemented in a complex 'reality' situation.

Another factor is that specific ideological tenets tend to be held with fervour and conviction for somewhat autonomous reasons. A danger that this poses is that they may become goals in themselves. Being 'democratic' or 'permissive' comes to be the *summum bonum*, and the more fundamental question of how such behaviour contributes to any patient's therapy may be lost sight of. This tendency is enhanced, in the Unit, because of the separate formulation of each idea as an independent, absolute principle—with no statement of their interrelationship as a guide in the resolution of any conflict between them. There tends to be an assumption that each is a 'good', worthy end in itself, more or less regardless of context.

While the humanistic-sounding goals described are now rather generally accepted in psychiatry, some psychiatrists advocate different degrees of firmness and control (even punishment) as therapeutic necessities for certain cases. Even where there is general agreement on broad orientation—e.g., democratization—there are differences in the type and degree of democratization considered therapeutic under different conditions. In some forms of 'patient government', the patients' participation in decision-making is restricted to a well-defined and comparatively narrow-range of administrative problems.[6] In other forms, the patients' role is limited to the formulation of opinions, which are then referred for decision to the staff who make no pretence of delegating their authority to patients.[7]

Aside from the overall means-ends problems, there are also problems of internal organization of ideological tenets which flow from their heterodox origin. Unlike more evolved systems of belief, the ideology as it stands does not contain a set of principles for hierarchizing these values at points in which they conflict with one another. Thereby, any member of the Unit who is faced with a situation, for example, in which it is 'unrealistic' to be 'permissive' must resolve the dilemma adventitiously or expediently. Thus, the ideology functions adequately in very simple situations, but furnishes fewer guiding principles as the complexity of situations increases.

As an experimental psychiatric treatment centre the Unit is not only dedicated to goals of therapy (to which the ideology is directed), but also to goals of scientific knowledge (which may conflict with therapeutic goals). We have observed that some of the qualities that have helped to make Unit ideology therapeutically effective—the staff's deep sense of conviction and emotional commitment[8]—are precisely those that transform treatment means into entrenched ends in themselves, with consequent resistance to objective appraisal and to changes in the system.

In this section we have examined some points intrinsic to the treatment ideology. On the basis of our observations of unit ideology in action, it seems possible to state several implications that might be helpful as general postulates for guiding the organization of a therapeutic milieu:

Postulate 1: It is important to make explicit the ideas that are held by members of the group about how the milieu should be developed and used.

Postulate 2: A higher degree of consensus than is necessary in most hospitals is desirable among practitioners of milieu therapy.

Postulate 3: The principles developed should be explicitly related to therapeutic goals and recognized as means towards the achievement of these goals. There are dangers in regarding ideological principles as ends in themselves which may frequently serve to contravene the larger goals.

Postulate 4: In order to avoid confusion and maintain consensus the staff should continuously try to clarify how abstract principles are to be related to concrete behaviour in specific situations.

Postulate 5: It is important that the ideology itself constitute a coherent, logical system so that confusion in conflict situations may be minimized. Continuous work on internal organization of the ideology should assist people in the system in choosing from among alternative courses of action in an acceptable way. Techniques must be developed for hierarchizing values in action situations.

Postulate 6: There is an advantage in developing a shorthand concise and simplified way of expressing the ideas about which consensus is sought. These concise, sloganish statements should be presented with enthusiasm and a sense of positive commitment.

Postulate 7: Dilemmas and conflicts, however, can be avoided if the staff remains aware of the implicit qualifications accompanying the shorthand statement of ideological tenets.

Postulate 8: The enthusiasm and positive endorsement of ideology must not close the minds of the practitioners to the necessity for continuous scrutiny, evaluation, and revision. These measures are required if the clinicians are to use their ideas for the development of a scientific treatment theory, as well as for achieving social integration in the particular therapy context.

Ideology itself only *partly* determines the staff's treatment, which in turn only partly affects the actual outcome for particular patients. We shall examine some of the other determinates of social processes and therapeutic outcomes for the light that they cast on larger issues in the field.

THE ORGANIZATION OF STAFF ROLES

In psychiatric hospitals there is a great deal of experimentation with redefinition of staff roles. Dissatisfaction with the rigid hierarchies and with the classic restriction of therapy to a narrow range of role relationships is growing. The type and degree of change, however, varies greatly. In some hospitals therapies are being developed in a wider variety of professional roles than heretofore. Group therapy may be conducted in a single hospital by doctors, nurses, social workers, or psychologists and patients may be assigned to any of the groups on a random basis. Each group therapist can, and sometimes does interchange his role with the others. Other hospitals do not display this interchangeability of function among staff, but have increased the joint participation of people from several roles in activities formerly considered the exclusive province of only one. Thus, a doctor may not yield his therapeutic group leadership to a nurse, but he may have nurses participate as co-leaders of groups that he formerly conducted himself. The emphasis given to any particular method varies from hospital to hospital, as does the degree of jointness or interchangeability of functions among personnel. But the overall trend is towards the overlapping of functions which previously were sharply differentiated by role.

The Unit advocates an extensive interchangeability and jointness of functions among staff members. Specialized role prescriptions are deemphasized and blurred as much as possible so as to stimulate an equalitarian community with a great deal of joint participation of staff and patients in both therapeutic and administration affairs. In addition to the elimination of bureaucratic formalities, the Unit seeks through the flattening of the power hierarchy to maximize the use of whatever skills and talents are present in the staff, regardless of anybody's formal position in the authority structure.

What are some of the difficulties observed in this revision of the conventional staff roles and what generalizations and implications may be derived from these observations?

First, we have noted discrepancies between the informal role conceptions promulgated by the Unit staff and those formally laid down in tradition and statute within the profession and the hospital structure. While the Unit wants its staff to be equalitarian and to have interchangeable functions, the hospital system prescribes a hierarchical and specialized organization of roles. In other words, a system of broadly diffused authority and responsibility is posed against formal requirements of highly differentiated authority and responsibility. The 'built-in' contradictions between these two sets of role conceptions and their associated expectations give rise to patterned dilemmas for the staff. These dilemmas vary according to specific role. Doctors, for example, tend to experience more acute dilemmas in the area of responsibility and authority, while nurses encounter conflicts in the area of affectual involvement with patients. All roles, however, have many common elements. People must work out for themselves ways of resolving the dilemmas of any particular position. Their modes of resolution vary somewhat by role according to such factors as transiency, formal authority, and the number of persons in the role. The choice of resolution also depends on the personality of the incumbent. Thus, an obsessional doctor on the permanent staff, one of the few people close to the pinnacle of the formal authority structure, may resolve strains by becoming unusually restrictive. He might rationalize this in terms of medical responsibility and reality pressures. Another doctor in the same position might tend to withdraw from the Unit and to spend time drinking in local bars with patients, rationalizing this on the grounds of permissiveness and communalism.[9]

In general, it may be observed that where deviating innovations occur within an established system which retains jurisdiction over the innovating sub-system, personnel will experience endemic strains. Conflict may develop in external relations; conflicts may arise between staff members who are more exposed to external controls (e.g., the director) and subordinates who are less exposed (e.g., a staff physician with tenure who does not immediately account for his activities to higher authorities outside the Unit); or personal strains may develop which reflect the chronic conflict between two incompatible sets of role obligations.

In the Unit, the staff's ideal role conceptions, which blur specialized skills and attributes, are not fully accepted by patients. There is a systematic tendency for patients to defer to doctors and other staff in accordance with the prevailing cultural definitions of hierarchical role authority. Indeed, it would seem that such differential deference may indicate good 'reality testing' and mental health as reflected in the superior improvement of those patients who act as if staff authority cohered with conventional patterns.

The de-emphasis of formal differences between staff positions is reflected in the conception that *untrained* personnel are best in the social therapist role. The social therapists are transient and drawn from the general population outside the hospital. They do not systematically return to any specific professional positions, though many of them do go into some form of social work. The use of untrained nurses avoids the difficulties of *inappropriately* trained staff and has some additional positive functions (e.g., creating a group of personnel comparable to the patients in transiency, but made up of healthy individuals). However, it does not develop a stable corps of competent, *appropriately* trained specialists within the Unit or for the profession at large. Conceivably the continuous recruitment of these 'healthy' transients represents the most satisfactory way to create and maintain therapeutic milieux although there is little evidence for this assumption. It seems more likely that this approach was effective in the transitional period when the new concepts of milieu therapy were being implemented.

The stimuli towards change, to which the social therapist role was one response, are generally being met in milieu therapy in at least two different ways. One approach is by modification of psychiatric nurses' training and practice. With increased professionalization of nursing, has come a trend towards their more active participation in medical treatment and rehabilitation.[10] This experimentation in the changing nurse's role includes their conduct of therapeutic groups, formerly the prerogative of doctors and/or clinical psychologists. The second new approach that parallels the Unit's conception of social therapists makes greater use of volunteers and untrained people in involving mental hospital patients in a normal-like round of activities.[11] A good deal of experimentation is under way on the effects of such people, under various conditions, upon the rehabilitation of patients.

From observations of the Unit's organization of staff roles, it seems possible to derive some implications that might be valuable as general postulates of staff organization in therapeutic communities:

Postulate 9: Role conflicts can be reduced by minimizing discrepant directives impinging on staff members. Among innovating institutions there is frequently a discrepancy between ideologically prescribed behaviour and role behaviour prescribed in the conventional system. The first step in minimizing contra-therapeutic potentials engendered by these discrepancies is to make them explicit.

Postulate 10: Where there is a radical discrepancy between formally prescribed conventional role obligations and informally prescribed ideological norms, which cannot be handled informally, a structural change in the social system may be required. Relevant structural changes might be a change in the formal requirements, a change in the ideological requirements, or a change in the relation between the two by disengaging the innovating system from the jurisdiction of the discrepant formal system (e.g., by establishing an autonomous institution).

Postulate 11: Where harmonization, neutralization, or disengagement of discrepant role directives are not possible, it is advisable to make explicit the effective limitations of the ideological prescriptions in the particular context. Where this is not done, role-incumbents may feel an unnecessary sense of failure or it may encourage the extensive use of denial. Both reactions tend to be antithetical to the goals of therapy.

Postulate 12: Continuous turnover of staff is a short-term expedient for abolishing tradition-bound rigidities and introducing therapeutic 'naturalness' and 'spontaneity'. However, the haphazard training and the flow of transient trainees to work outside the profession is inimical to the consolidation of milieu therapy methods in an experienced corps of practitioners. The development of professional practitioners with the new skills of milieu therapy will depend in part on systematic training and institutionalization of the therapeutic roles.

THE ORGANIZATION OF PATIENT ACTIVITIES

The organization of patient roles will vary within the capacities of different groups of patients. Psychiatrists generally agree that those with the greatest personality resources are easiest to work with, can accept the greatest responsibilities and do best therapeutically. Other things being equal, younger individuals, with comparatively strong egos, generally respond more favourably and with longer effects than do the older entrenched and deteriorated cases. These differences will affect institutional policy in defining the role of the patient.

One point emphasized by the Unit staff in structuring the role of patient is the importance of peer-group relationships. They feel that this is effective not only because psychopathic patients tend to resist the influence of staff authority figures, but also because of cultural gaps that exist between the majority of physicians and the majority of patients. Middle-class physicians must bridge sub-cultural differences in treating working-class patients. One way to improve patient-staff communications across this gap is to channel it through patient intermediaries. Thereby, possible barriers of class norms and language with individual patients may be hopefully moderated by translations of other more perceptive patients.

In the larger field, milieu therapists differ in the way they allow patients to participate in therapy. In some instances it is considered useful for patients to increase their interaction and 'socializing' without discussion of one another's psychological problems or motives; in other instances they are encouraged to comment on social consequences of one another's behaviour but not on motivation;[12] in only a few instances outside of formal group therapy are patients encouraged to analyse one another's motivations.[13] The only element apparently common to all approaches in psychiatry is the feeling that some degree of professional supervision is necessary.

Our findings indicate that collateral influences are indeed important, but as supportive factors rather than as major mechanisms of therapeutic change. Patients who improved tended to relate to their peers in a comparatively friendly and intimate way, but they were also the same patients who formed positive cathexes with staff figures. That is, they showed a higher *generalized* capacity to identify with and relate to others, and consequently they received therapeutic influence directly from staff members as well as from their peers.

The benefits of a levelled hierarchy, patient participation and collateral relationships are most effectively experienced by patients who can also identify with senior staff members. The latter presumably provide exemplars and ego ideal models. Fellow patients, on the other hand, afford group support during the period of disturbance sometimes entailed in psychotherapeutic confrontations. They also provide opportunities to work through problems specifically involving peer relationships. All would seem to be valuable, complementary elements of therapy.

A second point concerns the staff's view that the dominant culture of the Unit should be geared to the working-class norms to which patients must ultimately return. The actual culture of the patients tends to be a *tertium quid*, different from the staff culture or the culture of the working-class outside. This was symbolically expressed by the patient who, after striking one of his fellows, said: 'I'm only trying to therapeut this bloke', illustrating the blend of staff language and Cockney modes of interaction. Many patients show an even clearer misuse than this of psychiatric technique. For example, some patients carry over therapeutic techniques to their family settings after discharge and apply them inappropriately to family problems. Other patients introduce the technique of the therapist destructively to their intimate relationships, as in imputing certain distorted drives to the motivation of their spouses, and cite their Unit experience to legitimize the procedure. Whatever the merits of presenting therapeutic procedures in the idiom of the patients' sub-cultural groups, there can be no question of matching post-hospital modes of interaction in the milieu therapy situation. The latter is novel to most patients and will remain extraneous to the others in the patients' post-hospital life.

Another issue in the definition of the patient role is the extent to which 'anti-social' behaviour ought to be allowed. The Unit ideology stresses the importance of a permissive policy for diagnostic and therapeutic purposes. Our data partially bear out the value of this position, indicating that patients who show a *moderate* amount of destructiveness and nonconformity are considered more improved at discharge than those who were either inordinately rebellious or impeccably compliant. Strong conformists and 'actor-out', those who most intensely accept and reject Unit values, experience the greatest difficulties in making the transition to life outside the hospital. The former never effectively enter treatment, the latter use the Unit way to satisfy their immediate needs, but not as a means to learning how to fit them into a more ordinary social environment. The special tolerance of deviant behaviour within the therapeutic community does not correspond to the attitudes outside the Unit; similarly, the high value placed on expressiveness and discussion of 'problems' and motives has few counterparts in ordinary life, and communication in such terms often arouses antagonism. The type and degree of interest given to individuals in the Unit by idealized authority figures, likewise, is often lacking in the world outside. Though the Unit seeks to simulate the world of ordinary life (and approximates to it more than do the conventional mental hospitals), there is a profound discontinuity between the patients' roles during and after treatment which must be transcended if they are to adjust successfully in the outside world.

This suggests a more complex set of questions about the prediction of treatment results. What kind of patients does a therapeutic milieu actually help? The Unit claims that its method is the best for patients with personality disorders, but that it is also suitable for other kinds of patients. Data indicate that patients respond in a complex pattern to the treatment given. They tend to do so in proportion to their 'ego-strength'. The strong-ego patients presumably had fewer initial difficulties in role performance than those with weaker egos. It could be argued that because they had 'less room for improvement', one might, therefore, expect them to show less improvement. In fact, they are more frequently seen as 'better' at the end of treatment. This may reflect their greater resources in the therapeutic situation, or even the staff's satisfaction at their superior role performance in comparison with other patients. With level of ego strength held constant, the factor that is most related to improvement is the duration of treatment. Patients who stay more than six months get better much more frequently than those who stay less than six months. This raises the question whether the Unit should concentrate on fewer patients for longer periods rather than on many more who do not benefit from briefer treatment. Such a course would require instruments to predict the types of patients to be kept who would accept the necessary course of therapy. Such instruments, however, are notoriously difficult to develop because of the multiplicity of factors involved.

A further problem in defining the patient role inheres in patients' conceptions about the organization of a treatment institution. The Unit staff consider their values to be representative of 'normal' society and patient deviation from them to be evidence of personal pathology. Our data indicate that Unit values differ markedly from those of people outside. We have shown that new patients have a range of values *vis-à-vis* the Unit's treatment ideology, and these cannot be simply attributed to their psychopathology or even their background. New patients whose values resemble those of the Unit or who subsequently adopt them tend to adjust better in the hospital and are considered more improved on discharge than those with discrepant views. While congruent values were found to be predictors of success *within* the Unit, they are notably less successful predictors of good adjustment after discharge. Patients whose values came to resemble those of the Unit showed steady improvement in their post-hospital adjustment, while those with pro-U value shifts showed declining rates of improvement afterwards. The latter group apparently experienced a greater discontinuity in their transition to the world outside than did the former.

In any given hospital the administrative policies and milieu will interact with the personal proclivities of the patient to create unique patterns of response.

The organization of group activities as well as their composition and intended purposes affect the way they function and consequently their impact on participating individuals. The Unit's structure—i.e., the pattern of continuous reshuffling of groups with interlocking memberships—fosters both the desired high level of inter-group communication and also the less explicitly sought phenomena of emotional contagion. The latter, particularly in the context of a permissive staff policy and a patient population with predispositions to behave disruptively, contributes to frequent and great periodic surges between states of relatively good social organization and relative disorganization.

We have noted that the Unit is subject to variations that are oscillatory or cyclical. These affect the degree and type of patient participation, the staff's practices, and therapeutic results. Some concomitants of the oscillatory process seem to support the generally held notion that 'collective disturbances' in psychiatric hospitals are anti-therapeutic—e.g., premature discharges increase in number, patients change their orientation to one another and their leaders to more negative ones. On the other hand, some aspects of the oscillatory process seem therapeutic for individual patients—e.g., the reparative drives, the affective involvements stimulated by mounting crises.

It must be recognized that permissive and dynamic institutions provide different kinds of stimuli for patients at different times. When things are functioning smoothly, the organization may be able to assimilate patients with acting-out symptoms without much trouble. On the other hand, when disorganization is at its height, the institution cannot absorb too disruptive, acting-out patients and will tend to transfer or discharge them. This implies that a given individual might experience a different therapeutic fate if he were present at one stage rather than another. The Unit's arrangement entails the loss of patients who might otherwise be helped. Such transfers and discharges tend not to be easily readmitted, despite the formal policy favouring it. In some cases the patient's own attitudes constitute the barrier, particularly if he feels that he has been rejected; in other cases he may have developed a reputation that makes the organization reluctant to accept him back from a mental hospital or elsewhere.

Thus, the issue of patient participation in treatment and administration becomes more complex than the Unit staff suppose. We have already indicated that patients actually define doctors in their formal authority roles, however democratic and benign their manner. We have also noted that doctors in fact retain control over important decisions and this control is actively exercised in times of crisis and disorganization. On the other hand, it has also been noted that active patient participation in treatment may contribute to the Unit's therapeutic effect. It would seem that something between the Unit's ideal position and its more drastic expedients based on the conventional medical authority pattern might ultimately prove most effective with non-psychotic patients. In order to implement this modified approach, the staff would have to clarify the limits of and conditions under which democratic participation may apply, avoiding both the total commitment implied in current unit ideology and the inconsequential commitment implied in some superficial efforts at 'patient government'.

Democratization, like other aspects of the patients' ideological role prescriptions has the dual purpose of creating a milieu favourable for changing the patient's personality on the one hand and helping him learn to participate constructively in ordinary life, following discharge from the hospital, on the other. As we shall indicate again in a later section, these purposes do not always coincide. It cannot be said, therefore, that as patients improve they should be granted increasingly great participation in administrative and therapeutic decision-making. As the degree of such participation in the Unit is abnormally higher, this would only unfit patients for participation in their normal roles outside the hospital. It would seem that some plan of graduated involvement followed by progressive disengagement from participation in Unit modes of group interaction would be best.

Another issue is the choice between segregated groups of similar patients and mixed groups of heterogeneous patients. Some hospitals favour the sorting of patients into relatively homogeneous groups according to their behavioural capacities and tendencies. The advantage of this, aside from ease of administration, is in focusing of specific treatment efforts. The Unit's mixed group plan rests on the assumption that patients will benefit more from a broad diversity of stimuli and behaviour than from a fairly uniform group.[14] The mixed group also shows symbiotic elements suggestive of a 'balanced aquarium'. Patients in such groups somehow complement one another's needs in a fashion beneficial to individuals and to the group as a whole. Since the strengths and weaknesses vary widely from one person to another, the group has a range of resources, flexibility, and capacity for group support beyond that of homogeneous groups.

Mixed and homogeneous groups are not necessarily mutually exclusive alternatives. It seems possible to exploit the advantages of the 'balanced aquarium' while also providing more specialized experiences for those who need them. Specially sheltered structures might be developed for people who temporarily cannot function in the larger institution. When they achieve the capacity or when disturbances in the system subside so that they can be accommodated, they can then return to the larger group. Such group supports need not be left to chance nor to the spontaneous formation of informal groups. These informal groups do not necessarily arise when they are needed nor are they always therapeutic. It cannot be assumed that the mere existence of a spontaneous peer group is 'good' or that its possible harmful effects can safely be ignored. Systematic efforts should be made not only to provide opportunities for such grouping to emerge but to guide their activities in therapeutic directions. As knowledge develops about the peculiar needs of patients at different junctures in therapy, special roles can be devised to enable patients to advance from one stage of treatment to the next.

The Unit established an unstructured system in which each patient was expected to 'find his own' pattern in a universal round of communal activities. However, there seems to be a need to restore more explicit expectations and clearer structure. Patients' individual resources and needs require differential handling which the ideology of democratization and communalism tends to obscure. The implication of equal opportunity for treatment by the community as a whole is that any individual who cannot seize the opportunity tends to be discarded as 'too sick for the Unit method of treatment', 'not really wanting treatment', and so on. Although patients are *defined* as a mixed group, they are *handled* as a homogeneous group, or at least as one where deficient participation is regarded as pathological and deviant. Another approach would carefully assess individual needs and resources, fitting individuals to suitable social roles in the Unit—roles that are carefully prescribed for their therapeutic appropriateness to the individual patient. Under the present system, the Unit staff have developed roles which are blurred but still fundamentally differentiated. An important component, for example, in the way any staff member's participation is evaluated by others in the Unit is in reference to the formal role of which he is a member (e.g., social worker, psychologist, nurse, physician). Amongst the patients there are relatively few such roles, (reception committee member, entertainment committee chairman, etc.), and of these there is little systematic assignment with therapeutic rationality. In some cases patients are elected, in others they may volunteer, in others they are assigned. The ideology of democratization and permissiveness taken too uncritically here allows any of these procedures to be rationalized as therapeutic. The path to rational use of milieu therapy would seem to require more critical specification of patient roles within the overall structure than is at present possible or in practice.

On the basis of our observations of the patient role as it is developed in the Unit it seems possible to state some general postulates about the role of patients in therapeutic communities.

Postulate 13: The maximum therapeutic benefit to be derived from patients' participation in hospital life seems to depend on the provision of a variety of relationships. Effective influence in any given situation may flow from a patient's relationships with peers or seniors, with members of his own sex or of the opposite sex, or from some combination of these.

Postulate 14: Patients' administration of therapy to one another is fraught with hazards. It's success depends on the careful selection of patients, the close supervision, and their careful indoctrination in the dangers of indiscriminate, irresponsible 'therapizing', especially in their personal relations outside.

Postulate 15: Rigid coercion and conformity do not seem conducive to therapeutic reorientations, but this does not imply that complete permissiveness is. Permissiveness is not in and of itself an effective therapeutic policy, nor is it an adequate way of defining patients' role prescriptions. A modification of permissiveness, designed on explicit principles to suit the therapeutic requirements of particular situations, would seem most profitable.

Postulate 16 :A hospital milieu that is inordinately permissive poses different but comparably great problems for post-hospital adjustment as compared to a milieu that is extremely repressive. Neither prepares the patient for coping with the real world that awaits him. Thus, aside from the learning potential engendered by having the permissiveness policies operate within explicit limits, it would seem that a more moderate course during treatment would facilitate the transition between hospital and ordinary life.

Postulate 17: To the extent that a therapeutic institution engenders in its patients values that are at variance with those of the outside social world, patients who have successfully adapted to treatment must be 're-socialized' prior to their discharge. The very experience of socializing patients to the institution may entail important therapeutic gains, but these may be lost in the post-hospital period if the norms adopted for treatment are not appropriately revised in preparation for the world outside.

Postulate 18: Psychiatric hospitals with permissive policies can expect an unusually high level of periodic interpersonal disturbances. These disturbances will be greater to the extent that the social structure is a segmentary one, reshuffling its participants into groups with interlocking membership, and fostering great internal communication.

Postulate 19: Collective disturbances among patients are neither intrinsically desirable nor undesirable.

Postulate 19a: Collective disturbances contain social forces which can be potent therapeutic influences. One example would be the mobilization of individuals' tendencies to participate in a process of social reconstruction.

Postulate 19b: Collective disturbances may have harmful as well as beneficial effects on individuals. Patients may become personally disturbed, or the staff may feel that conditions favourable for some patients' therapy require the removal of other patients from the unit. But patient casualties are not the inevitable price of the survival and stability of a therapeutic community. Steps can be taken to diminish casualty rates by postponing admissions and by removing, sheltering, or otherwise protecting particularly vulnerable patients until such time as they can be absorbed in the community.

Postulate 20: While democratic procedures may be valuable therapeutically, a completely democratic system is neither possible within the framework of psychiatric medicine nor directly applicable to the goals of rehabilitation. Where democratic measures are used in modified form, it would seem valuable to arrange patient participation to take into explicit account both considerations—i.e., the real structure of formal authority and discrete requirements of treatment and rehabilitation.

Postulate 21: Each patient's treatment and rehabilitation plan should be made individually. Emphasis on shared community life does not necessarily imply that all patients must be uniformly exposed to all aspects of the therapeutic community. Thus, for example, patients, at different times in their therapeutic careers, could be assigned to different role relationships, different group activities, and different degrees of responsibility.

Postulate 21a: Where the therapeutic community constitutes only one phase of a therapeutic plan (other phases of which might be external to the facility in which the therapeutic community method is employed) overall perspective should be maintained so that whatever the therapeutic community has available can be used to fit with other efforts to fulfil the individual patient's long-term needs.

THE INVOLVEMENT OF INDIVIDUALS OUTSIDE THE HOSPITAL IN TREATMENT

Like any psychiatric centre, the Unit has external relationships that affect its internal functioning. We have at different places in this book considered some of these relationships—those governing the referral of patients, those governing the recruitment of staff, those governing the Unit's relations with its larger authority structure, and the family relations of patients.

The Unit maintains a flow of patients through its professional referral sources, which in turn make use of the Unit for different purposes. Interest in the Unit among leading psychiatric institutions grew in response to reports of its novel and experimental method. In time, the bulk of professional use of the Unit has shifted to more peripheral agencies. This may be due in part to the fact that leadership institutions which tried the Unit wanted more rigorous evaluation of treatment results than were forthcoming. The failure to produce satisfactory evaluative data probably accounts for some of the decline in use of the Unit by major institutions. In addition, despite the lack of precise evaluative evidence, the Unit's methods are spreading to many modern psychiatric centres, and are thereby losing their uniqueness. This makes it less necessary for the other hospitals to refer as many patients away for milieu therapy. The Unit itself has also in recent years solicited and drawn an increasing proportion of its patients from the courts. This reflects not only the general trend in penal reform but also the Unit's own special interest in treating sociopathic individuals.[15]

The necessity of recruiting certain categories of transient staff further involves the Unit staff in external relations. Aside from the social therapist discussed previously, the other major staff role involving transient personnel is the junior psychiatrist. Unlike the social therapists, doctors are recruited from a formally defined, qualified, and organized professional group. Doctors present themselves as applicants for National Health Service posts in the Unit, typically selecting these posts because of their special interests in milieu therapy. In contrast to the social therapists, who typically come for the purpose of getting valuable life-experience, junior doctors come to the Unit for the purpose of learning a technical skill. When they leave the Unit, doctors, in contrast to the social therapists, characteristically remain part of the same professional community and several of them have sought to apply therapeutic milieu methods to other settings.

The problem of what kind of a relationship an innovating therapeutic community should have to its larger authority external structure is a complex one. All innovating institutions face problems of opposition and resistance to some degree, no matter how sound their support in the formal structure within which they take form. Different types of innovations arouse different types of reaction, and for any particular innovation different strategies may be found to offset the disturbing effects of such reaction. Among experimental therapeutic communities external authority relationships have been handled in various ways. Some innovators, as in the Unit's case, form a sub-unit within a larger hospital. It seems to hold generally that such units tend to be 'snobbish', 'odd', 'cliquey' on the one hand, and on the other hand to consider the more conventional part of the hospital as 'reactionary', 'authoritarian', or 'rigid'. It has been noted that under some circumstances the sharing of antipathies may help to promote group cohesiveness, and that this may have a therapeutic affect.[16] However, our data indicate that such a strategy may have anti-therapeutic consequences as well. Many patients have a tendency to project negative feelings onto the established authorities; where this tendency is reinforced rather than counteracted in a hospital environment, the consequences are not therapeutically so desirable. In some innovating experiments, the innovation comes from the top of the authority structure. This pattern seems to entail other problems—factionalism, splitting of authority figures, critical areas of inertia within the system, etc. To some extent the type of problems experienced will also vary with whether or not the innovator is attempting to change an established hospital or set up a new one. In general, each innovating strategy seems to have certain advantages and a certain cost. The nuances of each innovating procedure must receive considerable systematic study before we shall be able to state the conditions under which one or another procedure will produce the greatest gains with the smallest cost.

Perhaps the most important external relations for workaday therapy are those that the patients have with persons significant to them, mainly their family members. The Unit staff believe that these relationships contain not only the roots and manifestations of the patient's pathology but also vital therapeutic forces which might be harnessed to contribute to the patient's ultimate recovery.

Within the Unit 'bringing the family into treatment' has become an ideological imperative comparable to the directives about democratization or permissiveness. Our analysis has brought out some of the complexities of involving patients' families in the treatment situation.

Psychiatric findings about the effects of family relations on patients are ambiguous. On the one hand, family members are sometimes represented as pathogenic forces to be excluded from the therapeutic enterprise, or at best neutralized. On the other hand, they are sometimes seen as persons relatively disengaged from the patient's pathogenesis who might be either irrelevant to therapy or potential allies of the therapist.[17]

The traditional psychoanalytical position has been to strengthen the relationship between therapist and individual patient and keep the family out. To the extent that therapy is effective for the patient, it is assumed that he will successfully work out his problems with other people. The therapist does not hold himself responsible for the functioning of a family but only of an individual patient.

The Unit's position seems to be somewhere between this view and the increasingly fashionable opinion that the family should be treated as a unit.[18] The Unit seems to use information and efforts from family members. Yet the primary focus is on the individual patient who was referred for treatment, and comparatively minor attention is given to others in his family.

When families visit the Unit some judgement is made about what assets and liabilities they contain relevant to the patient's therapy, and whether the family members are therapeutic resources or 'in need of treatment' themselves, or neither. Consequently, a policy crystallizes on whether relatives should be objects of treatment, sources of information, or co-therapists. This decision is made without explicit criteria or systematic procedures, and is quite inconsistently observed.

When patients' families do become involved in the treatment situation, particularly by being taken into the Unit as full-time patients themselves, they tend to be handled as individuals with their own problems, rather than as members of a family in treatment. Indeed, the Unit separates spouses, assigning them to male and female wards. Further, there are no situations comparable to the home itself in which family members work out a domestic division of labour and pattern of interaction. In fact, family members might have some of their centrifugal tendencies strengthened in the Unit. In some cases, the arrangements may even strengthen any incipient tendencies toward involvements outside the family. This may help some inwardly-turned families to function more satisfactorily, but it may serve to disintegrate other families. We have few data, however, to specify the probable outcome in any given situation.

The norms of Unit practice do not distinguish treatment goals and procedures which are appropriate for different family types. This parallels the failure to clarify differential needs of individual patients. The blurring of individual requirements under uniform treatment techniques misses the opportunity provided by having several members of a family in therapy together. The Unit staff's differentiation of family types and their needs is usually implicit and ambiguous. This makes for erratic operation and the neglect of theoretical and applied problems of family treatment.

Despite the fact that patients with stronger egos are more likely than those with weaker egos to marry and to improve during and after treatment, marital responsibility itself may be related to therapeutic outcome. We found empirically that married patients do better than the unmarried. Married patients, for example, recover in greater numbers than unmarried patients from the post-discharge setback that is generally experienced. But for many, particularly among the unmarried patients, family relationships serve not as a stimulus for responsible role performance, but as a buffer against the demands of the world. Then the Unit and the family pressures operate at cross-purposes, one towards the patient's adult role performance and the other towards his continued dependency and passivity. Where these counter-pressures exist, the Unit experience may not alter the patient's condition in the face of the family organization. This is less likely to occur in the case of married patients who are typically not insulated from adult role responsibility and who may be more influential in changing their overall family structure. It is also among the married patients that there is a greater tendency for the Unit and the family pressures to reinforce one another.

If the Unit were to treat whole families, it would have to conceptualize how its therapy contributes to the family's superior functioning. This cannot simply be inferred from the patient's effects upon the functioning of the Unit. Furthermore, the Unit would have to consider the family as a self-contained system of interacting members rather than as the social background for a patient who is kept in the foreground. The appropriate variables in this approach would emphasize the fit of personality, norms, and emotional reaction patterns in role relationships, as discussed earlier, rather than individual characteristics. These changes require a great deal of thought and exploration on the frontiers of psychiatry and a redefinition of the physician's role which expands his treatment focus from an individual to a group.

For all patients, whether they live with families or not, there exists the problem of how they are to articulate with their network of social relationships after discharge from the hospital. Our follow-up studies indicate that the therapeutic community approach, however closely it is geared ideally to being in continuous experience with ordinary life, presents characteristic problems of post-hospital rehabilitation for its patients. While these problems may differ in substance from the problems faced by patients discharged from other kinds of hospitals, they are similar in general type. Patients must revise the ways they learned to relate to others in the Unit in favour of modes more adaptive in the outside world. This usually entails an immediate post-discharge setback, particularly for those who had adapted themselves to the Unit's special conditions, and showed improvement therein.

Just as patients show a diverse pattern of improvement under therapy, they show a diverse pattern of post-hospital recovery. Given the limitations of some patients' regenerative capacities and psychiatrists' current methods, there is a sizeable group of patients who cannot sustain any enduring improvement, or who retain serious residual incapacities, regardless of how well they may have performed in the therapeutic community. For such patients the increasing tendency among psychiatrists is to attempt to work out some way of maintaining them in the community rather than in institutions. This means that both the individual and those who relate to him must adjust to some level of chronic incapacity in the ex-patient. Where the acceptance of chronicity is the most realistic goal, it need not be adopted by default or with a sense of failure. This form of ultimate adjustment where collaboratively worked out as an explicit goal by staff, patient, and significant others, is more likely to be a viable one for all concerned. It is an area that especially needs development of therapeutic techniques for following on through the handling of problems arising after discharge. It would be expected that sociological perspectives would be useful in restructuring family and other role relationships to accommodate an individual from whom only deviant forms of participation can ever be expected.

On the basis of our observations of the Unit's external relations as they effect the internal functioning of the therapeutic community, it is possible to state some further postulates:

Postulate 22: A number of pitfalls are attendant on the innovating character of most contemporary therapeutic communities. Innovators tend to arouse opposition in the more established segments of their network of external relationships. While this opposition may have some therapeutic value in promoting internal cohesion, it may also have some therapeutic dysfunctions.

Postulate 22a: One of the therapeutic dysfunctions, short of the termination of the experiment by authoritative action by opposing external authorities, is to foster in the patients stereotyped negative attitudes towards authority figures. One of the aims of therapy is to modify precisely such attitudes in patients.

Postulate 22b: Another more indirect dysfunction is to block the flow of communications and personnel from the experimental unit to the larger system which it perceives as embodying structured defects needing remedy. To the extent that the experiment thus fails to contribute to the remedy, it deals inadequately with some of its goals.

Postulate 22c: At some points in the development of an innovating unit, the best consensus with its external authority system may be to agree to disagree and to arrange an insulated form of functioning. This mode is usually not, however, the best permanent arrangement, and it tends not only to foster the pitfalls noted above, but to allow the innovators to beg many questions that more active professional interchanges would stimulate.

Postulate 23: Family members of patients often act as significant forces in their lives. If one wishes to understand a patient either to return him to functioning in his family context or to society generally, it is necessary to assess these forces and to plan therapy to take them into account.

Postulate 24: The goals may vary with any particular patient from treating his family as a whole system to treating him in isolation from his family.

Postulate 24a: One factor that affects the scope of the goal is the responsibility assumed by the therapist. Where responsibility is felt only for the individual patient, other members of the family tend to be seen as sources of information and possibly assistance, but not as objects of therapy. To the extent that responsibility towards the family as a whole is to be assumed, changes in the conventional medical way of defining therapeutic obligations will have to be developed.

Postulate 24b: Another factor affecting the involvement of other family members in the definition of therapeutic goals is the sociological status of the patient. With single patients of good prognosis, for example, the generally held goals of increasing mature independence seem to work against pressing for greater involvement of their (parental) families. With married patients of similarly good prognosis, the usual goal is towards improving family integration, and thus towards the attempt to include other family members in the definition of social dimensions of therapeutic goals.

Postulate 25: In addition to setting goals, an assessment of the actual situation will affect the planning for family involvement in any particular case.

Postulate 25a: In some cases the family members or the patient may not wish to have anyone besides the patient involved, or the others may be unable to become involved.

Postulate 25b: Where the family members are accessible, their participation in therapy may still be contra-indicated. The therapist may assess them as providing such negative or inflexible stimuli as best to be kept out of the therapeutic situation.

Postulate 26: Where participation of family members is possible and indicated, the development of an explicit though flexible therapeutic strategy is advisable. In formulating therapeutic strategies for whole families, it will be useful to assess how individuals 'fit' with one another as well as attempting to understand each individual as a psychodynamic entity. By understanding how the patient 'fits' with his family members—in terms of personality, norms, and emotional toning in the relationships—one can assess how family elements constitute assets or liabilities with reference to the therapeutic goals.

Postulate 26a: One of the first tasks of the therapist is to work toward consensus among the perspectives—his own, the patient's, the family members who become involved —as to the goals of therapy and how particular aspects of the family network of relationships constitute assets or liabilities in relation to these goals.

Postulate 26b: Changes in the asset-liability balance can be achieved by shifts in personality or norms of the patient or his family members, or by changes of emotional toning in the problematic areas of their interpersonal relationships.

Postulate 27: The problem of choice of techniques for dealing with families is to be considered independently of setting the goals and of assessing the family situation. Even with the choice of the goal of treating the family as a whole and with the assessment of their value and amenability for such treatment, there is no necessary implication that all the members of the family need be dealt with directly or simultaneously.

Postulate 27a: It may be judged that the healthy functioning of the family would be improved by dealing, at some stages at least, with only the patient; or with the patient and his family members separately; or only with the members of the family who were not initially referred to the hospital. To some extent these choices are functions of the therapists' styles of treatment, but circumstances may favour one or another approach. It is not necessary to consider that these segmental techniques imply an abandonment of the goals of family treatment.

Postulate 27b: If treatment is to take place in an institution rather than at home, it is valuable, diagnostically and therapeutically, to provide situations that replicate those the family members must deal with in their ordinary setting.

Postulate 27c: If treatment is to take place in an institution, follow-through techniques are important to assist with the transitions from performance in sheltered, somewhat unusual social role situations to performance in those of ordinary life. Help is needed for the transfer of learning and the 'working through' of emotional and interpersonal upheaval often consequent on therapy.

Postulate 27d: To the extent that consideration of the healthy functioning of whole families becomes a paramount therapeutic goal, the efficiency of transplanting the family into the hospital becomes increasingly questionable. Techniques for conducting therapy in the family's natural habitat will probably be preferable for this purpose wherever possible.

THE CONCEPTUALIZATION OF TREATMENT AND REHABILITATION

Some problems about the way therapeutic goals are conceptualized in the Unit have been discussed. The Unit staff state that they aim at the simultaneous maximization of treatment (reorganization of individual psycho-dynamics) and rehabilitation (the adjustment of the individual to his social roles). Our analysis indicates that this ideal of *simultaneously* implementing these goals is not always possible, though sometimes the same activities may be used to implement either goal.

We have provided data that indicate the advisability of distinguishing conceptually between activities oriented to treatment aims and activities oriented to rehabilitation aims. For example, we have shown how the special conditions of permissiveness, communalism, and democracy, which characterize the milieu of the Unit (and have a putative treatment value) may pose problems for the patient after his discharge because of the discontinuity between the Unit way and the way of the outside world. Thus, to the extent that the Unit provides a special treatment milieu, it may not be able simultaneously to provide a microcosm of the 'real' world. Another example was seen in the role of social therapist. The social therapists experience a number of dilemmas due to the potential conflict in the two sets of role directives; to the extent that a therapist is 'natural' and 'herself', she may not be able to maintain at the same time an impersonal distance that is prescribed for the detection and handling of transference phenomena. To be simply 'oneself' may not coincide with being 'therapeutic', and the reconciliation of these directives constitutes a fundamental and recurrent problem for social therapists.

Thus, current therapeutic strategies in the Unit, by emphasizing simultaneous implementation of both sets of goals, tend to obscure the numerous and important situations in which it would be advantageous to see them as conceptually distinct.

In formulating the kinds of refinements that may be made on the basis of our observations, we take as our point of departure the central cluster of assumptions made by the Unit staff—i.e., that treatment and rehabilitation goals can be pursued simultaneously by one set of activities directed uniformly towards all patients (who are conceived as having essentially a single type of nuclear personality problem). In actual fact, therapeutic outcomes are linked to personality proclivities of individual patients; different kinds of activities are sometimes rationalized by staff as required for treatment goals as contrasted with rehabilitation goals; and finally the actual characteristics of therapy vary with the state of the Unit and the particular network of relationships which the patient generates in it—so that different patients get different treatment, but not through design of the staff.

In part, the different needs of patients because of their differences in fundamental personality structure and/or their differences in capacity to participate in treatment at various points in time could be recognized by instituting phases in the treatment regimen. All patients have problems that are in some ways similar, requiring assistance at predeterminable points in the treatment career—e.g., at points of entry and exit—but it would be helpful also to recognize their differences. Some patients come with greater ego-strengths than others, and can participate more rapidly in the whole range of Unit activities. Other patients might require considerable attention in preparatory stages before they can tolerate the levels of expressiveness and confrontations in treatment groups as they function in the Unit. For these patients more sheltered phases could be used as anticipatory to the entry into the more advanced stages of therapy. The degree to which preparatory phases would be necessary before entering the more rigorous phases of therapy and the speed with which progression through the phases would be accomplished would depend on the particular patient's capacities.

While mental hospitals have always had different wards that partly reflect the patients' capacities and prospects for 'normal' behaviour, they have been essentially different from the phase concept advanced here. The phases would be part of a regular programme of expectations put forth for each patient to accomplish at his own speed. Great attention would be given to how supportive and rewarding incentives might be provided for each patient to advance through the system. The emphasis in providing these rewards might initially be on things not ordinarily available to the patient outside the hospital, but on the special conditions of communal life that a therapeutic community could offer. Then, when patients reach a suitable point of personality strength, emphasis might be placed on using the hospital for rehearsing ways of getting greater rewards from generally available life opportunities, as in friendships, social activities, or work.

Throughout the progression, the patient need not be transferred from one organized group or ward to another. Rather his changing therapy regimen might comprise changing his activities and changing his network of role relationships. Thus, neither the composition nor the timing of the phases need be standardized, but might vary according to the individual patient's needs. While the Unit ideology emphasizes the dual utility of all its activities—for treatment and rehabilitation—it is recognized informally that some activities and some relationships are closely geared to the goals of personality reorganization (e.g., the doctor-patient relationship in doctors' groups) while others are more closely geared to goals of social adjustment (e.g., the instructor-patient relationship in workshops). The failure to give these distinctions explicit recognition leads to certain limitations. For example, the view that treatment and rehabilitation should be simultaneously implemented makes the staff tend to take a position about workshops such that a choice is posed between a 'realistic' industrial type of workshop on the one hand, and 'diversionary' occupational therapy programme on the other. When the choice is made in favour of the industrial workshops, with the implication that these are better for treatment and rehabilitation than the other, opportunities are lost to use occupational therapy programmes for purposes to which they are especially adapted. For example, occupational therapy could be used to provide treatment channels for very disorganized personalities, allowing the rehabilitation goals to be pursued at a more advanced therapy stage through the later assignment of patients to industrial type workshops if appropriate. If each individual's therapy is to have a 'tailored' character, geared to his individual rehabilitative needs, it might be that in some cases both kinds of therapy—occupational and work—would be necessary, in other cases only one, and in some cases neither. The range of types of occupational and work therapy provided would be used, ideally not as a blanket and randomly assigned regimen, but provided as appropriate to the treatment and rehabilitation needs of each individual patient.

A similar re-deployment of the use of staff in therapy can be visualized. In blurring the role prescriptions within the Unit the staff effectively did away with many of the attributes of conventional roles that were undesirable in a therapeutic milieu. It is apparent, however, in the emergent pattern of role performances under the joint impact of conventional definitions and Unit ideology that a new kind of role differentiation has come into existence. Basically within the Unit there are two kinds of attributes in staff members that have proved useful, corresponding to the requirements of treatment on the one hand, and rehabilitation on the other. The physicians and experienced permanent staff, whatever their 'human' qualities or their acquaintance with the patients' sub-cultures, have a degree of training and skill in understanding psychodynamics that is not found reliably associated with other roles. Those who use the Unit successfully recognize this fact. The workshop instructors and D.R.O.s, whatever else they might have by way of therapeutic gifts, function reliably to present the patients with a realistic picture of the requirements of the outside industrial situation. The social therapists, representing an intermediate position, seem to function on the one hand as 'natural', 'good' female figures, and on the other hand they act as extensions of the physicians, serving as figures onto whom transferences of prior female relationships and fantasies are projected for psychodynamic interpretation. It seems clear that the physician's role is primarily a treatment role, that of the workshop instructors is primarily a rehabilitation role, and the social therapists have aspects of each.

The patients' involvement in treatment-rehabilitation seems also to have a mixed quality. Patients do seem to influence one another in ways that lead to personality change (as when, under supervision, they serve as channels for 'beaming' the doctors' view onto their peers). But on the other hand, another use of patients for therapy in the Unit is to gain information on the nature of one another's normal social network outside the hospital and to provide characteristic interaction patterns for rehearsing typical role relationships.

It would seem that there are two reasons for clarifying the definition of role obligations so as to distinguish between treatment and rehabilitation. First, incumbents in any given role would experience less conflict about what they should be doing if their primary commitment were clearer. Second, with a clearer concept of the responsibilities and capacities associated with any given role, it might be possible to use the different roles more strategically in planning each individual patient's therapy. Thus, rather than having a blanket prescription that each patient must have a doctor, a workshop instructor, etc., it might be possible to construct a 'tailored' social network of role relationships as each individual required it. For example, in the early stages it might be that one patient would only be exposed to a relationship with a physician and then only later with others who became concerned with his social behaviour as well as his intrapsychic state, while another patient might be assigned to a peer group and perhaps a social therapist before exposing him to the interpretations of a psychiatrist.

The notion of phases, then, need not involve the movement of patients from one totally organized set of groupings to another (as prevails in custodial mental hospital wards, or in movement from one institution to another). The phases might be conceptually distinguished by those administering therapy, but integration might be maintained by retaining the mixed group concept in the overall community life. Thus, a patient, once he had received his introductory communication (anticipatory socialization) and been absorbed into the Unit through the admission procedures, might live in the wards and participate in the informal and formal social activities of the Unit, but not be assigned to other therapy groups until it was felt that he was ready for them.

Then assignments of groups and role relationships could be made for each individual as his therapy requires it—in no fixed sequence, speed, or composition of phases. In general, a paradigm of the following kind might be used as an overall guiding plan, but the specifications of its use for each patient would be different.

anticipatory socialization (pre-entry phase)—e.g., letters, visits, information via referring person

entry—(e.g. new-patient groups, orientation, diagnosis)

treatment ◄——► | sheltered |

rehabilitation ◄——► | recovery |

re-settlement—(post-discharge)—(e.g., home visits, ex-patient clubs).

When the patient is perceived to be ready to be 'in treatment' assignments of groups and role relationships could be made that would serve treatment goals. There would be no necessary effort to rationalize resemblance between the milieu influences exerted here and those of ordinary life outside. They would be self-consciously geared to personality reorganization, regardless of their resemblance to other kinds of activities and relationships. If conflicts were to arise in this phase, they would be resolved in favour of treatment goals. The phase of rehabilitation, on the other hand, some elements of which might begin concurrently with the treatment phase, would be designed to fit patients into 'ordinary' networks or social relationships. The sub-phases of rehabilitation that occur within the Unit would be oriented to creating as much of a microcosm of the patients' probable outside environment as possible for the purpose of rehearsing appropriate social behaviour in a sheltered milieu. In the later sub-phases, stretching over into the re-settlement (post-discharge) phase, efforts would be made to adapt the patient's behaviour to the *specific* social network in which he is to live. Increasingly, real role relationships would replace role surrogates, and therapists gradually withdraw, but not precipitously at discharge.

In some hospitals the social behavioural dimensions of treatment are distinguished from the intra-psychic ones through recognizing the difference between the role of administrator and that of therapist. We have learned from studies of this type of system that its good functioning depends, in part, on the co-ordination of the activities of the individuals in these two roles. A similar point might be made about sequential as well as synchronic relationships to which a patient is exposed in the course of his therapy. Coordination of the activities of those engaged in treatment and those in rehabilitation of each patient should be dealt with by constant recognition of the essential inter-relationship of these tasks. Treatment goals can most effectively be served by incorporating a planned dimension of rehabilitation in the overall therapy programme and vice versa.

Considering the factors that we have indicated to be linked to therapeutic success, we would propose the following postulates:

Postulate 28: The distinction between goals of social adaptation (rehabilitation) and goals of personality change (treatment) helps to clarify changing requirements of patients at different therapeutic stages. This lays the basis for more systematic, less intuitive judgements about therapeutic strategies.

Postulate 29: One way in which the distinction between treatment and rehabilitation can be institutionalized would be by planning the therapeutic programme in terms of stages which are conceptualized as pathways towards the goals of therapy. Recognition could thus be given to the different requirements of patients at different phases of treatment and resettlement.

Postulate 29a: A relevant distinction in differentiating aspects of the therapy programme would be between groups or activities that are primarily oriented to treatment goals and groups that are primarily oriented to rehabilitation goals. Patients could then be assigned to groups according to their particular therapeutic needs at any given time. Within groups having mixed aims, conflicts could be resolved in terms of the goals of particular patients within the groups.

Postulate 29b: Another way of building more rational therapeutic strategies based on the distinction between treatment and rehabilitation would be to distinguish between roles primarily geared to one set of goals and roles primarily geared to the other. Formal recognition of this distinction would imply that some are authorized and expected to assume responsibility for treatment-oriented activities and others for rehabilitative activities.

Postulate 30: All the distinctions recommended can lead to a harmful fragmentation of therapeutic efforts unless integrative activities give recognition to their essential interdependence.

CONCLUSION

Many psychiatric centres today are using at least some of the innovating approaches advocated by the Unit. In some cases they use only a few of them, in other cases many. In some places, milieu therapy is the very heart of treatment, while elsewhere it is peripheral or ancillary to treatment. The Unit has been of interest because of its attempt to make pervasive, focused use of milieu techniques to the exclusion of other methods.

Our study has critically examined the Unit's functioning in order to probe any instructive pitfalls in the new methods. No new method is miraculous, nor does it appear full-blown in a perfect state. Almost inevitably, new and often unforeseen difficulties must be recognized and dealt with before the method can be refined to the point where its superiority to old methods can be established. Our analysis, however, is tentative and suggestive rather than final. Our postulates, while frequently deriving from a critical appraisal of the Unit's position, have grown out of the opportunity to study Unit experimentation. The abstract nature of our present postulates does not go very far towards giving practical directives for specific activity. On the other hand, they are perhaps less global and all-embracing than many current directives about milieu therapy. They must be taken with the same sceptical caution that we recommend in examining assertions of the Unit staff (or any other proponents of an idealistic programme of action). Perhaps the next step towards perfecting milieu therapy techniques should be based on a systematic evaluation of postulates like those we are able to make on the basis of the present study. Their implementation would indubitably entail new problems and pitfalls which, in turn, would require critical study and reformulation.

Our recommendations, of course, are by no means exhaustive, nor are they intended to be. The field is too large, complex, and rapidly changing to allow for this, and the problems too heterogeneous.

Different kinds of therapeutic milieux will probably be most effective for different kinds of patients, with different kinds of staffs under different administrative systems. There is no single, simple high road to the realization of potentials of therapeutic hospital milieux. Principles that are effective in the experience of one group cannot be taken as dogma. Myriad factors of personality, culture, and social structure establish the conditions, limits and potentials for any therapeutic programme, and these factors may differ significantly from one organization to another. No system realizes its goals completely, and most systems have by-products that are actually inimical to their major goals. These facts of social life must be understood and accepted if a realistic perspective is to be maintained.

In sum, milieu therapists face the problem of integrating the therapeutic needs of individual patients, the capacities of the treating institution, and the requirements of the patients' social networks outside. Under these circumstances, the therapeutic yield is always the resultant of a complex field of vectors—psychodynamic, institutional, familial, and cultural—*all* of which must be optimally managed if effectiveness is to be maximized. Travel along the road towards optimal management is made easier to the extent that light is thrown on where one's steps are actually (rather than ideally) falling, and on unrecognized pitfalls along the way.

NOTES AND REFERENCES

1. Taylor, F. Kräupl, 'A History of group and administrative therapy in Great Britain', *Brit. J. med. Psychol.*, **31**: No. 3, 1958, pp. 153–73.
2. Hamburg, David, 'Therapeutic hospital environments' in Symposium on Preventive and Social Psychiatry, Washington, D.C., Walter Reed Army Institute of Research, 1957, p. 489.
3. Many of the generalizations in this chapter about the field at large have been drawn from discussions with Dr Morris Schwartz and his associates of the Joint Commission for the study of Mental Illness and Health, and will be documented in their forthcoming publication.
4. In general, where data from the present study are used to discuss issues in this chapter, the same qualifications on usages and methodology are to be understood as were noted when the data were presented in Chapter 7.
5. Mannheim, Karl, *Ideology and Utopia*, New York, Harcourt, Brace, 1949; also Polanyi, Michael, 'The Stability of beliefs', *Brit. J. Philos. Sci.*, Nov. 1952, p. 217.
6. The formally organized 'patient governments' (cf. Robert Hyde and H. C. Solomon, 'Patient government: A new form of group therapy', *Digest Neurol. Psychiat.*, 1950, **18**: pp. 207–18) differ both from the Unit's more comprehensive

aspirations and the more limited goals of such an organization as Dr P. Howard's Patient-Personnel Committee at McLean Hospital. The latter is seen strictly as an 'opinion-forming' body.

7. For an analysis of the functioning of Dr Howard's groups, see Daniel Rosenblatt 'Formal voluntary organization among patients in a psychiatric hospital', unpublished Ph.D. Thesis, Harvard 1959.

8. In the opinion of at least one expert committee, the emotional climate created by the staff is the most important element in milieu therapy. *The Community Mental Hospital*, Geneva: Third Report of the Expert Committee on Mental Health of the W.H.O., 1953.

9. Rapoport, Robert, and Rapoport, Rhona, 'Permissiveness and treatment in a therapeutic community', *op. cit.* and Rapoport, Robert, and Rapoport, Rhona, 'Democratization and authority in a therapeutic community', *op. cit.*

10. For example, Schwartz, Morris, and Shockley, E. L., *The Patient and the Psychiatric Nurse*, New York, Russell Sage, 1956; Schwartz, Charlotte G., *Problems for Psychiatric Nurses in Playing a New Role on a Mental Hospital Ward*, p. 402–26; Greenblatt, M., Levinson, D., and Williams, R., *op. cit.*

11. *The Volunteer and the Psychiatric Patient*, Report of the Conference of Volunteer Services to Psychiatric Patients, American Psychiatric Association, Washington D.C., 1959.

12. Main, T., 'The Ailment', *Brit. J. med. Psychol.*, **30**: pp. 129–45, 1957. In this paper value of the distinction between management and treatment, also held in other psychoanalytic hospitals (such as Chestnut Lodge, McLean, Austen Riggs), is advocated.

13. Wilmer, Harry, *op. cit.*; Rundle *et al.*, *op. cit.*

14. Sivadon, Paul, 'Techniques of Sociotherapy' in *Symposium on Preventive and Social Psychiatry*, *op. cit.*, p. 458.

15. *Report of the Royal Commission on the Law Relating to Mental Illness and Mental Deficiency*, London, H.M.S.O., 1957.

16. Sivadon, *ibid.*

17. Freeman, Howard, and Simmons, Ozzie, 'Wives, mothers and post-hospital performance of mental patients, *Soc. Forces*, **37**: No. 2, Dec. 1958, Simmons, Ozzie, Davis, James A., and Spencer, Katherine, 'Interpersonal strains in release from a mental hospital', *Soc. Problems*, **4**: No. 1, July 1956. Meyer, Henry J., and Borgatta, Edgar F., *An Experiment in Mental Patient Rehabilitation*, Russell Sage Foundation, New York, 1959. Carstairs, G. Morris, 'The social limits of eccentricity: an English study', in M. Opler (ed.), *Culture and Mental Health*. New York, Macmillan, 1959. For refined analysis of some of the dynamics involved see Lidz, T.; Cornelison, A.; Fleck, E. S.; and Terry, D., 'The intra-familial environment of schizophrenic patients: II. Marital schism and marital skew', *Amer. J. Psychiat.*, **114**: pp. 241–8, Sept. 1957. Bowen, Murray; Dysinger, Robert H.; and Basamania, Betty, 'The role of the father in families with a schizophrenic patient', *Amer. J. Psychiat.* **115**: No. 11, May 1959, pp. 1,017.

18. Jackson, Don, 'The question of family homeostasis', *Psychiat. Quart.* (Supp.), **31**: pp. 79–90, 1957; Alexander, Thomas, *op. cit.*; Ackermann, Nathan, *op. cit.*; Spiegel, John, *op. cit.*

APPENDIX A

Letter Sent to New Patients before their Arrival at the Unit

BELMONT HOSPITAL
Sutton, Surrey
SOCIAL REHABILITATION UNIT

Before you come to the Social Rehabilitation Unit you would probably like to know something about it. The Unit has 100 beds (70 men
and 30 women) and is part of a larger hospital for nervous disorders. It
may be very different from what you expect. Although you will have
your own doctor most of your discussions will be in groups. You will
not be put to bed unless you are physically unwell and most of the
activities take place outside the ward.

These other activities are as follows:

TIMETABLE OF UNIT

You are called at 7.15 a.m.

Monday to Friday
8.30– 9.45 a.m.—Community meeting.
10.15–11.45 a.m.—Doctor's Group.
1.00– 3.45 p.m.—Work Group (except Wednesday).
4.00– 7.00 p.m.—You are free to go out if you wish or choose a
recreation, e.g. music, play reading, etc.
7.00– 8.30 p.m.—There is a social every evening which is held in
the clubroom (including Saturday and Sunday).
9.00 p.m.—Patients in pyjamas in wards.
10.00 p.m.—Lights out.

Monday, Tuesday, and Friday
12.30– 1.00 p.m.—There is a meeting in one of the four wards.

Saturday only
9.00–10.00 a.m.   A voluntary group in the clubroom.

You will note that there is an opportunity for you to go out of the hospital (if approved by the doctor) between 4–7 p.m., and in addition Wednesday is a half day from 1–7 p.m. and the week-ends are also free days. Those people who are able to go home for the week-end may leave on Saturday morning after breakfast and are asked to return by 7 p.m. on Sunday. If you remain you are, however, asked to be in the hospital by 9 p.m. on Saturdays and 7 p.m. on Sundays and in pyjamas by 9 p.m., for at this time the night staff come on duty. This 9 o'clock rule is a most important one.

Difficulties people may have in 'fitting in' may be discussed by the community, who deal to a large extent with all matters of Unit life and discipline. This sharing of responsibility and treatment in hospital is very important. It is designed to help you to face up to and accept the responsibility of your own life and your future from the very beginning of your stay in the Unit.

Work may have been a problem with you for some time. In the Unit your job future will be the concern of everyone, and there is a full-time Disablement Resettlement Officer of the Ministry of Labour to help with job placement when you leave. The workshops (Furniture Repair, Painting and Decorating, Tailoring and repairs, Building labouring, and Home Group or domestic) are important in helping you towards this goal. They are in no sense a training for work, but let us see you in a work situation and study your work problems at first hand. These can be discussed in the group which follows each work period. It is hoped that by these methods we can help you to overcome your difficulties at work (if any) and thus help you and your family when you leave here.

What is going to happen to your family while you are in hospital? You will be entitled to Sickness Benefit or National Assistance or both while you are in hospital, and this will help to take care of the financial side. But there are usually other worries for the family besides financial ones. To help with these we have a Family Group from 2.00 to 3.30 p.m. every Wednesday and also one on Saturday morning at 10.30

a.m. to which many patients come with friends and relatives and discuss difficulties which lie in the family. In addition there is a social worker who can visit your home and help in many other ways to see the families through during this period.

There will probably be many questions that remain unanswered by this letter, but you can find answers when you are admitted. Besides other patients who are helpful and well informed there is a staff of four psychiatrists, four trained nurses, ten social therapists, four workshop instructors, one psychologist, and one psychiatric social worker who will help you to get fit.

Before you come there are a few practical points:

a. Bring pyjamas, toilet things, and a towel and some clothing which you can use for work. Do not bring too much; we cannot be responsible for your belongings, and there is little cupboard space.

b. Your money will not come through to you for ten days, so a few shillings would be helpful.

c. If you come from a distance and need help with your fares, go to the National Assistance Board with your admission letter and this form and they will assess your need and give help if it is needed.

d. The use of the Hospital telephone number (VIGilant 0054) is for an emergency, as messages cannot be taken in the normal course of events. There is a telephone booth specifically for the use of patients (VIGilant 4526 or 5011) in the main hospital building near the patients' cafeteria.

e. The nearest station is Belmont (Southern Railway) which is only a few yards from the hospital gates. Frequent trains run from Victoria and London Bridge. You should go straight to the Unit, where you will be welcomed by one or two Unit patients who, like any members of the staff, will be pleased to answer any questions you may ask.

You are expected to take an active part in your own treatment and in helping other patients. This you can do by talking in the various groups and trying to understand the meaning of your behaviour, difficulties with people at home or at work, etc. This we believe will help you more than giving you sleeping pills or medicines.

Relationships Between Clinical and Sociological Characteristics of Patients

Our data indicate that there are at best only very weak relationships between demographic factors and ego-strength. *Table 42* shows that there is very little difference in the ego-strength of younger and older people, in this case those under 30 years and those 30 years and older.

TABLE 42   DIAGNOSIS OF AGE GROUPS

Diagnosis	Under 30 No.	Under 30 %	30 and Over No.	30 and Over %
Psychotic	11	11	5	8
PD Weak	55	54	28	48
PD Strong	31	31	22	34
Neurotic	4	4	9	10
Totals:	(101)	100	(64)	100

$$\chi^2 = 6\cdot5226, \text{3 d.f., } p > \cdot05$$

Among our patients, the older group has a very slightly greater incidence of stronger ego, but this falls well within the normal range of sampling error. It may also be affected by the tendency of our neurotics to be drawn from a somewhat older age group than the remaining patients. (cf. *Table 42*) Similarly, there is no significant difference in the ego-strength of men and women, as is evident from *Table 43*. A little more than half of each sex is in the two weaker diagnostic categories, although women appear a little more frequently as neurotics and men as psychotics. This might reflect a slight bias in the disposition of men and women patients in the referral channels to the Unit, or it may reflect sex-linked differences in psychiatrists' tendencies to use the psychotic or neurotic categories for borderline personality disorders. In any case, the diagnostic differences between the sexes are quite negligible.

TABLE 43   DIAGNOSIS OF SEX GROUPS

Diagnosis	Males No.	%	Females No.	%
Psychotic	15	12	1	2
PD Weak	60	50	23	52
PD Strong	39	32	14	32
Neurotic	7	6	6	14
Totals:	(121)	100	(44)	100

$\chi^2 = 5\cdot9803$, 3 d.f., $p > \cdot05$

Furthermore, we find a small but discernible relationship between diagnosis and social class, the extent of the relationship depending upon the class measures employed. As *Table 44* shows, if education is taken as a class index, then almost two-thirds (64%) of the patients with low education fall into the two weaker ego-strength diagnostic categories, as compared with about one-half (52%) of those with grammar school and university education. In other words, in our sample, the higher-class patients have slightly stronger egos than the lower-class, although the differences are by no means striking.

TABLE 44   DIAGNOSIS OF EDUCATION GROUPS

Diagnosis	Low (Elem. & Secondary) No.	%	High (Grammar & Univ.) No.	%
Psychotic	11	10	5	10
PD Weak	62	54	20	42
PD Strong	35	30	17	35
Neurotic	7	6	6	13
Totals:	(115)	100	(48)	100

$\chi^2 = 4\cdot5706$, 3 d.f., $p > \cdot05$

The same class trends appear a bit more pronounced when occupation is used as the class index in accordance with the Registrar-General's classification of occupations. Here the manual groups appear in our weaker diagnostic categories more than twice as frequently as in the stronger, although the non-manual occupations are distributed almost exactly as the higher educational group.

The relationship between ego-strength and adult role performance is not simply one of stronger egos performing at a higher level than those with weaker egos. There seems to be a timing factor as well. The weaker egos are apparently somewhat slower in accepting their adult responsibilities, reaching a level of performance comparable to the stronger egos only later in their lives. This is apparent if we examine the marital status of these people according to the different age groups, which is shown in *Table 45*.

TABLE 45   MARITAL STATUS OF DIAGNOSTIC GROUPS BY AGE

Diagnosis	Young (Under 30)*					Div.-Sept.		100% Σ
	Single		Married					
Psychotic	10	91	1	9		—	—	11
PD Weak	48	87	5	9		2	4	55
PD Strong	17	55	14	45		—	—	31
Neurotic	3	75	1	25		—	—	(4)
	Old (30 and Over)**							
Psychotic	—	—	2	40		3	60	(5)
PD Weak	11	39	12	43		5	18	28
PD Strong	9	41	7	32		6	27	22
Neurotic	7	78	1	11		1	11	9

* $\chi^2 = 17 \cdot 8905$, 6 d.f., $p < \cdot 01$
** $\chi^2 = 11 \cdot 4799$, 6 d.f., $p > \cdot 05$

Among the younger people, those under 30 years of age, less than 10% of the weakest-ego group are married, compared to significantly more among the patients with stronger egos. Thus, the groups with stronger egos apparently marry younger than those with weaker egos. Profiles of older patients, those 30 years of age or more, make it apparent that most of the weaker-ego people eventually marry, reducing the difference between married and unmarried in the various ego-strength groups to non-significant proportions. Among the older patients, except for the neurotics, roughly three patients try marriage for every two who remain single, but if the rate of marital dissolution by divorce or separation is any criterion, these marriages are not distinguished by any marked success.

A noteworthy datum in *Table 45* is the extent to which neurotics in our sample resist marriage. Roughly three-fourths of them in both age groups remain single. Despite the small number of cases, it is difficult to account for this finding. It may be that the weaker-ego people are contracting marriages for pathological reasons which the neurotics are loath to accept. The weaker-egos may be seeking highly sheltered relationships for their dependence needs, or may be establishing relatively safe outlets for aggression, or simply have hastened impulsively into a permanent relationship without being concerned with the problem of responsibility. Neurotics, on the other hand, may prefer different marital relationships, but of kinds to which they feel inadequate. Unfortunately, we have no data in this series on the patients' spouses or on the character of the marital relationship, which might cast light on these speculations. Some relevant data on comparable relationships are presented in Chapter 8, in which another series of Unit patients are studied in their family settings.

With regard to the problem of aetiology of ego-strength condition, our patients provide interesting data on Bowlby's 'separation hypothesis'.[1] Bowlby contends that the mother serves a function in the development of the child's character, such that separation from the mother during critical periods of the child's early years hypothetically has profound, permanent effects which impair the development of his ego and his capacity for affective relationships. Our data support this general line of analysis to the extent that patients who have histories of significant separation from parents before the age of 10 have perceptibly weaker egos proportionate to the degree of separation. These data appear in *Table 46*.

TABLE 46 EFFECT OF EARLY SEPARATION FROM PARENTS ON EGO-STRENGTH

Ego-Strength	None		Separation Moderate		Severe	
	No.	%	No.	%	No.	%
Weaker	41	54	46	62	12	80
Stronger	35	46	28	38	3	20
	(76)	100	(74)	100	(15)	100

$$\chi^2 = 3.8044,\ 2\ \text{d.f.},\ p > .05$$

Though not statistically significant, the data show differences that are consistent in their patterning. They indicate that the more severe early separation from parents, the greater is the chance for a child's ego to be weakened. Of those patients who were not separated from either parent, about half (54%) showed a relatively weak ego structure, compared with over three-fourths (80%) of those who were totally separated from either or both parents during their early childhood.

Within the limitations of quality in our data, we may examine the 'separation hypothesis' in such a way as to compare effects of separation from father with those stemming from mother separation. Among our patients who suffered separation from either parent, those separated from the mother were judged to have almost identically weak egos with those separated from the father (*Table 47*).

TABLE 47   DIAGNOSIS OF PATIENTS SEPAR-
ATED FROM MOTHER V. FATHER

| Diagnostic Group | Separated from: | | | |
| | Mother | | Father | |
	No.	%	No.	%
Psychotic	4	6	7	8
PD Weak	40	58	49	58
PD Strong	18	26	23	28
Neurotic	7	10	5	6
Totals:	(69)	100	(84)	100

$$\chi^2 = 1.2139,\ 3\ \text{d.f.},\ p > .05$$

Thus, while separation may generally have perceptibly ego-weakening effects on the child, apparently it makes little difference statistically in a given series of patients whether the absent parent is the father or the mother. Roughly two-thirds of both separation groups fall into the first two diagnostic categories, designated as 'weaker-ego'. On this basis, both parents would seem to have comparable importance for the normal character development of the child, without either parent being more crucial than the other. Accordingly, father separation seems to be comparably serious to mother separation in the crude determination of ego-weakness, at least in this statistical series.

But this finding must be qualified in the light of other data. Presumably, ego-strength is a function of the parents' relationship with the child, which should be reflected in his orientation to them. Consequently we would expect orientation to parents to be related to ego-strength, perhaps even more closely than actual separation, since the orientation would relate to subjective deprivation. Furthermore, because of the apparently equal importance of both parents for character development (*Table 47*), we should expect no significant difference in ego-strength when there is a similar orientation to the mother and to the father.

This expectation, however, is not borne out by our sample. To be sure, almost one-half of the patients reporting positive orientation to father (44%) and to mother (49%) are diagnosed in the stronger-ego group. But of those who are indifferent or negatively oriented to either parent, a negative orientation to mother makes a greater difference than negative orientation to father (*Table 48*).

TABLE 48   EGO-STRENGTH ACCORDING TO ORIENTATION TO EACH PARENT

| Ego-Strength | Orientation to Father* | | | | Orientation to Mother** | | | |
	Positive No. %		Negative No. %		Positive No. %		Negative No. %	
Weaker	52	56	29	61	58	51	25	86
Stronger	41	44	19	39	55	49	4	14
Totals:	(93)	100	(48)	100	(113)	100	(29)	100

$* \chi^2 = 0.1118$, 1 d.f., $p > .05$
$** \chi^2 = 10.1706$, 1 d.f., $p < .001$

Data in *Table 48* indicate that positive orientation to mother gives no significantly greater ego-strength than positive orientation to father. Conversely, of those with negative orientations to mother, only 14% fall in the stronger-ego group, compared with almost three times as many (39%) of those negatively oriented to their fathers. Further, the great importance of one's relation to mother can be more sharply seen in the different consequences of a positive or negative orientation to either parent. While 61% of those negatively disposed towards father are weak-egos, fully 56% of those positively disposed are also classified as weak—a net gain of only 5% for positive over negative orientations. However, in the case of mothers, the differences are decidedly greater.

Where one-half (51%) of the positively oriented have weak egos—this is true of 86% of the negatively oriented—a significantly greater gain in positive over negative response. Thus these data suggest that there is a vital difference in the role of the two parents such that conditions producing in the infant a negative orientation to mother is likely to be more critical for ego-weakness that those producing a negative orientation to father.

This difference, incidentally, is no artefact of orientation to parent of the *opposite* sex, which might perhaps appear in a sample of three times as many men as women. Controls on the sex of the parent reveal no consistent effects of cross-sexual attachments on ego-strength.

How, then, can we reconcile the contradictory implications of *Table 47*, where mother is *not* more important than father, and *Table 48*, where mother *is* more important? Our data, unfortunately, do not afford a definitive check on Bowlby's hypothesis. Clearly, while separation from parents and orientation to parents are both related to the quality of the parent-child relationship, they are not identically weighted indices of it. While our data do suggest that the father may be more important for prolonged separation situations than is sometimes acknowledged, we have no conclusive evidence to cast on the scales.

Even on the basis of these data, however, it would seem appropriate to suggest that the 'separation' proposition be put as follows:

Prolonged separation from mother is one experience that tends to lead to ego-weakness; but this experience does not exhaust the possibilities for developing weak egos, nor does it assure this outcome. Separation from father seems comparably effective, considering separations that occur over a sustained period. On the other hand, conditions that produce conscious negative orientation of the child to the mother appear to be more damaging than those that produce the comparable orientation to father. These orientations may be produced by other determinants than separation, and separation in and of itself does not assure a negative orientation.

An example of another type of determinant of ego weakness, within physically intact families, is seen in our data on the effects of parental relationships on ego-strength. The sheer quality of parents' relationship *to each other* is, in our limited range of data, more significantly related to ego-strength than the extent of the child's separation from his parents (*Table 49*).

TABLE 49 DIAGNOSIS ACCORDING TO
PARENTS' RELATIONSHIP TO EACH OTHER

| Diagnosis | Parental Relationship | | | |
| | Satisfactory | | Poor | |
	No.	%	No.	%
Psychotic	6	11	5	8
PD Weak	18	32	39	61
PD Strong	22	39	18	28
Neurotic	10	18	2	3
Totals:	(56)	100	(64)	100

$$\chi^2 = 13 \cdot 0857, \text{ 3 d.f., } p < \cdot 05$$

Clearly, how well the parents got on together is not completely independent of how much separation from either parent the patient experienced. None the less, *Table 49* shows that of those whose parents were perceived as having a poor relationship with each other, over two-thirds (69%) were judged as having weak egos, compared with 43% of those with parents whose relationship to one another was perceived as good or tolerable. Stated differently, the latter group was statistically significantly more likely than the former to emerge with a stronger-ego–diagnosis. Patients in the stronger-ego diagnostic groups are almost twice as likely as the weaker groups to have avoided psychiatric treatment altogether, while the weaker groups are over twice as likely as the stronger to have actually been admitted to a psychiatric hospital at some time in their lives. These differences in overall history make

TABLE 50 PSYCHIATRIC HISTORY OF DIAG-
NOSTIC GROUPS

| Psychiatric Treatment | Ego-Strength | | | |
| | Stronger | | Weaker | |
	No.	%	No.	%
Psychiatric Hospital	14	21	50	51
Psychiatric O.P.D.	11	17	16	16
No Psychiatric Treatment	41	62	33	33
Totals:	(66)	100	(99)	100

$$\chi^2 = 16 \cdot 0842, \text{ 2 d.f., } p < \cdot 0005$$

the two groups significantly different, though both groups report about equal proportions of out-patient contact with psychiatrists.

The most conspicuous association appears between ego-strength and a history of work difficulty. This is shown in *Table 51*, where fully one-half of the weaker-ego group have had chronic work problems and the bulk of the remainder have had intermittent work difficulties. By contrast, among the stronger-ego group, well over 40% of the patients have never had serious work problems of any kind and only a smattering have had chronic trouble.

TABLE 51   WORK DIFFICULTY OF DIAGNOSTIC GROUPS

Work Difficulty	Psychotic No. %		PD Weak No. %		PD Strong No. %		Neurotic No. %	
Chronic	8	50	39	47	8	15	1	8
Intermittent	8	50	34	41	24	45	5	38
None	—	—	10	12	21	40	7	54
Totals:	(16)	100	(83)	100	(53)	100	(13)	100

$\chi^2 = 33 \cdot 6998$, 6 d.f., $p < \cdot 0005$

This pattern of statistically significant relationship between work problems and overall clinical picture is repeated among the behavioural defence groups, where about one-half of the aggressives and the extreme withdrawers have had chronic work problems, as compared with much smaller percentages among those showing more socially acceptable behavioural defences.

Similarly, those with stronger egos are significantly more capable of sustaining satisfactory interpersonal relationships with friends (*Table 52*).

TABLE 52   DIAGNOSTIC GROUPS' RELATION TO FRIENDS

Personal Relations	Psychotic No. %		PD Weak No. %		PD Strong No. %		Neurotic No. %	
Good	4	25	21	25	32	60	8	62
Unstable	4	25	38	46	10	19	—	—
Isolated	8	50	24	29	11	21	5	38
Totals:	(16)	100	(83)	100	(53)	100	(13)	100

$\chi^2 = 28 \cdot 9849$, 6 d.f., $p < \cdot 0005$

At least 60% of these groups enjoy good interpersonal relationships, as compared with exactly one-fourth of the weaker-ego groups. This is again echoed among the behavioural-defence types, although not with quite the same incisiveness and regularity.

REFERENCE

1. Bowlby, J.: *Maternal Care and Mental Health*. Geneva, World Health Organization, 1951.

INDEX